HANDBOOK FOR

Focus on Adult Health

Medical-Surgical Nursing

Andrea Rothman Mann, RN, MSN, CNE
Instructor and Third Level Chair
Aria Health School of Nursing
Philadelphia, Pennsylvania

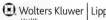
Wolters Kluwer | Lippincott Williams & Wilkins
Health

Philadelphia · Baltimore · New York · London
Buenos Aires · Hong Kong · Sydney · Tokyo

Acquisitions Editor: Julie Stegman
Product Manager: Helen Kogut
Editorial Assistant: Jacalyn Clay
Design Coordinator: Joan Wendt
Illustration Coordinator: Brett MacNaughton
Manufacturing Coordinator: Karin Duffield
Prepress Vendor: Aptara, Inc.

9 8 7 6 5 4 3 2 1

Printed in China

Library of Congress Cataloging-in-Publication Data

Mann, Andrea Rothman.
  Handbook for focus on adult health : medical-surgical nursing / Andrea Rothman
Mann.
    p. ; cm.
  Medical-surgical nursing
  Includes bibliographical references and index.
  ISBN 978-1-58255-887-5 (alk. paper)
  I. Title.   II. Title: Medical-surgical nursing.
  [DNLM: 1. Perioperative Nursing–methods–Handbooks.   2. Nursing Process–
Handbooks.   3. Primary Care Nursing–methods–Handbooks.   WY 49]
  617′.0231–dc23

                                                                    2011041458

PREFACE

Handbook for Focus on Adult Health: Medical-Surgical Nursing is a comprehensive yet concise clinical reference designed for use by nursing students and professionals. Perfect for use across multiple health care settings, the *Handbook* presents need-to-know information on over 170 commonly encountered diseases and disorders. The easy-to-use, colorful, consistent, and alphabetized format enables readers to gain quick access to vital information on

- Pathophysiology
- Risk Factors
- Clinical Manifestations and Assessments
- Diagnostic Methods
- Medical and Nursing Management
- Complications

For readers requiring more in-depth information, the *Handbook* is completely cross-referenced to chapters in *Focus on Adult Health: Medical-Surgical Nursing*.

Special Features

The *Handbook* places special emphasis on nursing management and includes the following special features:

- **Nursing Process sections** appear with many of the disorders and include all of the steps of the nursing process: Assessment, Diagnosis, Planning, Nursing Interventions, and Evaluation.
- **Nursing Alerts** offer brief tips or highlight red-flag warnings for clinical practice.
- **Gerontologic Considerations** highlight information that pertains specifically to the care of older adults, who comprise the fastest-growing segment of our population.

CONTENTS

A

Acquired Immunodeficiency Syndrome (HIV Infection)

Acquired immunodeficiency syndrome (AIDS) is defined as the most severe form of a continuum of illnesses associated with the retroviral human immunodeficiency virus (HIV) infection.

PATHOPHYSIOLOGY

HIV is a blood-borne pathogen, transmitted in body fluids containing HIV or infected CD4+ T lymphocytes. Infection with HIV occurs when it enters the host CD4 (T) cell, where viral RNA and viral proteins are replicated and released into the bloodstream, infecting other CD4+ cells.

The Centers for Disease Control and Prevention (CDC) standard case definition of AIDS categorizes HIV infection and AIDS in adults and adolescents on the basis of clinical conditions associated with HIV infection and CD4+ T-cell counts. Four categories of infected states have been denoted:

- Primary infection (acute/recent HIV infection, acute HIV syndrome also known as primary infection). High levels of HIV in the blood are accompanied by dramatic drops in CD4+ T-cell counts, normally between 500 and 1,500 cells/mm^3.
- HIV asymptomatic (CDC Category A: >500 CD4+ T lymphocytes/mm^3)

A

- HIV symptomatic (CDC Category B: 200 to 499 CD4$^+$ T lymphocytes/mm^3)
- AIDS (CDC Category C: <200 CD4$^+$ T lymphocytes/mm^3)

RISK FACTORS

HIV is transmitted through bodily fluids including:

- High-risk behaviors such as sexual intercourse with an HIV-infected partner or injection drug use
- Blood transfusion or blood products contaminated with HIV
- Children born to mothers with HIV infection, breastfed infants of HIV-infected mothers
- Health care workers exposed to needle-stick injury or transmucosal contamination from an infected patient
- Potentially infected body fluids, including blood, seminal fluid, vaginal secretions, amniotic fluid, and breast milk
- Estrogen and progesterone may increase a woman's risk for HIV infection through changes in the cervical mucosa.

CLINICAL MANIFESTATIONS AND ASSESSMENT

During the first stage of HIV infection, the patient may be asymptomatic. Patients who are in later stages of HIV infection may have a variety of symptoms related to their immunosuppressed state, including life-threatening opportunistic infections, malignancy, and the direct effect of HIV on body tissues.

Respiratory Manifestations

- Dyspnea, cough, chest pain, and fever are associated with opportunistic infections, such as those caused by *Pneumocystis jiroveci* (*Pneumocystis* pneumonia [PCP], the most common infection), *Mycobacterium avium-intracellulare,* cytomegalovirus (CMV), and *Legionella* species.
- *M. tuberculosis* tends to occur in IV/injection drug users and other groups with a preexisting high prevalence of tuberculosis

(TB) infection. HIV-associated TB occurs early in the course of HIV infection, often preceding a diagnosis of AIDS.

Gastrointestinal Manifestations

- Anorexia, nausea, and vomiting
- Oral and esophageal candidiasis or thrush causes white patches or oral lesions, painful swallowing, and retrosternal pain.
- Chronic diarrhea affects the majority of patients, causing profound weight loss, fluid and electrolyte imbalances, perianal skin excoriation, weakness, and inability to perform activities of daily living.

Wasting Syndrome (Cachexia)

- Multifactorial protein–energy malnutrition; a hypermetabolic state in which excessive calories are burned and lean body mass is lost.
- Profound involuntary weight loss exceeding 10% of baseline body weight
- Either chronic diarrhea for more than 30 days or chronic weakness and documented intermittent or constant fever with no concurrent illness
- Anorexia, diarrhea, gastrointestinal (GI) malabsorption, lack of nutrition

Oncologic Manifestations

Patients with AIDS have a higher than usual incidence of cancer; cancers are considered AIDS-defining conditions.

- Kaposi's sarcoma (KS) is the most common HIV-related malignancy; it involves the endothelial layer of blood and lymphatic vessels. KS in AIDS patients often begins with brownish-pink to deep purple cutaneous lesions that may become aggressive and disseminate to multiple organ systems.
- B-cell lymphomas are the second most common malignancy, often developing outside the lymph nodes. Most common areas include the brain, bone marrow, and GI tract. These types of lymphomas are characteristically high grade, indicating aggressive growth and resistance to treatment.

Neurologic Manifestations

An estimated 80% of all patients with AIDS experience some form of neurologic involvement during the course of HIV infection.

- HIV encephalopathy or HIV-associated dementia is a clinical syndrome characterized by a progressive decline in cognitive, behavioral, and motor functions.
- Symptoms of HIV encephalopathy include memory deficits, headache, difficulty concentrating, progressive confusion, psychomotor slowing, apathy, and ataxia. Later stages may include global cognitive impairments, delayed verbal responses, a vacant stare, spastic paraparesis, hyperreflexia, psychosis, hallucinations, tremor, incontinence, seizures, mutism, and death. May be difficult to distinguish from fatigue, depression, malignancy, or adverse effects of treatment.
- HIV-related peripheral neuropathy is thought to be a demyelinating disorder or an adverse effect of several HIV medications. Symptoms include pain and numbness in the extremities, weakness, diminished DTR, orthostatic hypotension, and impotence.
- Other common infections involving the nervous system include *Toxoplasma gondii,* CMV, *Mycobacterium tuberculosis,* and syphilis.

Depressive Manifestations

- Causes of depression are multifactorial and may include a history of preexisting mental illness, neuropsychiatric disturbances, psychosocial factors, or response to the physical symptoms.
- People with HIV/AIDS who are depressed may experience guilt and shame, loss of self-esteem, feelings of helplessness and worthlessness, and suicidal ideation.

Integumentary Manifestations

- KS, herpes simplex, herpes zoster viruses, and various forms of dermatitis
- Folliculitis, atopic dermatitis including eczema or psoriasis

- Patients treated with trimethoprim-sulfamethoxazole (TMP-SMZ) may develop a drug-related rash that is pruritic with pinkish-red macules and papules.

Gynecologic Manifestations

- Persistent recurrent vaginal candidiasis may be the first sign of HIV infection.
- Ulcerative sexually transmitted diseases, such as chancroid, syphilis, and herpes, are more severe in women with HIV.
- Human papillomavirus (HPV) causes venereal warts and is a risk factor for cervical intraepithelial neoplasia, a cellular change that is frequently a precursor to cervical cancer.
- Women with HIV are 10 times more likely to develop cervical intraepithelial neoplasia.
- Women with HIV have a higher incidence of pelvic inflammatory disease (PID) and of menstrual abnormalities including amenorrhea (bleeding between periods).

Immunological Manifestations

- Immune reconstitution inflammatory syndromes (IRIS) is characterized by fever and worsening of clinical manifestations of opportunistic infections, or the appearance of new manifestations.
- Develops weeks after the initiation of antiretroviral therapy

DIAGNOSTIC METHODS

- Enzyme immunoassay (EIA; formerly enzyme-linked immunosorbent assay [ELISA]) confirms presence of HIV antibodies.
- Western blot assay confirms seropositivity.
- Viral load tests can be measured by polymerase chain reaction (RTPCR), HIV RNA plasma levels, and nucleic acid sequence–based amplification (NASBA) and are used to track viral load and response to treatment.
- Home-based testing, using a small amount of blood or saliva is available; concerns exist due to lack of counseling and because of both false-positive and false-negative results.

A | MEDICAL AND NURSING MANAGEMENT

Protocols for treatment of HIV change frequently and are based on CD4$^+$ T-cell count, viral load, disease symptoms, and willingness to adhere to life-long treatment regimen.

Antiretroviral medications should be offered to individuals with a CD4$^+$ cell count of less than 350 cells/mm^3 or plasma HIV RNA levels exceeding 100,000 copies/mL.

Use of antiretroviral therapy preserves immune function, reduces the risk of opportunistic infections, and maintains quality of life.

Pharmacologic Therapy

Effective regimens contain at least three antiretroviral medications from at least two classes. Classes currently approved by the U.S. Food and Drug Administration (FDA) are the nucleoside/nucleotide reverse transcriptase inhibitors (NRTI), non-nucleoside reverse transcriptase inhibitors (NNRTI), protease inhibitors, fusion inhibitors, integrase inhibitors, and entry inhibitors.

- Many of the antiretroviral agents that prolong life may simultaneously cause lipodystrophy syndrome and place the person at risk for early-onset hypercholesterolemia, heart disease, and diabetes.
- Fat redistribution syndrome, an increase in fat loss in the legs, arms, and face, or a buildup of fat around the abdomen and at the base of the neck may develop.
- Vaccine research for HIV can potentially prevent new infections and treat those already infected with HIV (therapeutic vaccine).

Prevention and Treatment of Opportunistic Infections

Guidelines for the treatment of opportunistic infections should be consulted for the most current CDC recommendations

Pneumocystic Pneumonia

- People with HIV infection with a T-cell count less than 200 cells/mm^3 should receive chemoprophylaxis or treatment, when indicated, with trimethoprim-sulfamethoxazole (TMP-SMZ, Bactrim, Septra) to prevent PCP.

- PCP prophylaxis can be safely discontinued in patients who are responding to highly active antiretroviral therapy (HAART) with a sustained increase in T lymphocytes.
- Pentamidine (Pentacarinat, Pentam 300, NebuPent), an antiprotozoal medication, is used as an alternative to combat PCP.
- Adverse effects of pentamidine include fever, rashes, neutropenia, thrombocytopenia, renal dysfunction, hypotension, hepatic dysfunction and impaired glucose metabolism from damage to the pancreas.

Mycobacterium Avium Complex

Chemoprophylaxis for disseminated mycobacterium avium complex (MAC) disease is indicated for those with T-cell counts lower than 50 cells/mm^3, using clarithromycin (Biaxin) or azithromycin (Zithromax).

Cytomegalovirus Retinitis

- Prophylaxis with oral ganciclovir is considered for people who have CD4$^+$ T-cell counts of less than 50 cells/mm^3; intravitreal injections have been effective for patients who cannot tolerate systemic ganciclovir.
- Life-long treatment with ganciclovir (DHPG, Cytovene, Vitrasert) and foscarnet (Foscavir) offer effective treatment but not a cure for CMV retinitis.

Other Infections

- Herpes simplex or herpes zoster may be treated with oral acyclovir, famciclovir, or valacyclovir.
- Esophageal or oral candidiasis is treated topically with clotrimazole (Mycelex) oral troches or nystatin suspension.
- Chronic infection with candidiasis (thrush) or esophageal involvement is treated with ketoconazole (Nizoral) or fluconazole (Diflucan).

Antidiarrheal Therapy

Octreotide acetate (Sandostatin), a synthetic analog of somatostatin, has been shown to be effective in managing chronic severe diarrhea.

Chemotherapy

A

Kaposi's Sarcoma

- Antineoplastic medications are used to reduce symptoms by decreasing the size of the skin lesions, to reduce discomfort associated with edema and ulcerations, and to control symptoms associated with mucosal or visceral involvement.
- Radiation therapy is effective as a palliative measure; alpha-interferon can lead to tumor regression and improved immune system function.

Lymphoma

Combination chemotherapy and radiation therapy regimens may produce an initial response, but has limited success due to rapid progression of the malignancy.

Antidepressant Therapy

- Treatment of depression involves psychotherapy integrated with pharmacotherapy using antidepressants such as imipramine, desipramine, and fluoxetine, and possibly a psychostimulant (eg, methylphenidate) for fatigue and lethargy.
- Electroconvulsive therapy may be an option for patients with severe depression who do not respond to pharmacologic interventions.

Nutrition Therapy

- Malnutrition increases the risk for infection and may increase the incidence of opportunistic infections; nutrition is tailored to meet the needs of the patient, whether given orally, enterally, or parenterally. Megestrol acetate (Megace), a synthetic oral progesterone, promotes weight gain.
- Dronabinol (Marinol a synthetic tetrahydrocannabinol [THC]), the active ingredient in marijuana, has been used to relieve nausea and vomiting.
- Lactose-free oral supplements may be used to supplement diets that are deficient in calories and protein.
- Calorie counts should be obtained for patients experiencing unexplained weight loss. The goal is to maintain the ideal weight and, when necessary, to increase weight.

Complementary and Alternative Modalities

- Question patient about the use of alternative therapies; encourage patient to report any use of alternative therapies to primary health care provider.
- Adverse drug–drug interactions between certain complementary and alternative modality (CAM) therapies (eg, St. John's wort) and some antiretroviral medications may exist.

NURSING PROCESS

The Patient With AIDS

Assessment

- Identify potential risk factors, including sexual practices and IV/injection drug use history.
- Assess physical and psychological status and explore factors affecting immune system functioning.

Nutritional Status

- Obtain dietary history, identifying factors that may interfere with oral intake, such as anorexia, nausea, vomiting, oral pain, or difficulty swallowing.
- Assess patient's ability to purchase and prepare food.
- Measure nutritional status by weight, anthropometric measurements (triceps skinfold measurement), and blood urea nitrogen (BUN), serum protein, albumin, and transferrin levels.

Skin and Mucous Membranes

- Inspect daily for redness, breakdown, ulceration, and infection.
- Monitor oral cavity for and creamy-white patches (candidiasis).
- Assess perianal area for excoriation and infection.
- Obtain wound cultures to identify infectious organisms.

Respiratory Status

- Monitor for cough, sputum production, shortness of breath, orthopnea, tachypnea, and chest pain; assess breath sounds.

(continues on page 10)

A

- Assess other parameters of pulmonary function including chest X-rays, arterial blood gases (ABGs), pulse oximetry, pulmonary function tests.

Neurologic Status

- Perform baseline assessment of mental status as early as possible. Note level of consciousness and orientation to person, place, and time, and memory lapses.
- Observe for sensory deficits, such as visual changes, headache, and numbness and tingling in the extremities.
- Observe for motor impairments, such as altered gait, paresis, or paralysis.
- Observe for seizure activity.

Fluid and Electrolyte Status

- Examine skin and mucous membranes for turgor and dryness.
- Assess for dehydration by observing for increased thirst, decreased urine output, postural hypotension, weak and/or rapid pulse, or elevated urine specific gravity.
- Monitor for serum sodium, potassium, calcium, magnesium, and chloride imbalances, typically from diarrhea.
- Assess for signs and symptoms of electrolyte deficits, including decreased mental status, muscle twitching, muscle cramps, irregular pulse, nausea and vomiting, and shallow respirations.

Level of Knowledge

- Evaluate patient's knowledge of disease and transmission.
- Assess level of knowledge of family and friends.
- Explore patient's reaction to the diagnosis of HIV infection or AIDS, which may include denial, anger, fear, shame, withdrawal from social interactions, and depression.
- Identify patient's resources for support.

Nursing Diagnosis

- Impaired skin integrity related to cutaneous manifestations of HIV infection, excoriation, and diarrhea
- Diarrhea related to enteric pathogens, HIV infection, or antiretroviral medications
- Risk for infection related to immunodeficiency

- Activity intolerance related to weakness, fatigue, malnutrition, impaired fluid and electrolyte balance, and hypoxia associated with pulmonary infections
- Disturbed thought processes related to shortened attention span, impaired memory, confusion, and disorientation associated with HIV cognitive decline
- Ineffective airway clearance related to PCP, increased bronchial secretions, and decreased ability to cough related to weakness and fatigue
- Pain related to impaired perianal skin integrity secondary to diarrhea, KS, and peripheral neuropathy
- Imbalanced nutrition, less than body requirements, related to decreased oral intake
- Social isolation related to stigma of the disease, withdrawal of support systems, isolation procedures, and fear of infecting others
- Anticipatory grieving related to changes in lifestyle and roles and unfavorable prognosis
- Deficient knowledge related to HIV infection, means of preventing HIV transmission, and self-care

Planning and Goals

Goals for the patient may include achievement and maintenance of skin integrity, resumption of usual bowel patterns, absence of infection, improved activity tolerance, improved thought processes, improved airway clearance, increased comfort, improved nutritional status, increased socialization, expression of grief, increased knowledge regarding disease prevention and self-care, and absence of complications.

Nursing Interventions

Promoting Skin Integrity

- Assess skin and oral mucosa for changes in appearance, location and size of lesions, and evidence of infection and breakdown; encourage regular oral care.
- Encourage patient to balance rest and mobility whenever possible; assist immobile patients to change position every 2 hours.

(continues on page 12)

- Use devices such as alternating-pressure mattresses and low-air-loss beds, keeping linens wrinkle free.
- Encourage patient to avoid scratching, to use nonabrasive and nondrying soaps, and to use nonperfumed skin moisturizers on dry skin; administer antipruritic agents, antibiotic medication, analgesic agents, medicated lotions, ointments, and dressings as prescribed; avoid adhesive tape.
- Advise patient with foot lesions to wear cotton socks and shoes that do not cause feet to perspire; avoid tight or restrictive clothing.
- Assess perianal region for impaired skin integrity and infection.
- Instruct patient to keep the area as clean as possible, to cleanse after each bowel movement, to use sitz bath or irrigation, and to dry the area thoroughly after cleaning.
- Assist debilitated patient in maintaining hygiene practices.
- Promote healing with prescribed topical ointments and lotions.
- Culture wounds if infection is suspected.

Promoting Usual Bowel Patterns

- Assess bowel patterns for diarrhea; assess frequency and consistency of stool, abdominal pain or cramping with bowel movements.
- Assist patient in avoiding factors that exacerbate diarrhea.
- Measure and document volume of liquid stool as fluid volume loss; obtain stool cultures.
- To decrease diarrhea, recommend restricting oral intake for bowel rest and to avoid bowel irritants including raw fruits and vegetables, popcorn, carbonated beverages, and spicy food; encourage small, frequent meals.
- Administer antidiarrheal agents, anticholinergics, antispasmodics, opiates, antibiotics, and antifungal agents.

Preventing Infection

- Instruct patient and caregivers to monitor for signs and symptoms of infection: fever, chills, night sweats, cough, sputum production, difficulty breathing, creamy-white patches in the oral cavity, swollen lymph nodes, nausea, vomiting; persistent diarrhea; frequency, urgency, or pain on urination; drainage from skin wounds. Avoid others with active infections.

- Monitor WBC count and differential; culture wound drainage, skin lesions, urine, stool, sputum, mouth, and blood as ordered.

Improving Activity Tolerance

- Monitor ability to ambulate and perform daily activities.
- Assist in planning daily routines to maintain balance between activity and rest.
- Instruct patient in energy conservation techniques (eg, sitting while washing or preparing a meal).
- Decrease anxiety that contributes to weakness and fatigue by using measures such as relaxation and guided imagery.
- Collaborate with other health care team members to uncover and address factors associated with fatigue; administer epoetin alfa [Epogen] for fatigue related to anemia.

Maintaining Thought Processes

- Assess for alterations in mental status.
- Reorient to person, place, and time as necessary; maintain and post a regular daily schedule.
- Give instructions, and instruct family to speak to the patient in a slow, simple, and clear manner.
- Provide night lights for bedroom and bathroom. Plan safe leisure activities that patient previously enjoyed.

✴ NURSING ALERT

Provide around-the-clock supervision as necessary for patients with HIV encephalopathy.

Improving Airway Clearance

- Assess respiratory rate, rhythm, use of accessory muscles, cough and breath sounds; mental status, and skin color daily.
- Provide oxygen, suctioning, or mechanical ventilation as needed.
- Obtain sputum specimens as indicated.
- Encourage intake of 3 L of fluid if no renal or cardiac complications are present.

Relieving Pain and Discomfort

- Assess patient for quality and severity of pain associated with impaired perianal skin integrity, KS lesions, and peripheral neuropathy.

(continues on page 14)

A

- Explore effects of pain on elimination, nutrition, sleep, affect, and communication, along with exacerbating and relieving factors.
- Provide perineal care; encourage use of soft cushions or foam pads while sitting. Provide topical anesthetics, ointments, or systemic analgesics as prescribed.
- Administer analgesics including nonsteroidal anti-inflammatory agents and opiates; use nonpharmacologic approaches, such as relaxation techniques.
- Administer opioids, tricyclic antidepressants, and elastic compression stockings as prescribed to help alleviate neuropathic pain.

Improving Nutritional Status

- Assess weight, dietary intake, intake and output (I&O), serum albumin, BUN, protein, and transferrin levels.
- Based on factors interfering with oral intake, implement individualized measures to facilitate oral intake; consult dietitian to determine nutritional requirements.
- Administer antiemetics to control nausea and vomiting; encourage patient to eat easy-to-swallow foods; avoid spicy, extremely hot or cold foods; encourage oral hygiene before and after meals.
- Encourage rest before meals; do not schedule meals after painful or unpleasant procedures.
- Enhance nutrition and caloric intake with puddings, powders, milkshakes, or nutritional products for patients with HIV; avoid fiber-rich foods or lactose.
- Provide enteral or parenteral feedings to maintain nutritional status, as indicated.

Decreasing Sense of Social Isolation

- Provide an atmosphere of acceptance and understanding of AIDS patients, their families, and partners.
- Perform early baseline assessment of patient's usual level of social interaction; monitor for symptoms of social isolation such as decreased interaction with staff or family, hostility, noncompliance.
- Encourage patient to express feelings of isolation and aloneness; assure patient that these feelings are not unique or abnormal.

- Assure patients, family, and friends that AIDS is not spread through casual contact.

Coping With Grief

- Help patients explore and identify resources for support and mechanisms for anticipatory grieving and coping.
- Encourage patient to maintain contact with family, friends, and coworkers and to continue usual activities whenever possible.
- Encourage patient to use local or national AIDS support groups, hotlines, or mental health counselors to identify and address losses.

Monitoring and Managing Potential Complications

- Opportunistic infections: Report signs and symptoms including fever, malaise, difficulty breathing, nausea or vomiting, diarrhea, difficulty swallowing, and any occurrences of swelling or discharge to the health care provider. Teach patients to report these symptoms immediately.
- Respiratory failure: Monitor respiratory rate, pattern, and breath sounds, ABGs, and oxygen saturation; provide suctioning and oxygen therapy. Perform early assessment of patient wishes regarding mechanical ventilation; assess response to stress of intubation and mechanical ventilation.
- Cachexia and wasting: Monitor weight gain or loss, skin turgor and dryness, ferritin levels, hemoglobin and hematocrit, fluid and electrolyte balance. Assist in selecting foods that replenish electrolytes. Initiate measures to control diarrhea. Provide IV fluids and electrolytes as prescribed.
- Side effects of medications: Provide information about purpose, correct administration, side effects to report to physician, and strategies to manage or prevent side effects. Monitor laboratory test values and observe for drug interactions

Promoting Home- and Community-Based Care

Teaching Patients Self-Care

- Teach patient how to prevent disease transmission, including hand washing, delegating cleaning soiled pet areas to others, techniques and methods for safely handling and disposal of items soiled with body fluids.

(continues on page 16)

A

- Discuss precautions to prevent transmission of HIV: Use of condoms during vaginal or anal intercourse; using dental dam or avoiding oral contact with the penis, vagina, or rectum; avoiding sexual practices that might tear the lining of the rectum, vagina, or penis.
- Teach patient and family to clean kitchen and bathroom surfaces regularly with disinfectants to prevent growth of fungi and bacteria.
- Emphasize the importance of avoiding smoking, alcohol, and over-the-counter and street drugs. Instruct patients who are HIV positive or who inject drugs not to donate blood. Injection drug users who are unwilling to stop using should avoid sharing drug equipment with others.
- Teach medication administration, any IV preparation, techniques for enteral or parenteral therapies.

Providing Continuing Care
- Assist family and caregivers in providing supportive care.
- Refer patient to community programs, housekeeping assistance, meals, transportation, shopping, individual and group therapy, support for caregivers, telephone networks for the homebound, and legal and financial assistance.
- Refer patient and family for home care nursing or hospice for physical and emotional support.
- Encourage patient and family to discuss end-of-life decisions and provide care consistent with those decisions.

Evaluation

Expected Patient Outcomes
- Maintains skin integrity
- Resumes usual bowel habits
- Experiences no infections
- Maintains adequate level of activity tolerance
- Maintains usual level of thought processes
- Maintains effective airway clearance
- Experiences increased sense of comfort and less pain
- Maintains adequate nutritional status
- Experiences decreased sense of social isolation
- Progresses through grieving process

- Reports increased understanding of AIDS and participates in self-care activities as possible
- Remains free of complications

Emotional and Ethical Concerns

- Nurses are encouraged to examine their personal beliefs regarding fear of infection, manner in which AIDS was acquired, confidentiality, poor prognostic outcome.
- Values clarification and the American Nurses Association's Code of Ethics for Nurses can also be used to help resolve ethical dilemmas that might affect quality of care.
- Nurses who experience physical and mental distress in the form of fatigue, headache, changes in appetite and sleep patterns, helplessness, irritability, apathy, negativity, and anger may use interdisciplinary meetings, support groups, and spiritual advisors to solve problems.

For more information, see Chapter 37 in Pellico, L.H. (2013). *Focus on adult health: Medical-surgical nursing.* Philadelphia: Wolters Kluwer Health | Lippincott Williams & Wilkins.

Acute Coronary Syndrome and Myocardial Infarction

Acute coronary syndrome (ACS) is an emergent situation characterized by an acute onset of myocardial ischemia that results in unstable angina or myocardial infarction (MI).

PATHOPHYSIOLOGY

The underlying cause of ACS is atherosclerotic disease causing an imbalance between myocardial oxygen supply and demand. Unstable angina is caused by an incomplete occlusion of the coronary artery, an MI by complete occlusion; the term ACS is currently used to demonstrate progression of disease. Myocardial infarction may further be defined by the type (ST segment elevation or non-ST segment elevation), the location of the injury on the ventricular wall, or by the point in time in the process of infarction (acute, evolving, old).

Vasospasm, decreased oxygen supply from acute blood loss, anemia, or hypotension, or an increased demand for oxygen, from tachycardia, thyrotoxicosis, or cocaine use are other causes of MI. Each year in the United States, nearly 900,000 people have acute MIs; one-fourth of these people die.

RISK FACTORS

Uncontrollable risk factors:

- Age (men >45 years, women >55 years)
- Gender (men <55 years are at greater risk; after 55 years of age, men and women have the same risk)
- Race (African Americans, Mexican Americans, Native Americans, and some Asian Americans demonstrate increased risk)
- Family history of first-degree relative with premature diagnosis of heart disease

   Modifiable risk factors:

- Diabetes
- Hypertension
- Smoking
- Obesity
- Physical inactivity
- High blood cholesterol

   New and emerging risk factors:

- Inflammatory conditions such as periodontal disease and elevated C-reactive protein (CRP), influenza, sleep apnea, metabolic syndrome, and increased body mass index (BMI).
- Prothrombotic state (high fibrinogen)

※ N u r s i n g   A l e r t

C-reactive protein is a protein released in the blood during inflammatory states. The high-sensitivity CRP (hs-CRP) test is useful in assessing the risk of a cardiac event. A normal level is less than 0.1 mg/dL or less than 1 mg/L

CLINICAL MANIFESTATIONS AND ASSESSMENTS

In many cases, the signs and symptoms of MI cannot be distinguished from those of unstable angina.

- Classic signs and symptoms of myocardial ischemia include acute onset of crushing, substernal chest pain; pain in other areas of the chest, jaw, back, or arms; dyspnea, particularly in the elderly; tachycardia; extreme fatigue; diaphoresis; and nausea and vomiting.
- The pain of an MI may be differentiated from angina by persistence of pain despite rest and nitroglycerine.
- Women often complain of atypical chest pain and nonspecific signs and symptoms.
- Some patients have prodromal symptoms or a previous diagnosis of coronary artery disease (CAD), but about half report no previous symptoms.

DIAGNOSTIC METHODS

- Patient history of risk factors, description of presenting symptom; history of previous illnesses and family health history of heart disease
- Electrocardiography (ECG) upon onset of pain or arrival at the emergency department
- Cardiac biomarkers including creatine kinase-myocardial band (CK-MB), troponin, and myoglobin
- Exercise or pharmacologic stress test
- Cardiac catheterization, nuclear scan, or echocardiogram to evaluate ventricular function

A | MEDICAL AND NURSING MANAGEMENT

The objectives of the medical management are to decrease the oxygen demand of the myocardium and to increase the oxygen supply.

- Reduce myocardial oxygen demand and increase oxygen supply with medications, oxygen administration, and bed rest.
- Reperfusion via emergency use of percutaneous coronary intervention (PCI) and coronary artery bypass graft (CABG).
- Control risk factors

Pharmacologic Therapy

"Quality indicators" include an angiotensin-converting enzyme (ACE) inhibitors or angiotensin receptor blocker (ARB), ASA/aspirin, beta blockers, and statins; if not prescribed/ indicated, document the rationale.

- Beta-adrenergic blocking agents to reduce myocardial oxygen demand and cardiac mortality
- Aspirin as an antiplatelet agent
- Angiotensin-converting enzyme inhibitors or ARBs for ejection fraction of less than 40%.
- Statin medication prior to discharge
- Thrombolytics (alteplase [t-PA, Activase] and reteplase [r-PA, TNKase) to dissolve the thrombus in the coronary artery, permit reperfusion, minimize the size of the infarction, and preserve ventricular function; they must be given within 3 to 6 hours of onset of symptoms.
- Morphine sulfate intravenously to reduce pain, anxiety, and cardiac workload
- Nitrates (nitroglycerin) to reduce myocardial oxygen consumption
- Antiplatelet and anticoagulants, including aspirin, GPIIb/IIIa agent, or heparin

Reperfusion Procedures

Percutaneous Coronary Interventions

- Percutaneous coronary interventions to treat angina and CAD include percutaneous transluminal coronary angioplasty (PTCA) and intracoronary stent implantation.

- Because "time is muscle," door to balloon time (the time from arrival in the ED to PCI) should be less than 60 minutes.

☼ *N U R S I N G A L E R T*

It is imperative to assess patient's peripheral vascular system pre-procedure as a baseline for postprocedure assessment, especially distal pulses. Postprocedure, assess the affected extremity every 15 minutes for the first hour and then according to hospital protocol.

☼ *N U R S I N G A L E R T*

Renal failure is a complication of PCI; patients admitted with renal insufficiency are at a higher risk for renal failure. Monitor urinary output and renal function tests, and administer IV fluids to promote excretion of contrast media.

Cardiac Rehabilitation

- Targets risk reduction by means of education, individual and group support, and physical activity
- Begins in the hospital and continues with long-term conditioning

NURSING PROCESS

The Patient With ACS

Assessment

Obtain baseline data on current status of patient for comparison with ongoing status. Include history of chest pain or discomfort, dyspnea, palpitations, unusual fatigue, faintness (syncope), or diaphoresis.

- Evaluate chest pain, quality, duration, frequency, radiation.
- Assess heart rate and rhythm; assess for dysrhythmias.
- Evaluate 12-lead ECG.
- Assess heart and lung sounds; S_3 or crackles can be an early sign of impending left ventricular failure.

(continues on page 22)

A

- Measure blood pressure to determine response to pain and treatment; note pulse pressure, which may be narrowed after an MI, suggesting ineffective ventricular contraction.
- Assess peripheral pulses: rate, rhythm, and volume.
- Evaluate skin color and temperature.
- Observe urinary output and check for edema; an early sign of cardiogenic shock is hypotension with oliguria.
- Assess level of consciousness.

Nursing Diagnoses

- Ineffective cardiac tissue perfusion related to reduced coronary blood flow
- Risk for ineffective peripheral tissue perfusion related to decreased cardiac output from left ventricular dysfunction
- Pain related to decreased coronary blood flow
- Anxiety related to fear of death
- Deficient knowledge about post-ACS self-care

Planning and Goals

Balancing myocardial oxygen supply with demand as evidenced by the relief of chest pain, is the top priority for the patient with acute MI. Prevention of myocardial damage, absence of respiratory dysfunction, maintenance or attainment of adequate tissue perfusion, reduced anxiety, adherence to the self-care program, and absence or early recognition of complications are additional goals.

Nursing Interventions

Relieving Pain and Other Signs and Symptoms of Ischemia

- Administer 2 to 4 L of oxygen and medications to relieve pain associated with myocardial ischemia
- Assess vital signs frequently as long as patient is experiencing pain.
- Place the patient in semi-Fowler's position, rest with back elevated, or in a cardiac chair to decrease chest discomfort and dyspnea.

Improving Respiratory Function

- Assess respiratory function to detect early signs of complications.
- Monitor fluid volume status to prevent overloading the heart and lungs.

Promoting Adequate Tissue Perfusion

- Keep patient on bed or chair rest to reduce myocardial oxygen consumption until pain-free and stable.
- Check skin temperature and peripheral pulses frequently to determine adequate tissue perfusion.

Reducing Anxiety

Provide interventions to alleviate anxiety and fear, which increase sympathetic stress response and myocardial workload

Monitoring and Managing Complications

- Monitor signs and symptoms that signal complications such as dysrhythmia, hypotension, shock.
- Initiate emergency measures as indicated.

Evaluation

Expected Patient Outcomes

- Experiences relief of chest pain
- Has stable cardiac and respiratory status
- Maintains adequate tissue perfusion
- Exhibits decreased anxiety
- Complies with self-care program
- Experiences absence of complications

COMPLICATIONS

- Dysrhythmias and cardiac arrest
- Heart failure
- Cardiogenic shock

For more information, see Chapter 14 in Pellico, L.H. (2013). *Focus on adult health: Medical-surgical nursing.* Philadelphia: Wolters Kluwer Health | Lippincott Williams & Wilkins.

Acute Respiratory Distress Syndrome

Acute respiratory distress syndrome (ARDS) is a severe form of acute lung injury characterized by sudden and progressive non-cardiogenic pulmonary edema, increasing bilateral infiltrates, hypoxemia refractory to supplemental oxygen, and reduced lung compliance.

PATHOPHYSIOLOGY

ARDS occurs as a result of an inflammatory trigger that initiates the release of cellular and chemical mediators, which injure the alveolar capillary membrane. Protein-rich fluid leaks into the alveolar and interstitial spaces, impairing ventilation and surfactant. Without surfactant, the lungs become extremely stiff, the alveoli collapse, and severe hypoxemia develops. Blood returning to the lung for oxygen is shunted back to the heart markedly reduced in oxygen. ARDS has been associated with a mortality rate of 50% to 60%. Death results from multiple-system organ failure.

RISK FACTORS

Always secondary to another incident including:

- Direct injury to the lungs such as smoke inhalation, pulmonary contusion
- Indirect insult to the lungs such as septic shock or massive fluid resuscitation

CLINICAL MANIFESTATIONS AND ASSESSMENT

- Rapid onset of severe dyspnea, usually 12 to 48 hours after an initiating event

- Arterial hypoxemia not responsive to oxygen supplementation
- Lung injury then progresses to fibrosing alveolitis with persistent, severe hypoxemia
- Increased alveolar dead space and decreased pulmonary compliance
- Intercostal retractions and crackles

DIAGNOSTIC FINDINGS

A diagnosis of ARDS may be made based on the following criteria:

- History of systemic or pulmonary risk factors
- Acute onset of respiratory distress
- Bilateral pulmonary infiltrates, clinical absence of left-sided heart failure
- Ratio of PaO_2 to fraction of inspired oxygen (Fio_2) of less than 200 mm Hg (severe refractory hypoxemia)

MEDICAL AND NURSING MANAGEMENT

- Identify and treat the underlying condition; provide aggressive, supportive care using intubation and mechanical ventilation with positive end-expiratory pressure (PEEP).
- Monitor ABG values, pulse oximetry, and pulmonary artery pressures.
- Treat hypovolemia carefully, avoiding overload; inotropics or vasopressors may be required.

Pharmacologic Therapy

- There is no specific pharmacologic treatment for ARDS. The goal of the treatment is directed toward treating the underlying cause. Treatments under investigation include human recombinant interleukin-1 receptor antagonist, neutrophil inhibitors, pulmonary-specific vasodilators, surfactant replacement therapy, antisepsis agents, antioxidant therapy, and corticosteroids administered late in the course of ARDS.

A

- IV sedation with lorazepam, midazolam, dexmedetomidine, propofol, or short-acting barbiturates and analgesics combat anxiety and agitation from hypoxemia and intubation.
- Neuromuscular blockers such as pancuronium, vecuronium, atracurium, and rocuronium for continued inadequate oxygenation.

Nutritional Therapy

- Provide nutritional support (15 to 20 kcal/kg daily).
- Enteral feeding is considered first; however, parenteral nutrition may be required.

Nursing Management

General Measures

- Closely monitor the patient in the intensive care unit.
- Provide respiratory modalities including oxygen, nebulizer therapy, chest physiotherapy, endotracheal intubation or tracheostomy, mechanical ventilation, suctioning, bronchoscopy.
- Turn the patient frequently; prone position may be attempted.
- Reduce anxiety by explaining all procedures and providing care in a calm, reassuring manner.

Ventilator Considerations

- Identify any problems with ventilation that may cause anxiety: hypoxemia, sensations caused by PEEP, tube blockage, pneumothorax, pain, level of dyspnea, or ventilator malfunction.
- Closely monitor patients on paralytic agents: Ensure the patient is not disconnected from ventilator and that ventilator and patient alarms are on at all times, provide eye care, explain neuromuscular blockade to the family.

☼ NURSING ALERT

Neuromuscular blockade should be used with adequate sedation and analgesia; all skeletal muscles are paralyzed, which may result in fear, tachycardia, and increased O_2 demand.

For more information, see Chapter 10 in Pellico, L.H. (2013). *Focus on adult health: Medical-surgical nursing*. Philadelphia: Wolters Kluwer Health | Lippincott Williams & Wilkins.

A

Addison's Disease (Adrenocortical Insufficiency)

Addison's disease, or primary adrenocortical insufficiency, occurs when adrenal cortex function is inadequate to meet the patient's need for cortical hormones.

PATHOPHYSIOLOGY

Autoimmune or idiopathic atrophy of the adrenal glands is responsible for 80% to 90% of cases of Addison's disease. Inadequate secretion of adrenocorticotropic hormone (ACTH) from the pituitary gland or lack of cortisol from the adrenal cortex results in deficiency of glucocorticoids, mineralocorticoids, and androgens. Lack of cortisol results in inability to handle stress

RISK FACTORS

- Sudden cessation of exogenous adrenocortical hormonal therapy, which interferes with normal feedback mechanisms
- Bilateral adrenalectomy
- Infections of the adrenals, including TB and histoplasmosis
- Autoimmune destruction

CLINICAL MANIFESTATIONS AND ASSESSMENT

- Characterized by muscle weakness, anorexia, GI symptoms, fatigue, emaciation, dark pigmentation of the skin, hypotension, hyponatremia and hyperkalemia, and chronic dehydration

A

- Mental changes (depression, emotional lability, apathy, and confusion) are present in 60% to 80% of patients.
- In severe cases, disturbance of sodium and potassium metabolism may be marked by depletion of sodium and water and severe, chronic dehydration.

Addisonian Crisis

This medical emergency develops as the disease progresses. Signs and symptoms include:

- Cyanosis and classic signs of circulatory shock: Pallor, apprehension, rapid and weak pulse, rapid respirations, low blood pressure
- Headache, nausea, abdominal pain, diarrhea, confusion, restlessness
- Slight overexertion, exposure to cold, acute infections, or a decrease in salt intake may lead to circulatory collapse, shock, and death.
- Stress of surgery or dehydration from preparation for diagnostic tests or surgery may precipitate addisonian or hypotensive crisis.

DIAGNOSTIC FINDINGS

- Plasma ACTH >22.0 pmol/L in primary insufficiency
- Serum cortisol level lower than normal (<165 nmol/L) or in the low-normal range for primary insufficiency
- Hypoglycemia
- Hyponatremia
- Hyperkalemia
- Increased WBC count (leukocytosis)

MEDICAL AND NURSING MANAGEMENT

Immediate treatment is directed toward combating circulatory shock:

- Restore blood circulation, monitor vital signs, and place patient in a recumbent position with legs elevated.

- Administer IV hydrocortisone, followed by 5% dextrose in normal saline.
- Vasopressors may be required if hypotension persists.
- Antibiotics may be administered if infection has precipitated adrenal crisis.
- Assess patient to identify other factors that led to acute episode.

NURSING PROCESS

The Patient With Addison's Disease

Assessment

Assessment focuses on fluid imbalance and stress.

- Monitor blood pressure and pulse rate in lying, sitting, and standing positions to assess for inadequate fluid volume.
- Assess skin color, turgor, and pigmentation.
- Assess history of weight changes, muscle weakness, fatigue, and electrolytes.
- Ask patient and family about onset of illness or increased stress that may have precipitated crisis.

Diagnosis

- Alteration in fluids and electrolytes
- Impaired coping
- Alteration in protective mechanism
- Self-care deficit

Planning

Plan to restore fluid and electrolyte balance, assist with coping and stress reduction, protect the patient from complications, and promote self-care.

Nursing Interventions

Restoring Fluid Balance

- Administer IV fluids with sodium, glucose, corticosteroid, and vasopressors.

(continues on page 30)

- Along with the dietitian, help the patient to select foods high in sodium during GI tract disturbances and in very hot weather.
- Instruct the patient and family to administer hormone replacement as prescribed and to modify the dosage during illness and other stressful situations.
- Provide written and verbal instructions about the administration of mineralocorticoid (Florinef) or corticosteroid (prednisone) as prescribed.

Reducing Stress

- Avoid unnecessary activity and stress that could precipitate another hypotensive episode.
- Maintain a quiet, nonstressful environment and performs all activities, such as bathing and turning, for the patient.
- Provide supplemental glucocorticoids.

Maintaining Self-Care

- Give patient and family explicit verbal and written instructions about the rationale for replacement therapy and proper dosage.
- Teach patient and family how to modify drug dosage and increase salt intake in times of illness, hot weather, and stressful situations.
- Instruct patient to modify diet and fluid intake to maintain fluid and electrolyte balance.
- Provide patient and family with preloaded, single-injection syringes of corticosteroid for use in emergencies, and instruct when and how to use.
- Advise patient to inform health care providers (eg, dentists) of steroid use.
- Urge patient to wear a medical alert bracelet and to carry information at all times about the need for corticosteroids.
- Teach patient and family signs of excessive or insufficient hormone replacement.

Evaluation

Document assessment findings and response to interventions.

For more information, see Chapter 31 in Pellico, L.H. (2013). *Focus on adult health: Medical-surgical nursing.* Philadelphia: Wolters Kluwer Health | Lippincott Williams & Wilkins.

Alzheimer's Disease

Alzheimer's disease (AD) is a progressive, irreversible, degenerative neurologic disease that begins insidiously and is characterized by gradual losses of cognitive function and disturbances in behavior and affect.

PATHOPHYSIOLOGY

Alzheimer's disease can be classified into two types: familial or early-onset AD (which is rare, and accounts for <10% of cases) and sporadic or late-onset AD occurring in people over 65 years of age. Neuropathologic and biochemical changes found in patients with AD include neurofibrillary tangles (tangled masses of nonfunctioning neurons) and senile or neuritic plaques (deposits of amyloid protein) in the brain. The neuronal damage occurs primarily in the cerebral cortex and results in brain atrophy. The enzyme active in producing acetylcholine, which is specifically involved in memory processing, is decreased.

RISK FACTORS

The greatest risk factor for AD is increasing age

CLINICAL MANIFESTATIONS AND ASSESSMENT

Symptoms are highly variable; some include the following:

- In early disease, forgetfulness and subtle memory loss occur, with slight social or work difficulties, but patients are able to hide them.
- With progression of the disease, the patient forgets familiar faces and objects, gets lost in familiar environments, or repeats the same stories.
- Conversation becomes difficult and word-finding difficulties occur.

- Ability to formulate concepts and think abstractly disappears; patients have difficulty with everyday activities such as operating appliances or handling money.
- Patient may exhibit inappropriate impulsive behavior.
- Personality changes such as depression, suspicious or paranoid behavior, hostility, or combativeness may occur.
- Speaking skills deteriorate to nonsense syllables; agitation and physical activity increase, such as wandering at night.
- Eventually, patient requires help with all aspects of daily living, including toileting because incontinence occurs.
- The terminal stage finds the patient immobile and requiring total care; may last for months or years.

DIAGNOSTIC FINDINGS

The diagnosis, which is one of exclusion, is based on the clinical criteria and only confirmed on autopsy.

- Clinical symptoms are found through health history, including physical findings and results from functional abilities assessments such as Mini-Mental Status Examination and screening for depression.
- Electroencephalography (EEG)
- Computed tomography (CT) scan
- Magnetic resonance imaging (MRI)
- Complete blood cell count, chemistry profile, vitamin B_{12} and thyroid hormone levels, and examination of the cerebrospinal fluid (CSF) may refute or support the diagnosis of AD.

MEDICAL AND NURSING MANAGEMENT

The primary goal in management of AD is to manage the cognitive and behavioral symptoms. Cholinesterase inhibitors, such as donepezil hydrochloride (Aricept), rivastigmine tartrate (Exelon), galantamine hydrobromide (Razadyne [formerly known as Reminyl]), maintain memory skills for a period of time. Memantine (Namenda) may improve cognitive abilities for the duration of therapy.

NURSING PROCESS

The Patient With Alzheimer's Disease

Assessment

Obtain health history with mental status examination and physical examination, noting symptoms indicating dementia. Assist with diagnostic evaluation, promoting calm environment to maximize patient safety and cooperation.

Nursing Diagnoses

- Impaired cognitive function
- Risk for injury
- Alteration in nutrition
- Anxiety
- Impaired communication
- Activity intolerance, self-care deficit
- Risk for social isolation
- Caregiver role strain

Planning

Goals for the patient may include supporting cognitive function, physical safety, reduced anxiety and agitation, adequate nutrition, improved communication, activity tolerance, self-care, socialization, and support and education of caregivers.

Nursing Interventions

Supporting Cognitive Function

- Provide cues and guidance early in the disease; as cognitive ability declines, more assistance and supervision is required.
- A calm, predictable environment helps people with AD interpret their surroundings.
- Prominently display clocks and calendars, color-code doorways, encourage participation in activities.

(continues on page 34)

A

Promoting Physical Safety

- Remove fall hazards, install handrails, and provide adequate lighting to allow independence and relieve family's worry about safety.
- Use gentle distraction to reduce wandering.
- Prohibit driving.
- Allow smoking only with supervision.
- Secure doors leading from the house, supervise all activities outside the home. Ensure that patient wears an identification bracelet or neck chain in case of separation from caregiver.

Promoting Independence in Self-Care Activities

- Collaborate with occupational therapist to simplify daily activities into short, achievable steps.
- Maintain patient's personal dignity and autonomy.
- Encourage patient to make choices when appropriate and to participate in self-care activities as much as possible.

Reducing Anxiety and Agitation

- Provide emotional support to reinforce a positive self-image.
- When skill losses occur, adjust goals to fit patient's declining ability and structure activities to help prevent agitation.
- Keep the environment simple, familiar, and noise-free; limit changes.
- Remain calm and unhurried, particularly if the patient is experiencing a combative, agitated state known as *catastrophic reaction* (overreaction to excessive stimulation).

Improving Communication

- Reduce noises and distractions.
- Use easy-to-understand sentences to convey messages.

Providing for Socialization and Intimacy Needs

- Encourage visits, letters, and phone calls; visits should be brief and nonstressful, with one or two visitors at a time.
- Encourage patient to participate in simple activities or hobbies.
- A pet or plants can provide nonjudgmental stimulation, comfort, and contentment, satisfying activity, and an outlet for energy.

- Encourage spouse to talk about any sexual concerns; remind patient and partner that simple expressions of love, such as touching and holding, are often meaningful.

Promoting Adequate Nutrition

- Keep mealtimes simple and calm; provide familiar foods and avoid confrontations.
- Cut food into small pieces to prevent choking, and provide thickened liquids to prevent aspiration. Offer one dish at a time. Plan to feed the patient as it becomes necessary.
- Prevent burns by serving typically hot food and beverages warm.
- Provide adaptive equipment or suggest patient eat with a spoon or their fingers; use an apron or smock, rather than a bib.

Promoting Balanced Activity and Rest

- Sleep disturbances, wandering, and inappropriate behaviors are most likely to occur when there are unmet needs.
- Offer music, warm milk, or a back rub to help patient relax and fall asleep.
- To enhance nighttime sleep, provide sufficient opportunities for daytime exercise. Discourage long periods of daytime sleeping.

Supporting Caregiver

- Be sensitive to the emotional burden that the family is confronting.
- Observe for neglect or abuse due to caregiver fatigue or self-neglect.
- Refer family to the Alzheimer's Association for assistance with family support groups, respite care, and adult day care services.

Evaluation

Document assessment findings and response to interventions.

For more information, see Chapter 46 in Pellico, L.H. (2013). *Focus on adult health: Medical-surgical nursing.* Philadelphia: Wolters Kluwer Health | Lippincott Williams & Wilkins.

A

Amyotrophic Lateral Sclerosis

Amyotrophic lateral sclerosis (ALS), or Lou Gehrig's disease, is a degenerative disease characterized by loss of upper and lower motor neurons

PATHOPHYSIOLOGY

As the motor neurons die, the muscle fibers that they supply undergo atrophic changes. Theories about the cause of ALS include autoimmune disease, glutamate excitotoxicity, free radical injury, axonal strangulation, mitochondrial dysfunction, and oxidative stress.

CLINICAL MANIFESTATIONS AND ASSESSMENT

Clinical features of ALS depend on the location of the affected motor neurons. In most patients, the chief symptoms are fatigue, asymmetric, progressive muscle weakness, spasticity, and overactive deep tendon stretch reflexes.

- About 25% of patients experience weakness in muscles supplied by cranial nerves causing difficulty talking, swallowing, and ultimately breathing.
- Soft palate and upper esophageal weakness, causing liquids to be regurgitated through nose; weakness of posterior tongue and palate impair ability to laugh, cough, or blow the nose are noted.
- With bulbar muscle impairment, progressive difficulty in speaking and swallowing, nasal voice, unintelligible speech, and emotional lability develops.
- Eventually, aspiration, infection, and compromised respiratory function lead to death.
- Intellectual function is not impaired.

DIAGNOSTIC METHODS

Diagnosis is based on signs and symptoms because no clinical or laboratory tests are specific for this disease. Electromyographic (EMG) and muscle biopsy studies, MRI, and neuropsychological testing may be helpful.

MEDICAL AND NURSING MANAGEMENT

No specific treatment for ALS is available. Patients are managed at home and in the community, with hospitalization for acute problems.

Pharmacologic Therapy

- Riluzole (Rilutek), a glutamate antagonist, may have a neuro-protective effect in early stages.
- Baclofen, dantrolene sodium, or diazepam is given for spasticity.

Additional Interventions

- Enteral feedings via percutaneous endoscopic gastrostomy (PEG) tube
- Noninvasive positive-pressure ventilation or tracheostomy with invasive ventilation
- Decision about life support measures is based on patient's and family's understanding of the disease, prognosis, and implications of initiating such therapy.
- Encourage patient to complete an advance directive or "living will" to preserve autonomy.

Nursing Management

The nursing care of the patient with ALS is generally the same as the basic care plan for patients with degenerative neurologic disorders (see "Myasthenia Gravis" in Chapter M, page 483). Encourage patient and family to contact the ALS Association for information and support.

> For more information, see Chapter 46 in Pellico, L.H. (2013). *Focus on adult health: Medical-surgical nursing.* Philadelphia: Wolters Kluwer Health | Lippincott Williams & Wilkins.

Anaphylaxis

Anaphylaxis is an immediate type I hypersensitivity immunologic reaction between a specific antigen and antibody that induces a life-threatening allergic reaction.

PATHOPHYSIOLOGY

The reaction results from a rapid release of IgE-mediated chemicals toward a substance that is not normally toxic, such as food. Upon the first exposure to the substance, no physical reaction occurs; however, antibodies produced for that substance are stored, and reexposure causes release of chemical mediators such as histamine. Flushing, urticaria, angioedema, hypotension, and bronchoconstriction occur within seconds or minutes and may cause shock or death.

RISK FACTORS

Substances that most commonly cause anaphylaxis include foods, medications, insect stings, and latex.

- Foods that are common causes of anaphylaxis include peanuts, tree nuts, shellfish, fish, milk, eggs, soy, and wheat.
- Medications implicated in anaphylaxis include antibiotics (eg, penicillin), radiocontrast agents, IV anesthetics, aspirin and other nonsteroidal anti-inflammatory drugs (NSAIDs), and opioids.

CLINICAL MANIFESTATIONS AND ASSESSMENT

Anaphylaxis produces reactions that may be categorized as mild, moderate, or severe. The severity and onset depends on the degree of allergy and the dose of allergen.

- Mild reactions consist of peripheral tingling, a warm sensation, fullness in the mouth and throat, nasal congestion, periorbital swelling, pruritus, sneezing, and tearing eyes.
- Moderate reactions may include flushing, warmth, anxiety, and itching in addition to any of the milder symptoms. More serious reactions include bronchospasm and edema of the airways or larynx with dyspnea, cough, and wheezing
- Severe reactions have an abrupt onset and progress rapidly to bronchospasm, laryngeal edema, severe dyspnea, cyanosis, and hypotension. Dysphagia, abdominal cramping, vomiting, diarrhea, and seizures can also occur. Cardiac arrest and coma may follow.

DIAGNOSTIC METHODS

The diagnosis of risk of anaphylaxis is determined by skin testing. Skin testing for patients who have clinical symptoms consistent with a type I, IgE-mediated reaction is recommended

MEDICAL AND NURSING MANAGEMENT

Prevention

- Strict avoidance of potential allergens is essential.
- Patients at risk for anaphylaxis from insect stings should avoid areas populated by insects and should use appropriate clothing and insect repellent to avoid further stings.
- Instruct the patient to carry and administer epinephrine to prevent an anaphylactic reaction in the event of exposure to the allergen.
- Obtain history of sensitivity to any medications before administering, particularly in parenteral form, because this route is associated with the most severe anaphylaxis.

- Individuals predisposed to anaphylaxis should wear some form of identification, such as a medical alert bracelet, which identifies allergies to medications, food, and other substances.

Medical Management

- Respiratory and cardiovascular functions are evaluated and cardiopulmonary resuscitation (CPR) is initiated in cases of cardiac arrest.
- Oxygen is administered in high concentrations during CPR or when the patient is cyanotic, dyspneic, or wheezing.
- Patients with mild reactions need to be educated about the risk for recurrences. Patients with severe reactions need to be observed for 12 to 14 hours.

Pharmacologic Therapy

- Epinephrine, 1:1000, antihistamines, and corticosteroids are used to relieve urticaria and angioedema and airway patency.
- IV fluids (eg, normal saline solution), volume expanders, and vasopressor agents are administered to maintain blood pressure and hemodynamic status; glucagon may be administered.

Nursing Management

- Assess airway patency, wheezing, urticaria, angioedema, and vital signs.
- Prepare to initiate emergency measure including intubation, IV insertion, administration of fluids and medications, as well as oxygen.
- Explain the need to identify and avoid causative agent.
- Instruct the patient and family how to use preloaded syringes of epinephrine, and have the patient and family demonstrate correct administration.

For more information, see Chapter 38 in Pellico, L.H. (2013). *Focus on adult health: Medical-surgical nursing.* Philadelphia: Wolters Kluwer Health | Lippincott Williams & Wilkins.

Anemia

Anemia is a condition in which the hemoglobin concentration is lower than normal; it reflects the presence of fewer than the normal number of erythrocytes within the circulation.

PATHOPHYSIOLOGY

Anemia is not a specific disease state but a sign of an underlying disorder. Low concentrations of hemoglobin result in decreased oxygen delivery to the tissues or tissue hypoxia. As a result, anemia causes symptoms of poor tissue perfusion to the body.

RISK FACTORS

A physiologic approach classifies anemia according to whether the deficiency in erythrocytes is caused by a defect in their production (hypoproliferative anemia), by their destruction (hemolytic anemia), or by their loss (bleeding). Pernicious anemia is an inherited disorder caused by lack of intrinsic factor and inability to absorb vitamin B_{12} typically occurring in individuals of Mediterranean or Eastern European descent. Patients with alcoholism and pregnant women have a lack of dietary folate, causing anemia. Vitamin B_{12} deficiency may also occur in strict vegetarians.

CLINICAL MANIFESTATIONS AND ASSESSMENT

Symptoms of anemia will vary based on the severity of the anemia; rapidity of onset; the duration of the anemia (ie, its chronicity); the metabolic requirements of the patient; cardiac, pulmonary, or other underlying disease; and complications caused by the underlying disorder. In general, the more rapidly an anemia develops, the more severe its symptoms. Symptoms of anemia include:

- General symptoms: Dyspnea, chest pain, muscle pain or cramping, tachycardia, weakness, fatigue, general malaise, pallor of the skin and mucous membranes, conjunctival pallor, pale oral mucous membranes
- Megaloblastic or hemolytic anemia: Jaundice
- Iron deficiency: Brittle, ridged, concave nails, and pica (unusual craving for starch, dirt, ice); in patients with iron-deficiency anemia blood in stool, smooth, red tongue
- Megaloblastic anemia: Beefy, red, sore tongue
- Angular cheilosis (ulceration of the corner of the mouth)

DIAGNOSTIC METHODS

- Complete hematologic studies (eg, hemoglobin, hematocrit, reticulocyte count, and red blood cell (RBC) indices, particularly the mean corpuscular volume [MCV] and RBC distribution width [RDW])
- Iron studies (serum iron level, total iron-binding capacity [TIBC], percent saturation, and ferritin)
- Serum vitamin B_{12} and folate levels; haptoglobin and erythropoietin levels
- Bone marrow aspiration
- Other studies as indicated to determine underlying illness

MEDICAL AND NURSING MANAGEMENT

Management of anemia is directed toward correcting or controlling the cause of the anemia while treating the symptoms; if the anemia is severe, the erythrocytes that are lost or destroyed may be replaced with a transfusion of packed RBCs (PRBCs).

Gerontologic Considerations

Anemia is the most common hematologic condition affecting elderly patients. The impact of anemia on function is significant.

A review among the elderly has noted that increased fragility, decreased mobility and exercise performance, increased risk of falling, diminished cognitive function, increased risk of developing dementia and major depression, and lower skeletal muscle and bone density are associated with anemia.

NURSING PROCESS

The Patient With Anemia

Assessment

- Obtain a health history, perform a physical examination, and obtain laboratory values.
- Ask patient about extent and type of symptoms experienced and impact of symptoms on lifestyle; medication history; alcohol intake; athletic endeavors (extreme exercise).
- Ask about family history of inherited anemias.
- Perform nutritional assessment: Ask about dietary habits resulting in nutritional deficiencies, such as those of iron, vitamin B_{12}, and folic acid.
- Assess cardiac status (for symptoms of increased workload or heart failure): Tachycardia, palpitations, dyspnea, dizziness, orthopnea, exertional dyspnea, cardiomegaly, hepatomegaly, peripheral edema.
- Assess for GI function: Nausea, vomiting, diarrhea, melena or dark stools, occult blood, anorexia, glossitis; women should be questioned about their menstrual periods (eg, excessive menstrual flow, other vaginal bleeding) and the use of iron supplements during pregnancy.
- Assess for neurologic deficits (important with pernicious anemia): Presence and extent of peripheral numbness and paresthesias, ataxia, poor coordination, confusion.

Nursing Diagnoses

- Altered tissue perfusion related to inadequate hemoglobin and hematocrit

(continues on page 44)

- Altered nutrition, less than body requirements, related to inadequate intake of essential nutrients
- Fatigue related to decreased hemoglobin and diminished oxygen-carrying capacity of the blood
- Noncompliance with prescribed therapy

Planning and Goals

The major goals for the patient may include decreased fatigue, attainment or maintenance of adequate nutrition, maintenance of adequate tissue perfusion, compliance with prescribed therapy, and absence of complications.

Nursing Interventions

Managing Fatigue

- Assist patient to prioritize activities and establish a balance between activity and rest.
- Encourage patient with chronic anemia to maintain physical activity and exercise to prevent deconditioning.

Maintaining Adequate Nutrition

- Encourage a healthy diet, emphasizing nutrients lacking in the diet; folic acid, iron, vitamin B_{12}.
- Teach patient to avoid or limit intake of alcohol.
- Plan dietary teaching sessions for patient and family; consider cultural aspects of nutrition.
- Discuss nutritional supplements (eg, vitamins, iron, folate) as prescribed.

Maintaining Adequate Perfusion

- Monitor vital signs and pulse oximeter readings closely, and adjust or withhold medications (antihypertensives) as indicated.
- Administer supplemental oxygen, transfusions, and IV fluids as ordered.

Promoting Compliance With Prescribed Therapy

- Discuss the purpose of medication, how to take the medication and over what time period, and how to manage any side effects; ensure that the patient knows that abruptly stopping some medications can have serious consequences.

- Assist the patient to incorporate the therapeutic plan into everyday activities, rather than merely giving the patient a list of instructions.
- Provide assistance to obtain needed insurance coverage for expensive medications (eg, growth factors) or to explore alternative ways to obtain these medications.

Monitoring and Managing Complications

- Assess patient with anemia for heart failure.
- Perform a neurologic assessment for patients with known or suspected megaloblastic anemia.

Evaluation

Expected Patient Outcomes

- Reports less fatigue
- Attains and maintains adequate nutrition
- Maintains adequate perfusion
- Experiences no or minimal complications

COMPLICATIONS

- Heart failure
- Angina
- Paresthesias
- Confusion

For more information, see Chapter 20 in Pellico, L.H. (2013). *Focus on adult health: Medical-surgical nursing.* Philadelphia: Wolters Kluwer Health | Lippincott Williams & Wilkins.

Anemia, Aplastic

Aplastic anemia is a rare disease caused by a decrease in or damage to marrow stem cells, damage to the microenvironment within the marrow, and replacement of the marrow with fat.

A

PATHOPHYSIOLOGY

The precise etiology is unknown, but it is hypothesized that the body's T cells mediate an inappropriate attack against the bone marrow, resulting in bone marrow aplasia. Significant neutropenia and thrombocytopenia (ie, a deficiency of platelets) also occur; this is called *pancytopenia*. Most cases of aplastic anemia are idiopathic, but it can be congenital or acquired.

RISK FACTORS

Infections and pregnancy can trigger it, or it may be caused by certain medications, chemicals, or radiation damage. Agents that may produce marrow aplasia include benzene and benzene derivatives (eg, paint remover). Certain toxic materials, such as inorganic arsenic, glycol ethers, plutonium, and radon, have also been implicated as potential causes.

CLINICAL MANIFESTATIONS AND ASSESSMENT

- Infection and the symptoms of anemia (eg, fatigue, pallor, dyspnea)
- Retinal hemorrhages
- Purpura (bruising)
- Repeated throat infections with possible lymphadenopathy
- Splenomegaly sometimes occur.

DIAGNOSTIC METHODS

Diagnosis is made by a bone marrow aspirate that shows an extremely hypoplastic or even aplastic (very few to no cells) marrow replaced with fat.

MEDICAL AND NURSING MANAGEMENT

- Those who are younger than 60 years, who are otherwise healthy, and who have a compatible donor can be cured of the disease by a bone marrow transplant (BMT) or peripheral blood stem cell transplant (PBSCT).
- In others, the disease can be managed with immunosuppressive therapy, commonly using a combination of antithymocyte globulin (ATG) and cyclosporine or androgens.
- Supportive therapy plays a major role in the management of aplastic anemia. Any offending agent is discontinued. The patient is supported with transfusions of PRBCs and platelets as necessary.

Nursing Management

See "Nursing Management" under "Anemia" on pages 42–45 for additional information.

- Assess patient carefully for signs of infection and bleeding, as patients with aplastic anemia are vulnerable to problems related to erythrocyte, leukocyte, and platelet deficiencies.

Nursing Diagnoses
- Risk for infection
- Risk for altered tissue perfusion
- Risk for injury secondary to thrombocytopenia

Nursing Interventions
- Monitor for side effects of therapy, particularly for hypersensitivity reaction while administering ATG.
- If patients require long-term cyclosporine therapy, monitor them for long-term effects, including renal or liver dysfunction, hypertension, pruritus, visual impairment, tremor, and skin cancer.
- Carefully assess each new prescription for drug–drug interactions, as the metabolism of ATG is altered by many other medications.

- Ensure that patients understand the importance of not abruptly stopping their immunosuppressive therapy.

> For more information, see Chapter 20 in Pellico, L.H. (2013). *Focus on adult health: Medical-surgical nursing.* Philadelphia: Wolters Kluwer Health | Lippincott Williams & Wilkins.

Anemia, Iron Deficiency

Iron-deficiency anemia typically results when the intake of dietary iron is inadequate for hemoglobin synthesis. Iron-deficiency anemia is the most common type of anemia in all age groups, and it is the most common anemia in the world.

PATHOPHYSIOLOGY

- The most common cause of iron-deficiency anemia in men and postmenopausal women is bleeding from ulcers, gastritis, inflammatory bowel disease, or GI tumors.
- The most common causes of iron-deficiency anemia in premenopausal women are menorrhagia (ie, excessive menstrual bleeding) and pregnancy with inadequate iron supplementation.
- Patients with chronic alcoholism often have chronic blood loss from the GI tract, which causes iron loss and eventual anemia.
- Other causes include iron malabsorption, as is seen after gastrectomy or with celiac disease.

CLINICAL MANIFESTATIONS AND ASSESSMENT

Symptoms in more severe or prolonged cases include smooth, sore tongue; brittle and ridged nails; and angular cheilosis (mouth ulceration).

DIAGNOSTIC METHODS

- Bone marrow aspiration
- Laboratory values, including serum ferritin levels (indicates iron stores), blood cell count (hemoglobin, hematocrit, RBC count, MCV), serum iron level, and total iron-binding capacity

MEDICAL AND NURSING MANAGEMENT

- Assess and treat the underlying cause.
- Test stool specimens for occult blood.
- People aged 50 years or older should have periodic colonoscopy, endoscopy, or X-ray examination of the GI tract to detect ulcerations, gastritis, polyps, or cancer.
- Administer prescribed iron preparations (oral, intramuscular [IM], or IV).
- Have patient continue iron preparations for 6 to 12 months.

Nursing Management

See "Nursing Management" under "Anemia" on pages 42–45 for additional information.

- Administer IV iron in cases when oral iron is not absorbed, is poorly tolerated, or is needed in large amounts.
- Administer a small test dose before infusion with Imferon to avoid risk of anaphylaxis. Ferrlecit has largely replaced Imferon due to anaphylaxis.
- Advise patient to take iron supplements an hour before meals. If gastric distress occurs, suggest taking the supplement with meals and, after symptoms subside, resuming between-meal schedule for maximum absorption.
- Inform patient that iron salts change stool to dark green or black.
- Advise patient to take liquid forms of iron through a straw, to rinse the mouth with water, and to practice good oral hygiene after taking this medication.

- Teach preventive education because iron-deficiency anemia is common in menstruating and pregnant women.
- Educate patient regarding foods high in iron (eg, organ and other meats, beans, leafy green vegetables, raisins, molasses).
- Instruct patient to avoid taking antacids or dairy products with iron (diminishes iron absorption).
- Provide nutritional counseling for those whose normal diet is inadequate.
- Encourage patient to continue iron therapy for total therapy time (6 to 12 months), even when fatigue is no longer present.

For more information, see Chapter 20 in Pellico, L.H. (2013). *Focus on adult health: Medical-surgical nursing.* Philadelphia: Wolters Kluwer Health | Lippincott Williams & Wilkins.

Anemia, Megaloblastic (Vitamin B$_{12}$ and Folic Acid Deficiency)

In the anemias caused by deficiencies of vitamin B$_{12}$ or folic acid, identical bone marrow and peripheral blood changes occur because both vitamins are essential for normal DNA synthesis.

PATHOPHYSIOLOGY

Folic Acid Deficiency

Folic acid is stored as compounds referred to as *folates*. The folate stores in the body are much smaller than those of vitamin B$_{12}$, and they are quickly depleted when the dietary intake of folate is deficient (within 4 months). Folate deficiency occurs in people who rarely eat uncooked vegetables. Alcohol increases folic acid requirements; folic acid requirements are also increased in patients with chronic hemolytic anemias and in women who are pregnant. Some patients with malabsorptive diseases of the small bowel may not absorb folic acid normally.

Vitamin B$_{12}$ Deficiency

A deficiency of vitamin B$_{12}$ can occur in several ways. Inadequate dietary intake is rare but can develop in strict vegetarians who consume no meat or dairy products. Faulty absorption from the GI tract is more common, as with conditions such as Crohn's disease or after ileal resection or gastrectomy. Another cause is the absence of intrinsic factor. A deficiency may also occur if disease involving the ileum or pancreas impairs absorption. The body normally has large stores of vitamin B$_{12}$, so years may pass before the deficiency results in anemia.

RISK FACTORS

- Alcoholism
- European descent
- Inflammatory bowel disease or diseases of ileum or pancreas
- Strict vegetarians who do not consume meat or dairy

CLINICAL MANIFESTATIONS AND ASSESSMENT

Symptoms of folic acid and vitamin B$_{12}$ deficiencies are similar, and the two anemias may coexist. Symptoms are progressive, although the course of illness may be marked by spontaneous partial remissions and exacerbations.

- Gradual development of signs of anemia (dyspnea, weakness, listlessness, and fatigue)
- Possible development of a smooth, sore, red tongue and mild diarrhea (pernicious anemia)
- Mild jaundice, vitiligo, and premature graying
- Paresthesias in the extremities and difficulty keeping balance; loss of position sense; confusion may occur
- Lack of neurologic manifestations with folic acid deficiency alone

A

- Without treatment, patients die, usually as a result of heart failure secondary to anemia.

DIAGNOSTIC FINDINGS

- Schilling test (primary diagnostic tool) for vitamin B_{12} deficiency
- Complete blood cell count (Hgb value as low as 4 to 5 g/dL, WBC count 2,000 to 3,000 mm^3, platelet count <50,000 mm^3; very high MCV, usually exceeding 110 μm^3)
- Serum levels of folate and vitamin B_{12} (folic acid deficiency and deficient vitamin B_{12})

MEDICAL AND NURSING MANAGEMENT

See "Nursing Management" under "Anemia" on pages 42–45 for additional information.

Folic Acid Deficiency

- Increase intake of folic acid in patient's diet and administer 1 mg folic acid daily.
- Administer IM folic acid for malabsorption syndromes.
- Prescribe additional supplements as necessary, because the amount in multivitamins may be inadequate to fully replace deficient body stores.
- Prescribe folic acid for patients with alcoholism as long as they continue to consume alcohol.

Vitamin B_{12} Deficiency

- Provide vitamin B_{12} replacement: Vegetarians can prevent or treat deficiency with oral supplements with vitamins or fortified soy milk; when the deficiency is due to the more common defect in absorption or the absence of intrinsic factor, replacement is by monthly IM injections of vitamin B_{12}.

A

- A small amount of an oral dose of vitamin B$_{12}$ can be absorbed by passive diffusion, even in the absence of intrinsic factor, but large doses (2 mg/day) are required if vitamin B$_{12}$ is to be replaced orally.
- To prevent recurrence of pernicious anemia, vitamin B$_{12}$ therapy must be continued for life.

NURSING PROCESS

The Patient With Megaloblastic Anemia

Assessment

- Assess patients at risk for megaloblastic anemia for clinical manifestations (eg, inspect the skin, sclera, and mucous membranes for jaundice; note vitiligo and premature graying).
- Perform careful neurologic assessment (eg, note gait and stability; test position and vibration sense).
- Assess need for assistive devices (eg, canes, walkers) and need for support and guidance in managing activities of daily living and home environment.

Diagnosis

- Altered tissue perfusion
- Safety

Planning

Collaborate with interdisciplinary team to improve tissue perfusion, provide safety for neurologic deficits, and follow-up to detect complications.

Nursing Interventions

- Ensure safety when position sense, coordination, and gait are affected.
- Refer for physical or occupational therapy as needed.
- When sensation is altered, instruct patient to avoid excessive heat and cold.

(continues on page 54)

- Advise patient to prepare bland, soft foods and to eat small amounts frequently.
- Explain that other nutritional deficiencies, such as alcohol-induced anemia, can induce neurologic problems.
- Instruct patient in complete urine collections for the Schilling test. Also explain the importance of the test and of complying with the collection.
- Teach patient about chronicity of disorder and need for monthly vitamin B_{12} injections, even when patient has no symptoms. Instruct patient how to self-administer injections, when appropriate.
- Stress importance of ongoing medical follow-up and screening, because gastric atrophy associated with pernicious anemia increases the risk of gastric carcinoma.

Evaluation

Document assessment findings and response to interventions.

For more information, see Chapter 20 in Pellico, L.H. (2013). *Focus on adult health: Medical-surgical nursing.* Philadelphia: Wolters Kluwer Health | Lippincott Williams & Wilkins.

Aneurysm, Aortic

An aortic aneurysm is a localized sac or dilation formed at a weak point in the wall of the artery.

PATHOPHYSIOLOGY

An aneurysm may result from a congenital weakness in the arterial wall or atherosclerotic disease.

It may be classified by its shape or form. The most common forms of aneurysms are saccular and fusiform. A saccular aneurysm projects from only one side of the vessel. If an entire arterial segment becomes dilated, a fusiform aneurysm develops. Very small aneurysms due to localized infection are called *mycotic aneurysms*. The cause of abdominal aortic aneurysm (AAA), the most common type of degenerative aneurysm, is atherosclerosis. Occasionally, in an aorta diseased by arteriosclerosis, a tear develops in the intima or the media degenerates, resulting in a dissection. The thoracic area is the most common site of dissection. Aneurysms are serious because they can rupture, leading to hemorrhage and death.

RISK FACTORS

Abdominal Aortic Aneurysm (AAA)

- Age older than 50 years
- Dissection more common in men and in ages 50 to 70
- Male
- Tobacco use
- Hypertension
- Genetics

Thoracic Aneurysm

- Most caused by atherosclerosis
- Men between 40 and 70 years

CLINICAL MANIFESTATIONS AND ASSESSMENT

Thoracic Aortic Aneurysm

- Symptoms vary and depend on how rapidly the aneurysm dilates and affects the surrounding intrathoracic structures; some patients are asymptomatic.
- Constant, boring pain, and may occur only when the patient is in the supine position
- Dyspnea, cough (paroxysmal and brassy)

- Hoarseness, stridor, or weakness or complete loss of the voice (aphonia)
- Dysphagia
- Dilated superficial veins on chest, neck, or arms
- Edematous areas on chest wall
- Cyanosis
- Unequal pupils

Abdominal Aortic Aneurysm

- Some patients are asymptomatic.
- Pulsatile mass in the abdomen, patient complains of "heart beating" in abdomen when lying down or a feeling of an abdominal mass or abdominal throbbing.
- Cyanosis and mottling of the toes if aneurysm is associated with thrombus or embolus.

Dissecting Aneurysm

- Sudden onset with severe and persistent pain described as "tearing" or "ripping" in anterior chest or back, extending to shoulders, epigastric area, or abdomen (may be mistaken for acute MI)
- Low back pain may indicate pressure of AAA on lumbar nerves, a sign of rapidly expanding aneurysm and impending rupture.
- Pallor, sweating, and tachycardia
- Blood pressure elevated or markedly different from one arm to the other (thoracic)
- AAA rupture: Constant, intense back pain, falling blood pressure, and decreasing hematocrit

DIAGNOSTIC METHODS

- Thoracic aortic aneurysm: Chest X-ray, transesophageal echocardiography (TEE), and CT.
- Abdominal aortic aneurysm: Palpation of pulsatile mass in the middle and upper abdomen (a systolic bruit may be heard over the mass); duplex ultrasonography or CTA is used to determine the size, length, and location of the aneurysm.

- Dissecting aneurysm: Arteriography, CTA, TEE, duplex ultrasonography, and magnetic resonance angiography (MRA)

MEDICAL AND NURSING MANAGEMENT

Medical or surgical treatment depends on the type of aneurysm. When the aneurysm is small, ultrasonography is conducted at 6-month intervals.

Surgical Management

- For AAAs more than 5.5 cm wide or those that are enlarging, surgery is the treatment of choice.
- Thoracic aneurysms are treated by open surgical method or endovascular procedure.
- For a ruptured aneurysm, prognosis is poor and surgery is performed immediately.

Pharmacologic Therapy

- Strict control of blood pressure
- Systolic pressure maintained at 100 to 120 mm Hg with antihypertensive agents or beta blockers

N U R S I N G A L E R T

Constant intense back pain or tearing sensation, falling blood pressure, and decreasing hematocrit level are signs of a rupturing abdominal aortic aneurysm. Hematomas into the scrotum, perineum, flank, or penis indicate retroperitoneal rupture. Rupture into the peritoneal cavity is rapidly fatal.

For more information, see Chapter 18 in Pellico, L.H. (2013). *Focus on adult health: Medical-surgical nursing.* Philadelphia: Wolters Kluwer Health | Lippincott Williams & Wilkins.

Angina Pectoris

A

Angina pectoris is a clinical syndrome characterized by episodes of pain or pressure in the anterior chest.

PATHOPHYSIOLOGY

The cause of angina is insufficient coronary blood flow, usually caused by underlying atherosclerotic disease. Physical exertion or emotional stress increase myocardial demand for oxygen when supply cannot be increased, resulting in ischemia and pain.

RISK FACTORS

Same as for coronary atherosclerosis and ACS (see pp. 18-19).

CLINICAL MANIFESTATIONS AND ASSESSMENTS

- Pain varies from a feeling of indigestion to a choking or heavy sensation in the upper chest ranging from discomfort to agonizing pain.
- Angina is accompanied by severe apprehension and a feeling of impending death.
- The pain is usually retrosternal, deep in the chest behind sternum, and described as heavy, choking, strangling, or vise-like.
- Discomfort is poorly localized and may radiate to the neck, jaw, shoulders, and inner aspect of the upper arms (usually the left arm).
- Patients with diabetes mellitus may not have pain due to neuropathy; the elderly may experience weakness instead of pain.
- Associated symptoms include weakness or numbness in the arms, wrists, and hands, as well as shortness of breath, pallor, diaphoresis, dizziness, or lightheadedness. Nausea and vomiting may accompany the pain.

- An important characteristic of anginal pain is that it subsides with rest or nitroglycerin.

DIAGNOSTIC METHODS

- Evaluation of clinical manifestations of pain and patient history
- Electrocardiogram changes (12-lead ECG)
- Laboratory tests for biomarkers
- Echocardiogram, nuclear scan, or invasive procedures such as stress testing, cardiac catheterization, and coronary angiography

MEDICAL AND NURSING MANAGEMENT

The objectives of the medical management of angina are to decrease myocardial oxygen demand and increase oxygen supply. This is accomplished through pharmacologic therapy and control of risk factors. Alternatively, reperfusion procedures may be used to restore the blood supply to the myocardium. These include PCI procedures (eg, percutaneous transluminal coronary angioplasty [PTCA], intracoronary stents, and atherectomy) and CABG.

Pharmacologic Therapy

- Nitrates, the mainstay of therapy (nitroglycerin)
- Beta-adrenergic blocking agents (metoprolol and atenolol)
- Calcium channel blocking agents (amlodipine and diltiazem)
- Antiplatelet and anticoagulant medications (aspirin, clopidogrel, heparin, glycoprotein [GP] IIb/IIIa agents [abciximab, tirofiban, eptifibatide])

Oxygen Administration

Oxygen therapy

Percutaneous Coronary Intervention Surgical Treatments

See ACS on pages 20–21.

Surgical Procedures: Coronary Artery Revascularization

Coronary artery bypass graft is a surgical procedure in which a blood vessel is grafted to the occluded coronary artery so that blood can flow to the myocardium beyond the occlusion.

- Performed when coronary arteries are 60% to 70% occluded
- Vessels used for bypass include the saphenous veins, left internal mammary artery, or radial artery.
- Procedures are performed using extracorporeal bypass and heparin to prevent clotting; hypothermia is used to reduce metabolic oxygen demand.
- An alternate technique is "off pump," which decreases incidence of stroke, blood usage, and renal failure.
- Minimally invasive surgery (MIDCAB) is performed via thoracotomy for single-vessel disease.

Nursing Management

See ACS on pages 20–23.

For more information, see Chapter 14 in Pellico, L.H. (2013). *Focus on adult health: Medical-surgical nursing.* Philadelphia: Wolters Kluwer Health | Lippincott Williams & Wilkins.

Aortic Regurgitation (Insufficiency)

Aortic regurgitation is the backward flow of blood into the left ventricle (LV) from the aorta during diastole.

PATHOPHYSIOLOGY

When the aortic valve is incompetent, blood from the aorta returns to the LV during diastole. The LV dilates in an attempt to accommodate the blood volume, then hypertrophies. The LV expels more blood with greater force causing systolic blood pressure to rise. The peripheral arterioles relax, reducing peripheral resistance and diastolic blood pressure. Although compensatory mechanisms allow patients to remain asymptomatic for a time, when LV dysfunction develops, symptoms appear.

RISK FACTORS

- Rheumatic heart disease
- Infective endocarditis
- Marfan's syndrome
- Dissecting aortic aneurysm
- Bicuspid aortic valve

CLINICAL MANIFESTATIONS AND ASSESSMENT

- Asymptomatic for years; as disease progresses, symptoms related to increased stroke volume become apparent.
- Palpitations in supine position and visible neck vein pulsations
- Dyspnea, fatigue, angina, orthopnea and pulmonary congestion, signify decreased cardiac reserve and LV failure
- Systolic blood pressure in the lower extremities is higher than in the upper extremities.
- Widened pulse pressure
- Water-hammer (Corrigan's) pulse (pulse has rapid upstroke, then collapses)
- High pitched, blowing, decrescendo diastolic murmur (heard on the S_2), at the third or fourth intercostal space at the left sternal border; best heard with patient sitting up and leaning forward.

DIAGNOSTIC METHODS

- The diagnosis may be confirmed by echocardiography, valve morphology, degree of LV hypertrophy.
- Exercise stress testing will assess functional capacity and symptom response.

MEDICAL AND NURSING MANAGEMENT

Slowing disease progression, preventing complications, and optimizing the timing of surgery are the goals of medical management.

- Vasodilators for afterload reduction; avoid calcium channel blockers due to negative inotropic effects and beta blockers, which prevent compensatory tachycardia.
- Aortic valve replacement surgery with mechanical or tissue valve is advised when symptoms appear or if LV function begins to decrease. Acute AR is a surgical emergency.

Nursing Management

- Anticipate the patient will need long-term anticoagulation with mechanical valve replacement.
- Observe for postoperative complications, including thromboembolism, infection, arrhythmias, and hemolysis.
- Provide education to prevent infective endocarditis with antibiotic prophylaxis for patients with prosthetic valves.

See "Preoperative and Postoperative Nursing Management" in Chapter P on pages 531–554 for additional information.

For more information, see Chapter 16 in Pellico, L.H. (2013). *Focus on adult health: Medical-surgical nursing.* Philadelphia: Wolters Kluwer Health | Lippincott Williams & Wilkins.

Aortic Stenosis

Aortic stenosis is the narrowing of the valve opening between the left ventricle and the aorta, resulting in obstruction of blood flow across the valve.

PATHOPHYSIOLOGY

Progressive narrowing of the valve orifice usually occurs over several years to several decades. The LV overcomes this by contracting more slowly and more strongly than normal, forcibly squeezing the blood through the smaller orifice. The LV hypertrophies and dilates, with LV failure following. Elevated left atrial pressure, then pulmonary congestion occur, and ultimately right-heart failure develop.

RISK FACTORS

- Bicuspid aortic valve
- Advancing age
- Rheumatic valve disease
- Calcium deposits on valves
- Hypercholesterolemia

CLINICAL MANIFESTATIONS AND ASSESSMENTS

- May be asymptomatic for decades
- Triad of symptoms: Angina, dyspnea, and syncope with exertion
- A thrill or a vibration may be palpated in the aortic area (second intercostal space, right sternal border).
- A loud, systolic ejection murmur (heard on the S_1) may be heard over the aortic area and may radiate into the neck; auscultate with patient leaning forward.
- S_3 or S_4 gallop may be auscultated.

DIAGNOSTIC METHODS

- Echocardiography to diagnose and monitor progression
- Cardiac catheterization to measure severity, when noninvasive testing is inconclusive

A

MEDICAL AND NURSING MANAGEMENT

Most patients remain asymptomatic for years without intervention. The goal of medical therapy is to prevent complications.

- Nitrates are used if angina is present; use caution due to orthostatic hypotension and syncope.
- Digoxin may be used to treat LV dysfunction, and diuretics may be prescribed for dyspnea.
- With critical AS, strenuous exercise should be avoided.
- Surgery is recommended for patients with severe symptoms; note that once the patient develops angina, heart failure, or syncope, there is a significant decline in survival rate.
- Balloon valvuloplasty may be an option for older patients and those who are not surgical candidates.

Nursing Interventions

See "Preoperative and Postoperative Nursing Management" in Chapter P on pages 531–554 for additional information.

COMPLICATIONS

- Aortic regurgitation
- Embolization
- Ventricular perforation
- Rupture of the aortic valve annulus
- Ventricular arrhythmias
- Mitral valve damage
- Bleeding from the catheter insertion sites

For more information, see Chapter 16 in Pellico, L.H. (2013). *Focus on adult health: Medical-surgical nursing.* Philadelphia: Wolters Kluwer Health | Lippincott Williams & Wilkins.

Appendicitis

Appendicitis is an infection of the appendix, a small, finger-like appendage attached to the cecum just below the ileocecal valve.

PATHOPHYSIOLOGY

Because it empties into the colon inefficiently and its lumen is small, the appendix is prone to obstruction and infection. The obstructed appendix becomes inflamed, edematous, and eventually fills with pus. Appendicitis is the most common cause of acute inflammation in the right lower quadrant of the abdomen and the most common cause of emergency abdominal surgery.

RISK FACTORS

- Most common at 10 to 30 years of age, but may occur at any age.
- Winter months show most common presentation.
- Family history
- Male
- Patient with cystic fibrosis have higher risk.

CLINICAL MANIFESTATIONS AND ASSESSMENT

- Lower right quadrant pain usually accompanied by low-grade fever, nausea, and sometimes vomiting; loss of appetite; constipation can occur.
- Tenderness at McBurney's point, located halfway between the umbilicus and the anterior spine of the ilium.
- Rebound tenderness with pressure and rigidity of the lower portion of the right rectus muscle may be present; location of appendix dictates amount of tenderness, muscle spasm, and occurrence of constipation or diarrhea.

A

- Positive Rovsing's sign, elicited by palpating left lower quadrant, which paradoxically causes pain in right lower quadrant.
- With ruptured appendix, pain becomes more diffuse; abdominal distention develops from paralytic ileus, and sepsis may ensue.

DIAGNOSTIC METHODS

- Diagnosis is based on a complete physical examination and laboratory and imaging tests.
- Elevated WBC count with an elevation of the neutrophils
- Abdominal X-rays, ultrasound studies, and CT scans may reveal right lower quadrant density or localized distention of the bowel.
- Diagnostic laparoscopy may be used to rule out acute appendicitis in equivocal cases.

Gerontologic Considerations

Although acute appendicitis is uncommon in the elderly, signs and symptoms of appendicitis may vary greatly. Pain may be minimal or absent; leukocytosis and fever may not be present. Signs may be very vague and suggestive of bowel obstruction or another process; some patients may experience no symptoms until the appendix ruptures. The incidence of perforated appendix is higher in the elderly because many of these people do not seek health care as quickly as younger people.

MEDICAL AND NURSING MANAGEMENT

- Immediate surgery is indicated if appendix is ruptured.
- Administer antibiotics and IV fluids until surgery is performed.
- Plan to insert an NG tube for paralytic ileus.
- Avoid enemas, which may cause perforation.
- Abscess formation related to rupture may be treated with a drain placed into the abscess and antibiotic therapy, with subsequent surgical procedure to ensure complete drainage of the abscess.

- Postoperative care includes placing the patient in high-Fowler's position, administering analgesics, and reintroducing oral fluids as tolerated and after bowel sounds have returned.
- Discharge may occur on the day of surgery in uncomplicated patients; review incision care and dressing changes, activities, and follow-up care.
- If peritonitis develops, a drain may be left in and the patient monitored carefully for obstruction, hemorrhage, or abscess formation. Monitor the CBC and vital signs.

COMPLICATIONS

- Perforation
- Peritonitis
- Abscess formation (collection of purulent material)
- Portal pylephlebitis (septic thrombosis of the portal vein caused by vegetative emboli that arise from septic intestines)

For more information, see Chapter 24 in Pellico, L.H. (2013). *Focus on adult health: Medical-surgical nursing.* Philadelphia: Wolters Kluwer Health | Lippincott Williams & Wilkins.

Arthritis, Rheumatoid

Rheumatoid arthritis (RA) is an autoimmune, inflammatory arthritic condition.

PATHOPHYSIOLOGY

Rheumatoid factor (RF) antibodies develop in the synovium against the immunoglobulin IgG to form immune complexes. The activation of the complement system and release of lysosomal enzymes from leukocytes leads to inflammation. It is unknown why the body produces an antibody (RF) against its own antibody (IgG) and, in consequence, transforms IgG to an antigen or foreign protein that must be destroyed. Pannus, formation of vascular granulation tissue, is characteristic of RA and differentiates it from other forms of inflammatory arthritis. Pannus has a destructive effect on the adjacent cartilage and bone. Research has found that the inflammatory chemical messenger, tumor necrosis factor (TNF), is produced by cells at the cartilage–pannus junction and may also lead to cartilage destruction. The consequences are loss of articular surfaces and joint motion.

RISK FACTORS

- Autoimmune
- RA affects 1% of the population worldwide, affecting women two to four times more often than men.

CLINICAL MANIFESTATIONS AND ASSESSMENT

Clinical features are determined by the stage and severity of the disease and include:

- Joint pain, swelling, warmth, erythema, and lack of function are classic symptoms. Onset is usually acute.
- Joint involvement begins in the small joints of the hands, wrists, and feet. As the disease progresses, the knees, shoulders, hips, elbows, ankles, cervical spine, and temporomandibular joints are affected.
- Symptoms are usually bilateral and symmetric.
- Morning stiffness, indicating inflammation, lasts at least 30 to 45 minutes.
- Palpation of joints reveals spongy or boggy tissue.
- Rheumatoid nodules over bony prominences may be noted with more advanced RA.
- Deformities, such as hyperextension of proximal interphalangeal joint (PIP) joints (swan neck), flexion of PIP joints (Boutonniere), and ulnar deviation where fingers point ulnar, may be noted on examination.

- Fluid can usually be aspirated from the inflamed joint.
- Extra-articular features include arteritis, neuropathy, scleritis, pericarditis, splenomegaly, and Sjögren's syndrome (dry eyes and dry mucous membranes), weight loss, sensory changes, lymph node enlargement, and fatigue.

☀ Nursing Alert

Patients commonly have the inability to "wring out a wash cloth," need to hold a cup with both hands, and may complain of the sensation of having a "stone in my shoe."

DIAGNOSTIC FINDINGS

- Rheumatoid factor is present in about three-fourths of patients.
- Anticyclic citrullinated peptide (anti-CCP) is a marker that has similar sensitivity, but potentially has greater specificity to rheumatoid factor.
- Elevated erythrocyte sedimentation rate (ESR)
- High-sensitivity CRP testing may be done with or instead of ESR.
- Antinuclear antibody test results may be positive.
- RBC count and C4 complement component are decreased; ESR is elevated.
- Arthrocentesis shows abnormal synovial fluid that is cloudy, milky, or dark yellow and contains numerous inflammatory components, such as leukocytes and complement.
- Synovial biopsy for inflammatory cells
- X-rays, as disease advances, show bony erosions and narrowed joint spaces.

MEDICAL AND NURSING MANAGEMENT

Treatment begins with education, a balance of rest and exercise, pharmacologic therapy, and referral to community agencies for support.

A

- NSAIDs usually are the first choice in the treatment of RA to decrease inflammation and pain. Side effects such as gastric irritation, kidney damage, changes in liver function increase with age and long-term use.
- Cyclooxygenase-2 (COX-2) inhibitors decrease inflammatory process, with less GI complications that NSAIDs.

⚡ NURSING ALERT
COX-2 inhibitors must be used with caution because of the associated risk of cardiovascular disease.

- Disease-modifying antirheumatic drugs (DMARDs) are initiated if joint symptoms persist when using NSAIDs.
- Methotrexate (Rheumatrex, Trexall) is one of the first-choice DMARDs and has become the drug of choice due to its potency and its faster action than other DMARDs; improvement may develop in 3 to 6 weeks. Observe for sometimes fatal myelosuppression. Due to teratogenic effects, ensure patient has a negative pregnancy test.
- Another preferred DMARD, hydroxychloroquine (Plaquenil), an antimalarial agent, can be initiated early and used with mild symptoms, usually with methotrexate.
- Biologic agents or modifiers that interfere with TNF include etanercept (Enbrel), infliximab (Remicade), and adalimumab (Humira). Most recently golimumab (Simponi) and certolizumab pegol (Cimzia) have been approved for use in RA. Due to risk of serious infection, test the patient for TB before initiating therapy.
- Anakinra (Kineret) interferes with interleukin-1 (IL-1), which modulates immune and inflammatory responses.

⚡ NURSING ALERT
Do not give live vaccines to patients on a biologic agent. Nurses need to monitor for signs of infection (eg, fever, cough, flu-like symptoms, open sores on body). Nurses should also monitor for heart failure in patients on etanercept (Enbrel) or infliximab (Remicade).

- Small-molecule DMARDs include Leflunomide (Arava) and cyclosporine (Neoral, Sandimmune).

- Older DMARDs, gold salts, penicillamine, and azathioprine have limited use today and are reserved for progressive disease that has failed to respond to safer drugs.
- Glucocorticoids may be used during a "flare" or when "bridging" time for other medications to work. Long-term therapy can cause osteoporosis, gastric ulceration, adrenal suppression, and diabetes; use is limited to patients who have failed to respond to other treatment.
- Tetracycline derivatives minocycline (Minocin) and doxycycline (Vibramycin), are given to improve symptoms (morning stiffness, joint pain and tenderness, and activities of daily living).
- A protein A immunoadsorption column (Prosorba Column) that binds circulating immune system complex (IgG) is used in apheresis to remove RF from the blood.
- Low-dose antidepressant medications such as amitriptyline (Elavil), paroxetine (Paxil), or sertraline (Zoloft) are used to reestablish adequate sleep pattern and manage pain.

> For more information, see Chapter 39 in Pellico, L.H. (2013).
> *Focus on adult health: Medical-surgical nursing.* Philadelphia:
> Wolters Kluwer Health | Lippincott Williams & Wilkins.

Asthma

Asthma is a complex disease of the airways characterized by recurring and variable symptoms, airflow obstruction, and bronchial hyperresponsiveness. Inflammation is the key underlying feature and leads to recurrent episodes of asthma symptoms: cough, chest tightness, wheeze, and dyspnea.

PATHOPHYSIOLOGY

The underlying pathology in asthma is reversible and diffuse airway inflammation. Acute inflammation leads to airflow limitation and changes in the airways. Bronchoconstriction, the contraction of the smooth muscle of the airways, occurs; the airways become hyperresponsive. Airway edema becomes more progressive as asthma severity increases. Mucus hypersecretion and mucus plugs can occur. Advanced changes in the airways lead to airway narrowing and potentially irreversible airflow limitation.

An estimated 16 million American adults have asthma. Additionally, asthma accounts for 11 million outpatient visits, 2 million emergency room visits, approximately 500,000 hospitalizations and nearly 4,000 deaths per year.

RISK FACTORS

- Antigens: Pollens, molds, dust mites, animal dander, food
- Occupational exposure: Baking products, toluene
- Environmental factors: Tobacco smoke, air pollution, diet
- Viruses, sinus infections, postnasal drip
- Cold dry air
- Exercise, hard laughing, crying, yelling, emotions, and stress

CLINICAL MANIFESTATIONS AND ASSESSMENT

- Asthma is diagnosed based on history, physical examination, and spirometry with decreased forced expiratory volume (FEV_1).
- Asthma attacks frequently occur at night or in the early morning and may awaken patients.
- Asthma symptoms may occur suddenly or over days.
- Cough, productive or nonproductive, may be the only symptom reported.
- Exercise-induced asthma is common; it is defined as symptoms occurring during or soon after stopping exercise.
- Occupational asthma is worse on work days and improved on days off.
- Physical examination findings may reveal generalized wheezing initially heard during expiration. In between asthma episodes, physical exam findings may be normal.

NURSING ALERT

The occurrence of a severe, continuous reaction is referred to as *status asthmaticus* and is considered life-threatening. In more severe episodes, diaphoresis, wheezing heard on inspiration, tachycardia, and a widened pulse may occur along with hypoxemia. When airflow rates are very low, the "quiet chest" with minimal air movement may signal impending respiratory failure.

- As exacerbation progresses, central cyanosis secondary to severe hypoxia may occur.
- Additional symptoms, such as diaphoresis, tachycardia, and a widened pulse pressure may occur.
- A severe, continuous reaction, status asthmaticus, may occur. It is life-threatening.
- Eczema, rashes, and temporary edema are allergic reactions that may be noted with asthma.

DIAGNOSTIC METHODS

- ABGs
- Pulmonary function (FEV and forced vital capacity [FVC] decreased) tests are performed.
- Family, environment, and occupational history is taken to assess for allergic causes.
- Methacholine challenge, exercise challenge, or the administration of cold air to induce symptoms may be used to diagnose asthma when simple spirometry is normal and asthma is suspected.
- Sputum culture and blood test for eosinophilia and immunoglobulin E
- Chest X-ray to exclude alternate diagnosis; COPD and asthma may coexist.

MEDICAL AND NURSING MANAGEMENT

The goals of management are to prevent chronic and troublesome symptoms, maintain normal or near normal pulmonary function, maintain normal activity, prevent recurrent exacerbations, provide optimal pharmacotherapy, and meet patients' and families expectations of care.

Ongoing Assessment and Monitoring

- Perform physical assessment (similar to that for patient with COPD).
- Determine the patient's degree of risk for exacerbation.
- Assess ability to participate in normal activities, the frequency of exacerbations, and monitoring of pulmonary function by periodic spirometry or home peak flow monitoring.
- Perform a history of the patient's symptoms, self-care measures used, sequence of the current asthma episode, and response to medication and treatments used, including complementary and alternative therapy.
- Administer medications as prescribed and monitor the patient's response.
- Educate and prepare patient for discharge with focus on treatment, medication administration, management of asthma triggers, prevention and treatment of future exacerbations, and follow-up.

Patient Education

- Assist patients to identify and manage asthma triggers, monitor for early warning signs of acute episodes, and maintain proper medication management.
- Collaborate with patient to identify comorbid conditions, side effects, financial issues, living conditions, different beliefs about asthma, and other factors may influence the patient's adherence to the asthma management plan.

Pharmacologic Therapy

Quick-relief medications are used for the immediate treatment of asthma symptoms; long-acting medications are used to achieve and maintain control of persistent asthma. The lowest dose of medications to achieve control is recommended.

- Control of persistent asthma is accomplished primarily with regular use of anti-inflammatory medications; inhaled corticosteroids are treatment of choice. Patient should use a spacer and rinse the mouth after use to prevent thrush.

- Long-acting beta$_2$-adrenergic agonists (salbutamol and formoterol) with inhaled corticosteroid
- Leukotriene modifiers inhibitors/antileukotriene: Montelukast (Singulair), zafirlukast (Accolate), and zileuton (Zyflo)
- Cromolyn sodium and nedocromil stabilize mast cells; used for persistent asthma, exercise-induced asthma, and those not tolerating inhaled corticosteroids
- Omalizumab (anti-IgE) is used as an additional therapy for patients with severe, persistent asthma who have sensitivity to specific allergens.
- Occasionally used medications include methylxanthines, anticholinergic ipratropium.
- Oral corticosteroids regain quick control of asthma during exacerbations; long-term corticosteroid use may be needed with uncontrolled, severe, persistent asthma.

Environmental Control and Management of Triggers and Comorbid Conditions

- Skin testing is useful in some patients to identify specific allergens and in patients who may be candidates for immunotherapy.
- Help patients develop a trigger management plan.
- Comorbid conditions, particularly allergic bronchopulmonary aspergillosis (fungal infection), gastroesophageal reflux disease (GERD), obesity, obstructive sleep apnea, rhinitis, sinusitis, stress, and depression complicate asthma management and should be adequately treated to improve asthma control.

NURSING ALERT

Patients at high risk for asthma death need to seek medical care early during an exacerbation. High-risk situations include a history of previous severe exacerbation requiring intensive care and/or intubation, two or more hospitalizations or more than three emergency room visits in the past year, using more than two canisters of a short acting beta agonist (SABA) per month, difficulty perceiving worsening asthma, low socioeconomic status/inner-city residence, illicit drug use, severe psychiatric illness, and major comorbid conditions.

A

COMPLICATIONS

- Status asthmaticus
- Respiratory failure

For more information, see Chapter 11 in Pellico, L.H. (2013).
Focus on adult health: Medical-surgical nursing. Philadelphia:
Wolters Kluwer Health | Lippincott Williams & Wilkins.

Asthma: Status Asthmaticus

Status asthmaticus is a severe asthma episode that is refractory to
initial therapy. It is a medical emergency.

PATHOPHYSIOLOGY

See "Asthma" on pages 71–72.

RISK FACTORS

- Viral or respiratory infection
- Exposure to trigger or exercise in cold environment
- Nebulizer abuse
- Nonadherence to controller medications
- See Asthma for other triggers.

CLINICAL MANIFESTATIONS AND ASSESSMENT

- Similar to those in asthma; however, increased in severity, without recovery with usual treatments

- Wheezing, tachycardia, diaphoresis, and a widened pulse may occur along with severe hypoxemia.
- Progresses to minimal air movement, and the "quiet chest" reflects impending respiratory failure.

☀ **N U R S I N G   A L E R T**

A quiet chest is worrisome; the nurse considers that airflow can be so limited that wheezing cannot be detected. Sounds may begin to be audible with bronchodilator treatment when the airways are dilated enough to detect a wheeze.

DIAGNOSTIC METHODS

- See "Asthma" on page 73.

MEDICAL AND NURSING MANAGEMENT

- For status asthmaticus, actively assess patient's airway and response to treatment; administer fluids, systemic corticosteroids, bronchodilators, and energy conservation.
- Intubation and mechanical ventilation may be needed to keep saturation over 95%.
- Administer heliox, magnesium sulfate, and leukotriene modifiers.
- Ensure patient's room is quiet and free of respiratory irritants (eg, flowers, perfumes, or odors of cleaning agents); nonallergenic pillows should be used.

See additional nursing interventions under "Asthma" on pages 73–75.

For additional information, see Chapter 11 in Pellico, L.H. (2013). *Focus on adult health: Medical-surgical nursing.* Philadelphia: Wolters Kluwer Health | Lippincott Williams & Wilkins.

B

Back Pain, Low

Low back pain is one of the most common reasons for a visit to the provider. This condition is caused by one of many musculoskeletal problems, including acute lumbosacral strain, unstable lumbosacral ligaments and weak muscles, osteoarthritis of the spine, spinal stenosis, intervertebral disk problems, and unequal leg length.

PATHOPHYSIOLOGY

The spinal column can be considered as an elastic rod constructed of rigid units (vertebrae) and flexible units (intervertebral disks) held together by complex facet joints, multiple ligaments, and paravertebral muscles. Its unique construction allows for flexibility while providing maximum protection for the spinal cord. Obesity, disuse, postural problems, structural problems, and overstretching of the spinal supports may result in back pain.

The intervertebral disks change in character as a person ages. A young person's disks are mainly fibrocartilage with a gelatinous matrix. As a person ages, the fibrocartilage becomes dense and irregularly shaped. Disk degeneration is a common cause of back pain. The lower lumbar disks, L4–L5 and L5–S1, are subject to the greatest mechanical stress and the greatest degenerative changes. Disk protrusion (herniated nucleus pulposus) or facet joint changes can cause pressure on nerve roots as they leave the spinal canal, which results in pain that radiates along the nerve.

RISK FACTORS

- Obesity
- Aging
- Disuse, postural problems, structural problems, overstretching of the spinal supports
- Stress
- Occasionally, depression
- Back pain due to musculoskeletal disorders usually is aggravated by activity, whereas pain due to other conditions is not.

Gerontologic Consideration

Older patients may experience back pain associated with osteoporotic vertebral fractures, osteoarthritis of the spine, spinal stenosis, and spondylolisthesis, among other conditions.

CLINICAL MANIFESTATIONS AND ASSESSMENT

- Acute or chronic back pain, muscle spasm, sciatica, and fatigue
- Pain that radiates down the leg (sciatica) or a nerve root (radiculopathy); presence of this symptom suggests nerve root involvement
- Gait, spinal mobility, reflexes, leg length, leg motor strength, and sensory perception may be affected.
- Paravertebral muscle spasm (greatly increased muscle tone of back postural muscles) occurs with loss of normal lumbar curve and possible spinal deformity.

DIAGNOSTIC METHODS

- Health history and physical examination (back examination, neurologic testing)
- Spinal X-ray
- Bone scan and blood studies
- Computed tomography (CT) scan
- Magnetic resonance imaging (MRI)
- Electromyogram (EMG) and nerve conduction studies
- Myelogram
- Ultrasound

MEDICAL AND NURSING MANAGEMENT

Management focuses on relief of pain and discomfort, activity modification, use of back-conserving techniques of body mechanics, improved self-esteem, and weight reduction. Most back pain is self-limited and resolves within 4 weeks with analgesics, rest, stress reduction, and relaxation.

Relieving Pain

- Encourage patient to reduce stress on the back muscles and to change position frequently.
- Teach reduction of muscular and psychological tension using diaphragmatic breathing and relaxation, diversion, or guided imagery with other pain-relief strategies.
- Application of heat and cold provides temporary relief.
- Nonprescription analgesics may be used; additional muscle relaxants or opioids may be needed.
- In the absence of symptoms of disease (radiculopathy of the roots of spinal nerves), spinal manipulation performed by a chiropractor or an osteopath may be helpful.
- Massage, biofeedback, yoga, and acupuncture may be therapeutic.

Improving Physical Mobility

- As the back pain subsides, self-care activities are resumed with minimal strain on the injured structures.
- Position changes should be made slowly and carried out with assistance as required.
- The patient should avoid twisting and jarring motions.
- Encourage the patient to alternate lying, sitting, and walking; advise the patient to avoid sitting, standing, or walking for long periods.
- Sitting in a chair with arm rests to support some of the body weight and a soft support at the small of the back provides comfort.
- With severe pain, the nurse instructs the patient to limit activities for 1 to 2 days. Extended periods of inactivity are not effective and result in deconditioning

- A firm, nonsagging mattress (a bed board may be used) is recommended.
- Lumbar flexion is increased by elevating the head and thorax 30 degrees using pillows or a foam wedge and slightly flexing the knees, which are supported on a pillow; or patient may assume a lateral position with knees and hips flexed (curled position).
- Instruct the patient to get out of bed by rolling to one side and placing the legs down while pushing the torso up, keeping the back straight.
- Gradually resume activities; after 2 weeks, conditioning exercises for the abdomen and trunk are started. If there is no improvement within 1 month, additional assessments for physiologic abnormalities are performed.

Using Proper Body Mechanics

Good body mechanics and posture are essential to avoid recurrence of back pain.

- Encourage the patient to wear low heels with good arch support.
- The patient who must stand for long periods should shift weight frequently and should rest one foot on a low stool, which decreases lumbar lordosis.
- Patients who stand in place for a long period of time (eg, cashiers) should stand on a foot cushion made of foam or rubber.
- The proper posture can be verified by looking in a mirror to see whether the chest is up, the abdomen is tucked in, and the shoulders are down and relaxed.
- Instruct the patient in the safe and correct way to lift objects—using the strong quadriceps muscles of the thighs, with minimal use of weak back muscles. Place feet hip-width apart, bend the knees, tighten the abdominal muscles, and lift the object close to the body with a smooth motion, avoiding twisting and jarring motions.

Modifying Nutrition for Weight Reduction

- Obesity contributes to back strain by stressing the relatively weak back muscles.

- Weight reduction through diet modification may prevent recurrence of back pain using a sound nutritional plan that includes a change in eating habits to maintain desirable weight.
- Monitoring weight reduction, noting achievement, and providing encouragement and positive reinforcement facilitate adherence.
- Frequently, back problems resolve as optimal weight is achieved.

> For more information, see Chapters 40 and 42 in Pellico, L.H. (2013). *Focus on adult health: Medical-surgical nursing.* Philadelphia: Wolters Kluwer Health | Lippincott Williams & Wilkins.

Bell's Palsy

Bell's palsy causes unilateral facial paralysis due to peripheral involvement of the seventh cranial nerve, which results in weakness or paralysis of the facial muscles on the ipsilateral side.

PATHOPHYSIOLOGY

The cause is unknown, but possible theories about causes include vascular ischemia, viral disease (herpes simplex, herpes zoster), autoimmune disease, or a combination of all of these factors. Bell's palsy may be a type of pressure paralysis. The inflamed, edematous nerve becomes compressed to the point of damage, or its blood supply is occluded, producing ischemic necrosis of the nerve.

CLINICAL MANIFESTATIONS AND ASSESSMENT

- Facial distortion from paralysis; when asked to smile, weakness of the involved nerve will be noted, there will be an absence of

wrinkling on the forehead, the affected side will appear mask-like.
- Increased lacrimation
- Pain in face, behind the ear, and in the eye of the affected side
- Ear pain may precede paralysis by 24 to 48 hours.
- Speech difficulties and inability to eat on affected side
- Disturbance of taste

MEDICAL AND NURSING MANAGEMENT

The objectives of management are to maintain facial muscle tone and to prevent or minimize denervation.

Pharmacologic Therapy

- Corticosteroid therapy (prednisone) may be prescribed to reduce inflammation and edema; this reduces vascular compression and permits restoration of blood circulation to the nerve. Early administration of corticosteroids appears to diminish severity, relieve pain, and minimize denervation.
- Facial pain is controlled with analgesic agents or heat applied to the involved side of the face.
- Additional modalities may include electrical stimulation applied to the face to prevent muscle atrophy.
- If the eye does not close completely or the blink reflex is diminished, protect it from injury with a protective shield at night. Teach the patient to close the eye manually before going to sleep or applying eye shield.
- Wrap-around sunglasses or goggles may be worn during the day to decrease normal evaporation from the eye.

For more information, see Chapter 46 in Pellico, L.H. (2013). *Focus on adult health: Medical-surgical nursing.* Philadelphia: Wolters Kluwer Health | Lippincott Williams & Wilkins.

B

Bone Tumors

Neoplasms of the musculoskeletal system may include osteogenic, chondrogenic, fibrogenic, muscle (rhabdomyogenic), and marrow (reticulum) cell tumors, as well as nerve, vascular, and fatty cell tumors. They may be primary tumors or metastatic tumors; metastatic bone tumors are more common than primary bone tumors.

TYPES

Benign Bone Tumors

Benign tumors of the bone and soft tissue are more common than malignant primary bone tumors. Benign bone tumors are slow growing, well circumscribed, and encapsulated, present few symptoms, and do not cause death. Benign primary neoplasms of the musculoskeletal system include osteochondroma, enchondroma, bone cyst (eg, aneurysmal bone cyst), osteoid osteoma, rhabdomyoma, and fibroma. Some benign tumors, such as giant cell tumors, have the potential to become malignant.

Malignant Bone Tumors

Primary malignant musculoskeletal tumors are relatively rare and arise from connective and supportive tissue cells (sarcomas) or bone marrow elements (myelomas). Malignant primary musculoskeletal tumors include osteosarcoma, chondrosarcoma, Ewing's sarcoma, and fibrosarcoma. Soft tissue sarcomas include liposarcoma, fibrosarcoma, and rhabdomyosarcoma. Osteogenic sarcoma (osteosarcoma) appears most frequently in males between 10 and 25 years of age, and is the most common and most fatal primary bone tumor. It is also seen in older people with Paget's disease of the bone and in persons with a prior history of radiation exposure. Common sites are distal femur, the proximal tibia, and the proximal humerus.

Chondrosarcoma is a malignant tumor of the hyaline cartilage. It is the second most common primary malignant bone tumor characterized by large, bulky, slow-growing lesions of the pelvis, femur, humerus, spine, scapula, and tibia. Metastasis to the lung occurs; tumors may recur after treatment.

Metastatic Bone Disease

Metastatic bone disease (secondary bone tumors) is more common than any primary malignant bone tumor. Tumors arising from tissues elsewhere in the body may invade the bone and produce localized bone destruction (lytic lesions) or bone overgrowth (blastic lesions). The most common primary sites of tumors that metastasize to bone are the kidney, prostate, lung, breast, ovary, and thyroid. Metastatic tumors most frequently attack the skull, spine, pelvis, femur, and humerus, and often involve more than one bone.

PATHOPHYSIOLOGY

A tumor in the bone causes the normal bone tissue to react by osteolytic response (bone destruction) or osteoblastic response (bone formation). Primary tumors cause bone destruction, which weakens the bone, resulting in bone fractures. Adjacent normal bone responds to the tumor by altering its normal pattern of remodeling. The bone's surface changes and the contours enlarge in the tumor area.

Malignant bone tumors invade and destroy adjacent bone tissue. Benign bone tumors, in contrast, have a symmetric, controlled growth pattern and place pressure on adjacent bone tissue. Malignant invading bone tumors weaken the structure of the bone until it can no longer withstand the stress of ordinary use; pathologic fracture commonly results.

CLINICAL MANIFESTATIONS AND ASSESSMENT

Bone tumors present with a wide range of associated problems:

- Asymptomatic or mild, occasional to constant, severe pain; tumor may be diagnosed only after pathologic fracture

B

- Varying degrees of disability; at times, obvious bone growth
- Weight loss, malaise, and fever may be present.
- Spinal metastasis may result in cord compression with neurologic deficits (eg, progressive pain, weakness, gait abnormality, paresthesia, paraplegia, urinary retention, loss of bowel or bladder control).

DIAGNOSTIC FINDINGS

- May be diagnosed incidentally after pathologic fracture.
- CT scan, bone scan, myelography, MRI, arteriography, biopsy, X-ray studies
- Elevated alkaline phosphatase levels (osteogenic sarcoma), acid phosphatase (metastatic carcinoma of the prostate), hypercalcemia (with breast, lung, and kidney cancer bone metastases)
- Surgical biopsy is performed for histologic identification. Extreme care is taken during the biopsy to prevent seeding and resultant recurrence after excision of the tumor.

MEDICAL AND NURSING MANAGEMENT

The goal of treatment is to destroy or remove the tumor. This may be accomplished by surgical excision (ranging from local excision to amputation and disarticulation), radiation, or chemotherapy.

Primary Bone Tumors

- Limb-sparing (salvage) procedures are used to remove the tumor and adjacent tissue; prosthesis, total joint arthroplasty, or bone tissue from the patient (autograft) or from a cadaver donor (allograft) replaces the resected tissue.
- Chemotherapy is started before and continued after surgery in an effort to eradicate micrometastatic lesions.
- Soft-tissue sarcomas are treated with radiation, limb-sparing excision, and adjuvant chemotherapy.

- Complications may include infection, loosening or dislocation of the prosthesis, allograft nonunion, fracture, devitalization of the skin and soft tissues, joint fibrosis, and recurrence of the tumor.

Secondary Bone Tumors

- The treatment of metastatic bone cancer is palliative. The therapeutic goal is to relieve the patient's pain and discomfort while promoting quality of life.
- Structural support and stabilization may be needed to prevent pathologic fracture; large bones with metastatic lesions may be strengthened by prophylactic internal fixation, arthroplasty, or methylmethacrylate (bone cement) reconstruction to minimize associated disability and pain.
- Patients with metastatic disease are at higher risk than other patients for postoperative pulmonary congestion, hypoxemia, deep vein thrombosis (DVT), and hemorrhage.
- Hypercalcemia resulting from breakdown of bone must be recognized and treated promptly. Intravenous hydration with normal saline solution, diuresis, mobilization, and medications such as bisphosphonates, pamidronate, and calcitonin are used.
- Assist the patient to increase activity and ambulation to prevent loss of bone mass due to inactivity.
- Hematopoiesis may be disrupted by tumor invasion of the bone marrow or by treatment (chemotherapy or radiation). Blood component therapy restores hematologic factors.
- Pain can result from multiple factors, including the osseous metastasis, surgery, chemotherapy or radiation side effects, and arthritis. Opioid, nonopioid, and nonpharmaceutical interventions including external beam radiation to involved metastatic sites using systemically administered "bone-seeking" isotopes (eg, strontium 89) for multiple metastases may be used.
- Chemotherapy is used to control the primary disease.

NURSING MANAGEMENT

The nursing care of a patient who has undergone excision of a bone tumor is similar in many respects to that of other patients who have had skeletal surgery. Vital signs are monitored, blood

B

loss is assessed, and observations are made to assess for the development of complications such as DVT, pulmonary embolus (PE), infection, contracture, and disuse atrophy. The affected part is elevated to reduce edema, and the neurovascular status of the extremity is assessed.

Providing Patient Education

- Patient and family teaching about the disease process and diagnostic and management regimens is essential. Explanation of diagnostic tests, treatments (eg, wound care), and expected results (eg, decreased range of motion, numbness, change of body contours) helps the patient deal with the procedures and changes.

Relieving Pain

- Accurate pain assessment is the foundation for pain management.
- Pharmacologic and nonpharmacologic pain management techniques are used to relieve pain and increase the patient's comfort level.
- Intravenous or epidural analgesics are used during the early postoperative period. Later, oral or transdermal opioid or nonopioid analgesics are indicated to alleviate pain.
- External radiation or systemic radioisotopes may be used to control pain.

Preventing Pathologic Fracture

- Bone tumors weaken bone to a point at which normal activities or even position changes can result in fracture.
- The affected extremities must be supported and handled gently. External supports (eg, splints) may be used for additional protection.
- Elective surgery (eg, open reduction with internal fixation, joint replacement) may prevent pathologic fracture.
- Prescribed weight-bearing restrictions must be followed. The nurse and physical therapist teach the patient how to use assistive devices safely and how to strengthen unaffected extremities.

Promoting Coping Skills

- The nurse encourages the patient and family to verbalize their fears, concerns, and feelings, while offering support.
- Referral to psychiatric advanced practice nurse, psychologist, counselor, or spiritual advisor may be indicated.

Promoting Self-Care

- Assist the patient in dealing with changes in body image due to surgery and possible amputation; provide realistic reassurance about the future and resumption of role-related activities, and encourage self-care and socialization.
- Encourage the patient to be as independent as possible.

Monitoring and Managing Potential Complications

Delayed Wound Healing

Wound healing may be delayed because of tissue trauma from surgery, previous radiation therapy, inadequate nutrition, or infection.

- Assess the patient's nutritional status by monitoring weight, percentage of weight loss, and evaluating the serum albumin or prealbumin level.
- An unintentional weight loss of 10% of usual body weight in 3 months is a risk factor for malnutrition.
- Wound healing will increase the patient's requirements for calories, protein, vitamins, and minerals.
- Minimize pressure on the wound site to promote circulation to the tissues. Reposition the patient at frequent intervals to reduce the incidence of skin breakdown and pressure ulcers.
- Therapeutic beds may be needed to prevent skin breakdown and to promote wound healing after surgical reconstruction and skin grafting.

Inadequate Nutrition

- Anorexia, nausea, and vomiting are frequent side effects of chemotherapy and radiation therapy; these may interfere with adequate nutrition.

- Antiemetics and relaxation techniques reduce the adverse gastrointestinal (GI) effects of chemotherapy.
- Stomatitis is controlled with anesthetic or antifungal mouthwash.
- Adequate hydration is essential.
- Nutritional supplements, enteral or parenteral nutrition, may be prescribed to achieve adequate nutrition.

Osteomyelitis and Wound Infections

- Prophylactic antibiotics and strict aseptic dressing techniques are used to diminish the occurrence of osteomyelitis and wound infections.
- Monitor the white blood cell (WBC) count and instruct the patient to avoid contact with people who have colds or other infections during chemotherapy.

Hypercalcemia

Observe for muscular weakness, incoordination, anorexia, nausea and vomiting, constipation, electrocardiographic changes (eg, shortened QT interval and ST segment, bradycardia, heart blocks), and altered mental states (eg, confusion, lethargy, psychotic behavior). See Chapter 16, Table 16-12 in Pellico: *Focus on Adult Health: Medical-Surgical Nursing* for a discussion of hypercalcemia and its management.

> For more information, see Chapter 41 in Pellico, L.H. (2013). *Focus on adult health: Medical-surgical nursing.* Philadelphia: Wolters Kluwer Health | Lippincott Williams & Wilkins.

Bowel Obstruction, Large

Intestinal obstruction occurs when blockage prevents the forward flow of contents through the intestinal tract.

PATHOPHYSIOLOGY

Large bowel obstruction results in an accumulation of intestinal contents, fluid, and gas proximal to the obstruction. Obstruction in the colon can lead to severe distention and perforation unless gas and fluid can flow back through the ileal valve. Large bowel obstruction, even if complete, may be without catastrophic issue if the blood supply to the colon is not disturbed. However, if the blood supply is cut off, intestinal strangulation and necrosis (ie, tissue death) occur; this condition is life threatening. Adenocarcinoid tumors account for the majority of large bowel obstructions. Most tumors occur beyond the splenic flexure, making them accessible with a flexible sigmoidoscope.

RISK FACTORS

- Cancers (most common), polyps, benign tumors
- Diverticulitis
- Irritable bowel disease (IBD)
- Adhesions
- Hernias
- Volvulus, intussusception
- Neurologic disorders (Parkinson's)
- Abscesses
- Manipulation of bowel during surgery

CLINICAL MANIFESTATIONS AND ASSESSMENT

Symptoms develop and progress relatively slowly.

- Constipation may be the only symptom for months (obstruction in sigmoid colon or rectum).
- Shape of the stool is altered as it passes the obstruction that is gradually increasing in size.
- Blood is lost through the stool, which may result in iron-deficiency anemia.
- The patient may experience weakness, weight loss, and anorexia.
- Abdomen eventually becomes markedly distended, loops of large bowel become visibly outlined through the abdominal wall, and patient has crampy lower abdominal pain.
- Fecal vomiting develops rarely; symptoms of shock may occur.

DIAGNOSTIC METHODS

Symptoms plus imaging studies (abdominal X-ray and abdominal CT scan or MRI; barium studies are contraindicated due to risk of perforation)

MEDICAL AND NURSING MANAGEMENT

- Restoration of intravascular volume, correction of electrolyte abnormalities, and nasogastric (NG) aspiration and decompression are instituted immediately.
- Colonoscopy to untwist and decompress the bowel, if obstruction is high in the colon.
- Cecostomy may be performed for patients who are poor surgical risks and urgently need relief from the obstruction.
- A rectal tube may be used to decompress an area that is lower in the bowel.
- Usual treatment is surgical resection to remove the obstructing lesion; a temporary or permanent colostomy may be necessary; an ileoanal anastomosis may be performed if entire large bowel must be removed.

Nursing Management

- Monitor symptoms indicating worsening intestinal obstruction.
- Provide emotional support and comfort.
- Administer IV fluids and electrolyte replacement.
- Prepare patient for surgery if no response to medical treatment.
- Provide preoperative teaching as patient's condition indicates.
- After surgery, provide general abdominal wound care and routine postoperative nursing care.

For more information, see Chapter 24 in Pellico, L.H. (2013). *Focus on adult health: Medical-surgical nursing.* Philadelphia: Wolters Kluwer Health | Lippincott Williams & Wilkins.

Bowel Obstruction, Small

Small bowel obstruction refers to blockage of the small intestine including the duodenum, ileum, and jejunum. Most bowel obstructions occur in the small intestine.

PATHOPHYSIOLOGY

Intestinal contents, fluid, and gas accumulate above the intestinal obstruction. The abdominal distention and retention of fluid reduce the absorption of fluids and stimulate more gastric secretion. With increasing distention, pressure within the intestinal lumen increases, causing a decrease in venous and arteriolar capillary pressure. This causes edema, congestion, necrosis, and eventual rupture or perforation of the intestinal wall, with resultant peritonitis.

Reflux vomiting may be caused by abdominal distention, causing metabolic alkalosis. Dehydration and/or hypovolemic shock may occur.

RISK FACTOR

- Adhesions (most common)
- Hernias
- Neoplasms
- Intussusception
- Volvulus (twisting of the bowel)
- Paralytic ileus

CLINICAL MANIFESTATIONS AND ASSESSMENT

- Initial symptom is usually crampy pain that is wavelike and colicky. Patient may pass blood and mucus but no fecal matter or flatus. Vomiting occurs.

- If the obstruction is complete, peristaltic waves become extremely vigorous and assume a reverse direction, propelling intestinal contents toward the mouth.
- If the obstruction is in the ileum, fecal vomiting takes place.
- Dehydration results in intense thirst, drowsiness, generalized malaise, aching, and a parched tongue and mucous membranes.
- Abdomen becomes distended; the lower the obstruction in the GI tract, the more marked the distention.
- If uncorrected, hypovolemic shock occurs due to dehydration and loss of plasma volume.

DIAGNOSTIC FINDINGS

- Symptoms and imaging studies; abdominal X-rays reveal abnormal quantities of gas and/or fluid in intestines.
- Laboratory studies, electrolytes, and complete blood count show dehydration and possibly infection.

MEDICAL AND NURSING MANAGEMENT

Decompression of the bowel through a NG tube is successful in most cases. When the bowel is completely obstructed, the possibility of strangulation warrants surgical intervention. Before surgery, IV therapy is necessary to replace the depleted water, sodium, chloride, and potassium. Surgical procedures include, repairing a hernia, dividing an adhesion, or removing a portion of affected bowel.

Nursing Management

- Maintain the function of the NG tube.
- Assess and measure NG output.
- Assess for fluid and electrolyte imbalance.
- Monitor nutritional status and assess improvement (eg, return of normal bowel sounds, decreased abdominal distention, subjective improvement in abdominal pain and tenderness, passage of flatus or stool).

- Report discrepancies in intake and output, worsening of pain or abdominal distention, and increased NG output.
- If patient's condition does not improve, prepare him or her for surgery.
- Provide postoperative nursing care similar to that for other abdominal surgeries (see "Preoperative and Postoperative Nursing Management" in Chapter P on pages 531–554 for additional information).

For more information, see Chapter 24 in Pellico, L.H. (2013). *Focus on adult health: Medical-surgical nursing.* Philadelphia: Wolters Kluwer Health | Lippincott Williams & Wilkins.

Brain Tumors

A brain tumor is a localized intracranial lesion that occupies space within the skull.

PATHOPHYSIOLOGY

The effects of brain tumors, including seizure activity and focal neurologic signs, are caused by the compression or infiltration of tissue, or both. Tumors may be benign or malignant. Benign tumors are slow growing but can occur in a vital area where they can cause serious effects as they grow. Malignant tumors are rapidly growing in nature, can spread into surrounding tissue, and are considered life threatening. Primary brain tumors rarely spread to other areas of the body.

TYPES OF TUMORS

- Gliomas are tumors originating within brain tissue.
- Meningiomas, the most common brain tumor, arise from the coverings of the brain.

B

- Acoustic neuroma or vestibular schwannoma is a benign tumor of the eighth cranial nerve.
- Pituitary adenomas are usually benign, but in rare cases may be malignant.
- Tumors of the pituitary and pineal glands and of cerebral blood vessels are also considered types of brain tumors.
- Angiomas are masses composed largely of abnormal blood vessels and are found in or on the brain's surface. They may be asymptomatic or cause symptoms of brain tumor, such as seizure and headaches due to thin blood vessel walls. There is increased risk for hemorrhagic stroke.
- Cerebral metastasis, the spread of cancer cells from their primary site to the brain, occur four times more often than do primary tumors. Primary sites of cancers that commonly metastasize to the brain include the lung and breast.

RISK FACTORS

- Unknown
- Exposure to ionizing radiation and cancer-causing chemicals
- Possible risks requiring further investigation include nonionizing radiation, physical and acoustic trauma, dietary factors, and certain genetic syndromes.
- Higher risk in females than males

CLINICAL MANIFESTATIONS AND ASSESSMENT

Brain tumors can produce focal (localized) symptoms such as weakness, sensory loss, aphasia, visual dysfunction, and other site-specific manifestations. Generalized neurologic symptoms such as seizures, nausea and vomiting, cognitive impairment, and visual disturbances may also occur.

Increased ICP

- Headache, nausea with or without vomiting; most common in the early morning and is made worse by coughing, straining, or sudden movement

- Vomiting, often unrelated to food intake, may occur and may be projectile; headache may be relieved by vomiting.
- Papilledema (edema of the optic nerve) is associated with visual disturbances.
- Personality changes and a variety of focal deficits, including motor, sensory, and cranial nerve dysfunction, are common.
- New-onset seizure, whether simple partial seizures, complex partial seizures, or generalized tonic–clonic seizures, occur in approximately 50% of patients.
- Late symptoms include hypertension with widening pulse pressure, bradycardia, and respiratory depression, also known as Cushing's triad.

✳ N U R S I N G   A L E R T

Morning headaches are suggestive of a tumor. The nurse assesses for fever associated with the headache, which points to an infectious process such as meningitis or encephalitis. Headache without fever is associated with a tumor or intracerebral bleeding.

Localized Symptoms

The most common focal or localized symptoms are hemiparesis, seizures, and mental status changes.

- When specific regions of the brain are affected, additional focal signs and symptoms occur, such as sensory and motor abnormalities, visual alterations, changes in hearing, alterations in cognition, and language disturbances may occur. For example, if a tumor is present in the cerebellar area, the nurse might expect to see changes in balance and coordination.
- The progression of the signs and symptoms is important because it indicates tumor growth and expansion.
- Personality changes, difficulty concentrating, memory loss, confusion, and changes in temperament may occur.
- Fatigue may occur with malignant or nonmalignant brain tumors; a constant feeling of exhaustion, weakness, and lack of energy may occur and should be differentiated from stress, depression, and anxiety.

B

DIAGNOSTIC METHODS

- History of the illness and manner in which symptoms evolved
- Neurologic examination indicating areas involved
- Magnetic resonance imaging is the gold standard for detecting brain tumors.
- CT with contrast, positron emission tomography (PET), computer-assisted stereotactic (three-dimensional) biopsy, cerebral angiography, electroencephalogram (EEG), and cytologic studies of the cerebrospinal fluid

MEDICAL AND NURSING MANAGEMENT

A variety of medical treatments, including chemotherapy and radiation therapy, are used alone or in combination with surgical resection.

Surgical Management

Surgical intervention provides the best outcome for most tumors. The goal is to remove part of the tumor or the entire tumor without increasing the neurologic deficit The specific approach depends on the type of tumor, its location, and its accessibility.

Radiation Therapy

- Radiation therapy, the cornerstone of treatment for many brain tumors, decreases the recurrence of incompletely resected tumors.
- External beam radiation, or stereotactic radiation therapy using a linear accelerator or gamma knife may be used.
- Brachytherapy, implanting radiation seeds close to or into the tumor may be done, but is not standard.

Pharmacologic Therapy and Chemotherapy

- Chemotherapy may be given intravenously, orally, or intrathecally (injected directly into the subarachnoid space).

- Corticosteroids are used to reduce cerebral edema and side effects of treatment, such as nausea and vomiting. They may help relieve headache and alterations in level of consciousness.
- Antiseizure medications will be used if seizures occur.
- Pain is managed by means of a stepped progression with regard to the dosing, delivery method, and type of analgesic agents needed for relief.

Medical Management of Metastatic Brain Cancer

Treatment of metastatic brain cancer is palliative and designed to eliminate or reduce uncomfortable symptoms to improve the quality of life for patients and families.

☀ N U R S I N G   A L E R T

Although DVT and PE occur in approximately 15% of patients and can cause significant morbidity, anticoagulants avoided due to risk for central nervous system (CNS) hemorrhage.

Other Therapies

- Intravenous autologous bone marrow transplantation for marrow toxicity associated with high doses of drugs and radiation
- Gene-transfer therapy (currently being tested)

For more information on care of the patient undergoing neurosurgery, see Chapters 44 and Chapter 45 in Pellico, L.H. (2013). *Focus on adult health: Medical-surgical nursing.* Philadelphia: Wolters Kluwer Health | Lippincott Williams & Wilkins.

Bronchitis, Chronic

Chronic bronchitis, a type of chronic obstructive pulmonary disease (COPD), results in airflow limitation. It is defined as the presence of cough and sputum production for at least 3 months in each of 2 consecutive years.

PATHOPHYSIOLOGY

Chronic mucus hypersecretion, thickening of the epithelium, smooth muscle hypertrophy, and airway inflammation are implicated in remodeling of the airways and decreasing the size of the airway lumen. In later stages of COPD, gas exchange is impaired. Chronic hypoxemia increases pulmonary artery pressure, increasing the workload of the right ventricle. Right ventricular hypertrophy and failure (*cor pulmonale*) may result. Additionally, decreased carbon dioxide elimination results in increased carbon dioxide tension in arterial blood (hypercapnia) and leads to respiratory acidosis and chronic respiratory failure. In acute illness, worsening hypercapnia can lead to acute respiratory failure. Altered function of the alveolar macrophages make the individual more susceptible to respiratory infection. Most patients will have elements of both emphysema and chronic bronchitis.

RISK FACTORS

- Cigarette smoking, tobacco smoke, second-hand smoke, fetal exposure to smoke
- Occupational dust and chemicals (organic dusts, inorganic dusts, chemical agents, fumes)
- Indoor and outdoor air pollution (biomass cooking in poorly ventilated areas, heating in poorly ventilated areas)
- Infection (history of severe respiratory infections, history of tuberculosis in those >40 years old)
- Viral, bacterial, and mycoplasmal infections can produce acute exacerbations.

CLINICAL MANIFESTATIONS AND ASSESSMENT

- Diagnosis is based on history, physical exam, and pulmonary function testing.
- Characterized by three primary symptoms: dyspnea, chronic cough, and sputum production.

DIAGNOSTIC TESTS

- Pulmonary function tests
- Arterial blood gas (ABG)
- Chest X-ray, CT scan

> For more information, see Chapter 11 in Pellico, L.H. (2013). *Focus on adult health: Medical-surgical nursing.* Philadelphia: Wolters Kluwer Health | Lippincott Williams & Wilkins.

Burn Injury

Burns are caused by a transfer of energy from a heat source to the body and are categorized as thermal (including electrical burns), radiation, electrical, or chemical.

PATHOPHYSIOLOGY

Local effects of burns includes the denaturation of protein, which results in the disruption and potential destruction of cells, liberation of vasoactive substances, and the formation of edema. As a result of cellular injury, osmotic and hydrostatic pressure gradients are disrupted and intravascular fluid leaks into interstitial spaces. Shock and renal impairment occur from loss of capillary integrity and release of chemical mediators, with subsequent fluid shift from intravascular to interstitial spaces. Massive edema, electrolyte imbalances, lactic acidosis, and compartment syndrome may result. Severe inhalation injuries lead to carbon monoxide poisoning, airway edema, bronchospasm, and loss of surfactant.

RISK FACTORS

- Age over 60 years
- Smoking

B

- Individuals with disabilities, neurological illness, substance abuse, and psychiatric illness

Gerontologic Considerations

Elderly people are at higher risk for burn injury because of reduced coordination, strength, sensation, and changes in vision. The skin of the elderly is thinner and less elastic, which affects the depth of injury and its ability to heal. Morbidity and mortality are higher in the elderly.

☼ *NURSING ALERT*
Education on the prevention of burn injury is especially important among the elderly. Assess an elderly patient's ability to safely perform activities of daily living (ADLs), assist elderly patients and families to modify their environment to ensure safety, and make referrals as needed.

CLASSIFICATION OF BURNS

Burn injuries are classified by the depth of the injury and the extent of the total body surface area (TBSA) burned. Burns that exceed 25% TBSA may produce a local and a systemic response and are considered major burn injuries.

Depth

The depth of a burn injury depends on the type of injury, causative agent, temperature of the burn agent, duration of contact with the agent, and the skin thickness. Burns are classified according to the depth of tissue destruction:

- Superficial burns, formerly first-degree burns, are similar to sunburn: The epidermis is damaged, pink or red, dry with slight swelling but no blister.
- Superficial partial-thickness burns, one of two types of second-degree burns: The epidermis and a small portion of the dermis is injured. It is very painful, pink and moist, often blistered, and hair follicles are intact.

- Deep partial-thickness burns, the second type of second-degree burns, extends into the reticular layer of the dermis. They are red or white, mottled, and can be moist or fairly dry; the patient is in severe pain.
- Full-thickness burns, formerly third-degree or fourth-degree burns, involve total destruction of the dermis and extend into the subcutaneous fat. It can also involve muscle and bone. Wound color ranges widely from mottled white to red, brown, or black. The wound appears leathery, hair follicles and sweat glands are destroyed.

Extent of Body Surface Area Injured

Estimating total body surface area burned is determined by one of the following methods:

- Rule of Nines: An estimation of the total body surface area burned by assigning percentages in multiples of nine to major body surfaces (Fig. B-1, p. 104).
- Lund and Browder method: A more precise method of estimating the extent of the burn; takes into account that the percentage of the surface area represented by various anatomic parts (head and legs) changes with growth.
- The Severity Grading System (Box B-1, p. 105) adopted by the ABA includes minor, moderate, and major burns.

MEDICAL AND NURSING MANAGEMENT

Burn care is divided into three phases: emergent/resuscitative phase, acute/intermediate phase, and rehabilitation phase. The phases may overlap with assessment and management of problems and complications taking place throughout burn care.

Emergent/Resuscitative Phase

Nursing Assessment

- Airway, breathing, and circulation: It is important to support the *airway* and protect the cervical spine.

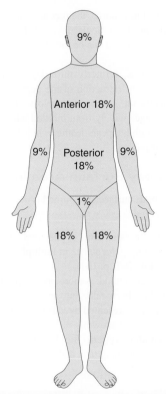

FIGURE B-1 **The rule of nines.** Estimated percentage of total body surface area (TBSA) in the adult is arrived at by sectioning the body surface into areas with a numerical value related to nine. (Note: The anterior and posterior head total 9% of TBSA.)

- Observe for signs of inhalation injury: Blistering of lips or buccal mucosa; singed nostrils; burns of face, neck, or chest; increasing hoarseness; or soot in sputum or respiratory secretions
- Monitor vital signs and pulse oximetry frequently; initiate cardiac monitoring, especially if evidence of electrical injury.
- Insert urinary catheter, monitor output hourly.
- Assess for decreasing level of consciousness, including restlessness, confusion, or difficulty attending to questions, which may indicate cerebral hypoxia.

BOX B-1

Classification of Extent of Burn Injury

Minor Burn Injury
- Second-degree burn of <15% total body surface area (TBSA) in adults or <10% TBSA in children
- Third-degree burn of <2% TBSA not involving special care areas (eyes, ears, face, hands, feet, perineum, joints)
- Excludes all patients with electrical injury, inhalation injury, or concurrent trauma, and all poor-risk patients (ie, extremes of age, intercurrent disease)

Moderate, Uncomplicated Burn Injury
- Second-degree burns of 15% to 25% TBSA in adults or 10% to 20% in children
- Third-degree burns of <10% TBSA not involving special care areas
- Excludes all patients with electrical injury, inhalation injury, or concurrent trauma, and all poor-risk patients (ie, extremes of age, intercurrent disease)

Major Burn Injury
- Second-degree burns >25% TBSA in adults or >20% in children
- All third-degree burns ≥10% TBSA
- All burns involving eyes, ears, face, hands, feet, perineum, joints
- All patients with inhalation injury, electrical injury, or concurrent trauma; all poor-risk patients

From Morton & Fontaine. *Critical care nursing: A holistic approach* (9th ed.). Philadelphia: Lippincott Williams & Wilkins, 2008.

- Assess the time of the burn injury, source of the burn, treatment provided at the scene, and history of falling with the injury. History of preexisting diseases, allergies, medications, and the use of drugs, alcohol, and tobacco is obtained.
- Assess the TBSA burned, the depth of the burn; consider whether the burn occurred in a closed space, the possibility of inhalation of noxious chemicals, and any related trauma.
- Check peripheral pulses on burned extremities hourly; use Doppler as needed.

B

- Assess body temperature, body weight, history of preburn weight, allergies, tetanus immunization, past medical-surgical problems, current illnesses, and use of medications.
- Arrange for patients with facial burns to be assessed for corneal injury.
- Assess psychological status, pain and anxiety levels, and behavior.
- Assess patient's and family's understanding of injury and treatment. Assess patient's support system and coping skills.

Nursing Interventions

Promoting Gas Exchange and Airway Clearance

- Provide 100% humidified oxygen; monitor ABGs, pulse oximetry, and carboxyhemoglobin levels. If airway edema develops, endotracheal intubation and ventilation may be necessary.
- Report labored respirations, decreased depth of respirations, or signs of hypoxia to physician immediately; prepare to assist with intubation and escharotomies.

Restoring Fluid and Electrolyte Balance

- Initiate fluid resuscitation using resuscitation formulas as a guideline. Lactated Ringer's is most frequently used to achieve urine output of 30 to 50 mL/hr (or .5 to 1 mL/kg/hr).
- Monitor vital signs and urinary output (hourly), central venous pressure (CVP), pulmonary artery pressure, and cardiac output. Note and report signs of hypovolemia or fluid overload.
- Elevate the head of bed and burned extremities.
- Hourly assess warmth, capillary refill, pulses, sensation, and movement as compared to the unaffected extremity to detect compartment syndrome. Plan for escharotomy if necessary.
- Monitor serum electrolyte levels (eg, sodium, potassium, calcium, phosphorus, bicarbonate); recognize developing electrolyte imbalances.
- Notify physician immediately of decreased urine output; blood pressure; central venous, pulmonary artery, or pulmonary artery wedge pressures; or increased pulse rate.

Minimizing Pain and Anxiety

- Administer IV opioid analgesics as prescribed and assess response to medication; observe for respiratory depression in patient who is not mechanically ventilated.

- Assess patient and family understanding of burn injury, coping strategies, family dynamics, and anxiety levels.

Potential Complications

- Acute respiratory failure
- Distributive shock
- Acute renal failure
- Paralytic ileus: Insert NG tube for burns of more than 25% TBSA.
- Curling's ulcer: Assess stools for occult blood; administer antacids and histamine blockers (eg, ranitidine [Zantac]) as prescribed.

Acute/Intermediate Phase

The acute or intermediate phase begins 48 to 72 hours after the burn injury. The focus during this phase includes preventing infection, burn wound care, pain management, and nutritional support. Continue assessment and maintenance of respiratory and circulatory status, fluid and electrolyte balance, and GI function.

Nursing Assessment

Pulmonary complications may develop due to fluid resuscitation and smoke inhalation; pneumonia is the most frequent complication.

- Monitor ABGs; assesses breath sounds and respiratory rate, rhythm, depth, and chest symmetry. Notify providers with concerns over pulmonary deterioration such as increasing dyspnea, stridor, and changes in respiratory pattern.
- Assess renal function and for early symptoms of heart failure.
- Monitor temperature and wound for signs and symptoms of infection.

Nursing Interventions

Restoring Normal Fluid Balance

Blood components are administered as needed to treat blood loss and anemia.

Preventing Infection

- Wear cap, gown, mask, and gloves while caring for the patient with burn wounds. Clean technique is used when caring directly for burn wounds.

B

- Apply topical antimicrobials; silver sulfadiazine (Silvadene), mafenide acetate (Sulfamylon), silver nitrate, and Acticoat are used to reduce the number of bacteria.
- Assist with wound débridement to remove contaminated tissue or eschar.
- Administer systemic antibiotics only for documented positive cultures in urine, sputum, or blood.
- Cover wounds with dressings. Maintain autografts, homografts, or dermal substitutes to decrease the risk of infection, prevent further loss of fluid and electrolytes through the wound, minimize heat loss through evaporation, and to keep the area moist and promote granulation.

Pain Management

- Administer analgesics for the three types of burn pain: background or resting pain, procedural pain, and breakthrough pain.
- Recognize that opioid tolerance is not addiction; provide analgesics when there is a clinical need. Remain mindful that wound care is necessary and carries with it the anticipation of pain and anxiety.

Nutritional Support

Burn injuries produce profound metabolic abnormalities fueled by the exaggerated stress response to the injury

- Feedings are started as soon as possible; the enteral route is superior to parenteral.
- Administer vitamin and mineral supplements.
- Collaborate with the dietician to plan a protein- and calorie-rich diet acceptable to patient.

Promoting Mobility

- Prevent atelectasis, pneumonia, edema, pressure ulcers, and contractures by deep breathing, turning, and proper repositioning.
- Modify interventions to meet patient's needs. Low-air-loss and rotation beds may be useful, and early sitting and ambulation are encouraged.
- Apply elastic pressure bandages before assisting patient to upright position when lower extremity burns are present.

Providing Psychological and Emotional Support

Family functioning is disrupted with burn injury; the nurse provides support to the patient and family.

- Instruct family in ways to support patient's adaptation.
- Make psychological or social services referrals as appropriate.
- Provide information about burn care and expected course of treatment.

Rehabilitation Phase

Rehabilitation begins immediately after the burn has occurred and often extends for years after injury. Wound healing, psychosocial support, and restoration of maximum functional activity remain priorities; reconstructive surgery may be needed.

- The wound is in a dynamic state for 1.5 to 2 years after the burn occurs. Hypertrophic scarring may occur, requiring the patient to wear a pressure garment.
- Assess response to losses of body image due to disfigurement, and to loss of personal property or home, loved ones, and ability to work.
- Assess need for follow-up care with burn support groups.

For more information, see Chapter 53 in Pellico, L.H. (2013). *Focus on adult health: Medical-surgical nursing.* Philadelphia: Wolters Kluwer Health | Lippincott Williams & Wilkins.

C

Cancer

Cancer is a disease process that begins when an abnormal cell is transformed by the genetic mutation of the cellular DNA.

PATHOPHYSIOLOGY

- The abnormal cell forms a clone and begins to proliferate abnormally, ignoring growth-regulating signals in the environment surrounding the cell. Cancer is the second leading cause of death in the United States and occurs more frequently in industrialized areas, with most cancers occurring in men and in people older than 65 years.
- Carcinogenesis is the process by which cancer arises. Categories of agents or factors implicated in carcinogenesis include viruses and bacteria, physical agents, chemical agents, genetic or familial factors, dietary factors, and hormonal agents. Patients who are immunoincompetent are also at risk for cancers.
- Cancer cells, or malignant neoplasms, grow in patterns that follow no physiologic demand, acquiring invasive characteristics. Cells infiltrate body tissues, lymph, and blood vessels, which carry the cells to other areas of the body; this is called metastasis. Initially, malignant cells in a tumor look alike; over time, the differences increase, with ongoing random mutations during tumor progression. Cancerous cells are classified and named by tissue of origin.

RISK FACTORS

- Primary prevention includes avoiding known carcinogens, maintaining a normal weight, and consuming a prudent diet, low in fat and including cruciferous vegetables such as broccoli.
- Secondary prevention focuses on early detection and screenings that focus on the highest detection rates such as mammography, digital rectal exam for prostate cancer screening, and colonoscopy.

CLINICAL MANIFESTATIONS AND ASSESSMENT

- Manifestations are related to the system affected and to tissue destruction with replacement by nonfunctional cancer tissue or overproductive cancer tissue (eg, bone marrow disruption, pressure on surrounding structures, increased metabolic demands, and disruption of production of blood cells). (See the specific type of cancer.)
- Generally, cancer symptoms are related to the area affected and may cause anemia, weakness, anorexia weight loss, and pain, often in late stages.

DIAGNOSTIC METHODS

A complete history and physical examination is performed. Knowledge of suspicious symptoms and of the behavior of particular types of cancer assists in determining which diagnostic tests are most appropriate.

Patients with suspected cancer undergo extensive testing to:

- Determine the presence and extent of tumor
- Identify possible spread (metastasis) of disease or invasion of other body tissues
- Evaluate the function of involved and uninvolved body systems and organs

- Obtain tissue and cells for analysis, including evaluation of tumor stage and grade

Diagnostic tests may include tumor marker identification, genetic profiling, imaging studies (mammography, magnetic resonance imaging [MRI], computed tomography [CT], fluoroscopy, ultrasonography, endoscopy, nuclear medicine imaging, positron emission tomography [PET], PET fusion, radioimmunoconjugates), and biopsy.

Tumor Staging and Grading

- Staging determines the size of the tumor and the extent of disease and is used to plan treatment and determine prognosis. Several systems exist for classifying the disease stage. The TNM system is frequently used for many solid tumor types. In this system, "T" refers to the extent of the primary tumor, "N" refers to lymph node involvement, and "M" refers to the extent of metastasis.
- Grading refers to the classification of the tumor and the degree to which the tumor cells retain the functional and histologic characteristics of the tissue of origin. A scale of I to IV is used; grade I tumors most closely resemble the cells of origin and respond well to treatment, whereas grade IV tumors are poorly differentiated (dissimilar) and tend to be aggressive and less responsive to treatment.

Gerontologic Considerations

Due to an increased life expectancy and the increased risk of cancer with age, cancer-related care involves a growing number of elderly patients. More than 58% of all cancers occur in people older than 65 years of age, and about two-thirds of all cancer deaths occur in people 65 years of age and older. Concerns in the elderly include:

- Chemotherapy-related toxicities, such as renal impairment, myelosuppression, fatigue, and cardiomyopathy, which may increase as a result of declining organ function and diminished physiologic reserves

- Delayed recovery of normal tissues after radiation therapy and more severe adverse effects, such as mucositis, nausea and vomiting, and myelosuppression
- Slower recovery from surgery due to decreased tissue healing capacity and declining pulmonary and cardiovascular functioning
- Higher risk for complications such as atelectasis, pneumonia, and wound infections

MEDICAL AND NURSING MANAGEMENT

Treatment goals may include complete eradication of malignant disease (cure), prolonged survival and containment of cancer cell growth (control), or relief of symptoms associated with the disease (palliation).

Surgical Management

- Surgery may be the primary method of treatment, or it may be prophylactic, palliative, or reconstructive. Diagnostic surgery is the definitive method of identifying the cellular characteristics that influence all treatment decisions.
- A biopsy is performed to obtain a tissue sample for analysis of cells suspected to be malignant.

Surgery as Primary Treatment

When surgery is the primary approach in treating cancer, the goal is to remove the entire tumor or as much as is feasible. Local excision refers to removing the tumor and a small margin of tissue surrounding it; wide excision refers to removing the tumor and any surrounding tissue that is involved or may be at high risk for tumor spread, including regional lymph nodes. Disfigurement or altered function may result; however, this method is considered when the chance of cure and control are good.

Prophylactic Surgery

Prophylactic surgery involves removing nonvital tissues or organs that are likely to develop cancer. Recent ability to identify genetic markers and predispositions to certain cancers contribute to decisions to undergo prophylactic surgery. Mastectomy and colostomy are examples of surgeries.

Palliative Surgery

When cure is not possible, the goals of treatment are to make the patient as comfortable as possible and to improve quality of life as defined by the patient. Palliative surgery is performed in an attempt to relieve complications of cancer, such as ulcerations, obstructions, hemorrhage, pain, and malignant effusions.

Nursing Management in Cancer Surgery

The nurse's role in caring for the patient undergoing cancer surgery is much like caring for all surgical candidates. In addition to focusing on the typical effects of surgery, caring for patients with cancer include:

- Addressing effects of surgery on body image, self-esteem, and functional abilities
- Observing for complications related to radiation and chemotherapy in addition to surgery, which may cause infection, impaired wound healing, or altered pulmonary or renal function
- Focus on prevention of venous thromboembolism (VTE) or deep vein thrombosis (DVT), which is more common in cancer due to an increase in circulating procoagulants

Radiation Therapy

Radiation is delivered to tumor sites by external or internal means.

- External radiation uses a machine to deliver X-rays to the affected area.
- Internal radiation implantation, or brachytherapy, delivers a high dose of radiation to a localized, internal area using radioactive needles, seeds, beads, or catheters inserted into body cavities (eg, vagina, abdomen, pleura) or interstitial compartments (eg, breast).
- Brachytherapy may also be administered orally, as with the isotope iodine-131, which is used to treat thyroid carcinomas.

Intracavitary Radiation

Intracavitary radioisotopes are frequently used to treat gynecologic cancers. The radioisotopes are inserted into applicators positioned in the cervix and vagina, and the position is verified by X-ray. These radioisotopes remain in place for a prescribed time period and then are removed. The patient is maintained on bed rest and log-rolled to prevent displacement.

Safety

Patients receiving internal radiation emit radiation while the implant is in place. Contact with the health care team is guided by principles of *time, distance,* and *shielding* to minimize exposure of personnel to radiation.

NURSING ALERT

For safety in brachytherapy, assign the patient to a private room and post appropriate notices about radiation safety precautions. Pregnant staff members should not be assigned to this patient. Staff members wear dosimeter badges. Children or pregnant women should not visit, and others should visit only 30 minutes daily. Instruct and monitor visitors to ensure they maintain a 6 foot distance from the radiation source.

Toxicity

- Toxicity is related to the area receiving radiation; symptoms may be increased if chemotherapy is concomitantly administered.
- Local reactions such as altered skin integrity, alopecia (hair loss), erythema, and shedding of skin (desquamation) may occur. Reepitheliazation occurs after treatments have been completed.
- Alterations in oral mucosa secondary to radiation therapy include stomatitis, xerostomia (dryness of the mouth), change and loss of taste, and decreased salivation.
- The entire gastrointestinal (GI) mucosa may be involved, and esophageal irritation with chest pain and dysphagia may result. Anorexia, nausea, vomiting, and diarrhea may occur if the stomach or colon is in the irradiated field. Symptoms subside and GI reepithelialization occurs after treatments have been completed.

- If sites containing bone marrow (eg, the iliac crest, sternum) are included in the radiation field, anemia, leukopenia (decreased white blood cells [WBCs]), and thrombocytopenia (a decrease in platelets) may result, putting the patient at increased risk for infection and bleeding. Chronic anemia may occur due to the cumulative effects of radiation, causing shortness of breath, dizziness, fatigue, decreased oxygen saturation, and decreased activity tolerance.
- Systemic side effects, secondary to substances released due to tumor destruction, include fatigue, malaise, and anorexia.

Chemotherapy

Chemotherapy uses antineoplastic agents to destroy tumor cells by interfering with cellular functions, including replication. Chemotherapy is used primarily to treat systemic disease rather than localized lesions that are amenable to surgery or radiation. Chemotherapy may be combined with surgery, radiation therapy, or both, to reduce tumor size preoperatively (neoadjuvant), to destroy any remaining tumor cells postoperatively (adjuvant), or to treat hematologic malignancies such as lymphoma and leukemia. The goals of chemotherapy (cure, control, palliation) define the medications to be used and the aggressiveness of the treatment plan.

- Chemotherapy kills rapidly dividing cells.
- Each cycle of chemotherapy kills a certain percentage of tumor cells. The goal of treatment is eradication of enough of the tumor so that the remaining tumor cells can be destroyed by the body's immune system.
- Chemotherapy drugs are often given in combinations, referred to as a *protocol* or *regimen*. Combination chemotherapy overcomes drug resistance and uses the synergistic effects of some drugs while minimizing toxicity of others.
- Chemotherapy is administered in the hospital, clinic, or home setting by a variety of routes including topical, oral, IV, intramuscular, subcutaneous, arterial, intracavitary, and intrathecal. Intrathecal chemotherapy is the administration of medication into the cerebrospinal fluid to prevent central nervous system (CNS) metastasis. This can be accomplished through a lumbar puncture or through the placement

of an intraventricular catheter with the tip lying in the fourth ventricle of the brain.

Classification of Chemotherapy

- Chemotherapy can be classed as cell cycle-specific or -nonspecific. Cell cycle-specific drugs destroy cancer cells in a certain phase of the cell cycle (ie, S phase). Cell cycle-nonspecific drugs act independently of the cell cycle and may have a prolonged effect on cells.
- Classification of chemotherapeutic agents include alkylating agents, nitrosoureas, antimetabolites, antitumor antibiotics, plant alkaloids, hormonal agents, and those that are miscellaneous.
- Dosage of antineoplastic agents is based on the patient's total body surface area and weight, previous response to chemotherapy or radiation therapy, function of major organ systems, and performance status.
- Central venous access devices may be recommended for frequent or prolonged treatment.

☀ *N U R S I N G   A L E R T*
Because of the high potential for error with chemotherapy dosing, the standard expectation is that two nurses verify the chemotherapy dose for accuracy.

☀ *N U R S I N G   A L E R T*
- Carefully assess the patient for infusion-related events such as hypersensitivity and extravasation.
- Common symptoms of hypersensitivity reactions include anxiety, flushing, rash, bronchospasm, and hemodynamic collapse. Be prepared to stop the infusion, maintain airway patency, and administer O_2 and emergency medications such as epinephrine.

- Vesicants are agents that, if extravasated into the subcutaneous tissue, cause tissue ulceration and necrosis, and may damage underlying tendons, nerves, and blood vessels. Stop infusion immediately and obtain an order for neutralizing agents. If frequent, prolonged administration of antineoplastic vesicants is anticipated, central venous access devices may be inserted.

> **NURSING ALERT**
>
> If extravasation is expected, stop the infusion immediately, aspirate any residual medication, obtain orders for a neutralizing solution or antidote, apply ice per policy, and notify the provider. Treatment of extravasation varies based on the individual medication.

Chemotherapy Toxicity

Cells with rapid growth rates (eg, epithelium, bone marrow, hair follicles, sperm) are most susceptible to the effects of chemotherapy.

- GI system: Nausea, vomiting, anticipatory vomiting
- Hematologic system: Anemia, thrombocytopenia, leukopenia
- Reproductive system: Abnormal ovulation, early menopause, azoospermia (absence of spermatozoa) or permanent sterility may develop. Chromosomal abnormalities in offspring may occur. Banking of sperm is recommended for men before treatments are initiated.
- As chemotherapy kills rapidly dividing cells and may damage the fetus, reliable methods of birth control must be used.

Bone Marrow Transplantation (BMT)

Hematopoietic Stem Cell Transplantation (HSCT)

- Bone marrow or stem cells from the patient (autologous) or from a donor (allogeneic) allow the bone marrow to be "rescued" from the toxic effects of the chemotherapy.
- Allogenic cells come from a related donor (family member), a matched unrelated donor (national bone marrow registry/cord blood registry), or are syngeneic (from an identical twin).
- Donor cells can be obtained by harvesting large amounts of bone marrow tissue under general anesthesia or, peripheral blood stem cell transplantation using apheresis may be used.
- The donor's healthy immune system is able to recognize the patient's malignancy as foreign and destroys tumor cells (graft vs. tumor effect).
- The infused cells travel to the bone marrow, where the cells mature and proliferate, producing RBCs, WBCs, and platelets

(2 to 4 weeks). Chemotherapy or radiation may be administered before the transplant to prevent destruction of the transplanted, foreign cells.

- Patients are at high risk for infection, sepsis, and bleeding. Side effects of high-dose chemotherapy and total body irradiation include alopecia, hemorrhagic cystitis, nausea, vomiting, diarrhea, and severe stomatitis. Chronic side effects include sterility, pulmonary dysfunction, cardiac dysfunction, and liver disease.
- Graft versus host disease (GVHD) occurs in allogeneic transplant when transplanted T lymphocytes view the recipient's tissue as "foreign" and mount an immune response against it. GVHD may be acute or chronic.

Nursing Care for HSCT

- Monitor vital signs and blood oxygen saturation.
- Assess for adverse effects, such as fever, chills, shortness of breath, chest pain, cutaneous reactions (hives), nausea, vomiting, hypotension or hypertension, tachycardia, anxiety, and taste changes.
- Maintain strict aseptic technique; until engraftment of the new marrow occurs, the patient is at high risk for death from sepsis and bleeding.
- Administer blood products, hematopoietic growth factors, and antibiotics, while observing for side effects including nephrotoxicity from chemotherapy and antibiotics.
- Monitor for GVHD. Effects on the skin, liver, and GI tract include red maculopapular rash commonly found on the palms of the hands and soles of the feet, elevated liver function tests (LFTs), weight gain, jaundice, right upper quadrant pain, diffuse abdominal pain, early satiety, and diarrhea.
- Provide ongoing support and patient teaching.

Targeted Therapies

The mechanisms of action of targeted therapies include stimulation or augmentation of immune responses through the use of biologic response modifiers (BRMs), targeting of cancer cell growth factors and proteins, promotion of apoptosis (programmed cell death), and genetic manipulation through gene therapy.

Nursing Management for Targeted Therapies

- Observe for flu-like symptoms such as fever chills, myalgia, nausea, hypotension, and pulmonary edema.
- Teach patient and family subcutaneous injection technique for self-administration, when appropriate.

Nursing Management for the Patient With Cancer

Patients with cancer may have signs and symptoms of varying severity depending on the site of the cancer, stage, and treatments. Goals for the patient may include:

- Management of stomatitis
- Maintenance of tissue integrity
- Maintenance of nutrition
- Relief of pain and fatigue
- Improved body image
- Progression through the grieving process
- Absence of complications

Nursing Interventions

- Minimize fatigue with anticipatory guidance that fatigue may accompany treatment; alternate periods of rest and planned activity/exercise. Continue with enjoyable activities. Manage pain, dyspnea, constipation, and fear/anxiety.
- Maintain nutrition and caloric intake encouraging small frequent meals. Monitor H&H and administer Erythropoiesis-stimulating agents (ESAs) for anemia

Prevent and Treat Sepsis

- Monitor the WBCs for leukopenia and the differential for neutropenia (a decrease in the number of neutrophils) and the absolute neutrophil count (ANC). The lowest point or nadir of the WBCs occurs 7 to 10 days after the patient receives chemotherapy.
- Monitor the temperature and central venous access device sites to detect early signs of infection.
- Obtain cultures of blood, sputum, urine, stool, catheters, and wounds if a fever of 38°C (100.4°F) develops. Collaborate with the physician to obtain orders for antibiotic therapy.

- Teach patients and families proper hand hygiene, signs and symptoms of infection.
- Administer hematopoietic growth factors when indicated.

Monitor and Manage Bleeding and Hemorrhage

- Monitor for thrombocytopenia; platelet counts between 20,000 and 50, 000 are associated with increased risk for bleeding; less than 20,000 is associated with spontaneous bleeding. Transfuse platelets prior to invasive procedures and as ordered.
- Avoid ASA, NSAIDs, warfarin, heparins.
- Observe for bleeding, bruising, petechiae, hematuria, epistaxis, hemoptysis, blood in the stools, oozing at injection sites. Have the patient use a soft toothbrush or sponge, and electric razor. Avoid unnecessary invasive procedures (eg, rectal temperatures, intramuscular injections, catheterization), and remove environmental hazards that may lead to falls or other trauma. Soft foods, increased fluid intake, and stool softeners may be indicated to reduce trauma to the GI tract. The joints and extremities are handled and moved gently to minimize the risk of spontaneous bleeding. Following venipuncture, pressure must be applied for 3 to 5 minutes.

Manage Stomatitis

Observe for inflammation, redness, or edema of the oral cavity. Encourage good oral hygiene, including brushing with a soft-bristled toothbrush or swab, flossing, and rinsing with saline or tap water.

Manage Nausea and Vomiting

- Nausea is subjective. Assess precipitating and alleviating factors, and previous experiences with nausea. Physical assessment should include signs of associated symptoms including sweating, tachycardia, dizziness, pallor, excessive salivation, weakness, gastric distention, abdominal tenderness, and evaluation of bowel sounds.
- Monitor laboratory values, including electrolytes and renal function.
- Administer serotonin receptor antagonists, such as odansetron, around the clock with breakthrough doses if needed, also corticosteroids, antianxiety medications. Consider nonpharmacologic interventions.

Maintain and Manage Alterations in Skin Integrity

- Observe for site-specific tissue reactions to cancer, surgery, chemotherapy, and radiation.
- Apply sulfadiazine cream for moist desquamation (painful, red, moist skin).
- Manage malignant skin lesions by reducing bacteria, controlling bleeding, preventing trauma, and relieving pain.
- Assist in coping with alopecia; the extent of alopecia depends on the extent and duration of radiation or chemotherapy. Hair loss usually begins 2 to 3 weeks after initiation of the therapy and begins to regrow within 8 weeks after the last treatment; radiation to the head may lead to permanent hair loss. Encourage the patient to obtain a wig before the hair falls out, and to use scarves or hats. Support the patient though the hair loss, which can interfere with coping, interpersonal relationships, and sexuality.

Improve Nutritional Status

- Monitor weight, anorexia, nausea, vomiting. Observe for cachexia (muscle wasting). Monitor diagnostic tests, serum protein, iron, electrolytes, lymphocytes, H&H.
- Anorexia typically results from altered taste, which may result from zinc or mineral deficiencies. Feelings of fullness develop. An aversion to food may develop secondary to nausea and vomiting:
  - Teach the patient to avoid unpleasant smells, consider patient preference, consume larger amounts of food earlier in the day, and avoid fluids with meals.
  - Provide oral hygiene prior to meals.
- Corticosteroids or progestational medications (ie, megestrol) may be used as appetite stimulants. Metoclopramide may promote gastric emptying.
- TPN, enteral nutrition, or vitamin replacement may be needed.

Relieve Pain

- Pain may be secondary to the tumor, diagnostic tests, or the treatment.
- Assess pain including physical and psychosocial influences. A comprehensive pain assessment is completed, including onset,

duration, location, quality or characteristics, quantity, aggravating and alleviating factors, associated symptoms, and those treatments that the patient has used to relieve pain.
- Assess for factors that increase the perception of pain, such as fear and apprehension, fatigue, anger, and social isolation. Encourage adequate sleep and rest, empathy.
- Administer analgesics with additional medication for breakthrough pain and adjuvants, such as antidepressants and antianxiety medications.
- Help improve body image by assisting patient to retain control and positive self-esteem. Encourage independence, and discuss negative feelings related to body image and sexuality.

Evaluation
- Maintains integrity of oral mucous membranes
- Maintains adequate tissue integrity
- Maintains adequate nutritional status
- Achieves relief of pain and discomfort
- Demonstrates increased activity tolerance and decreased fatigue
- Exhibits improved body image and self-esteem
- Demonstrates positive progression through the grieving process
- Experiences no complications, such as infection, or sepsis, and no episodes of bleeding or hemorrhage

END-OF-LIFE CONSIDERATIONS

- When cure or control of the disease is no longer possible, use a comprehensive multidisciplinary program that focuses on quality of life, palliation of symptoms, and provision of psychosocial and spiritual support for patients and families.
- Hospice care may be provided in the hospital or at home, with the nurse coordinating physicians, social workers, clergy, dietitians, pharmacists, physical therapists activities.
- The nurse helps patients and families with grief and loss, as well as providing bereavement counseling and family support for survivors.

For more information, see Chapter 6 in Pellico, L.H. (2013). *Focus on adult health. Medical-surgical nursing.* Philadelphia: Wolters Kluwer Health | Lippincott Williams & Wilkins.

Cancer of the Bladder

Cancer of the urinary bladder is more common in people older than 55 years, affects men more often than women (4:1), and is more common in Caucasians than in African Americans.

PATHOPHYSIOLOGY

Bladder tumors usually arise at the base of the bladder and involve the ureteral orifices and bladder neck. Transitional cell carcinoma of the bladder is the most common form of bladder cancer. Cancers arising from the prostate, colon, and rectum in males and from the lower gynecologic tract in females may metastasize to the bladder.

RISK FACTORS

Tobacco use continues to be a leading risk factor for all urinary tract cancers. People who smoke develop bladder cancer twice as often as those who do not smoke.

CLINICAL MANIFESTATIONS AND ASSESSMENT

- Painless, gross hematuria is the most common symptom.
- Infection of the urinary tract is common and produces frequency and urgency.
- Any alteration in voiding or change in the urine is indicative.
- Pelvic or back pain may occur with metastasis.

DIAGNOSTIC METHODS

Biopsies of the tumor and adjacent mucosa are definitive, but the following procedures are also used:

- Cystoscopy (the mainstay of diagnosis)
- Excretory urography
- CT scan
- Ultrasonography
- Bimanual examination under anesthesia
- Cytologic examination of fresh urine and saline bladder washings for staging
- Newer diagnostic tools, such as bladder tumor antigens, nuclear matrix proteins, adhesion molecules, cytoskeletal proteins, and growth factors are being studied.

MEDICAL AND NURSING MANAGEMENT

Treatment of bladder cancer depends on the grade of tumor, the stage of tumor growth, and the multicentricity of the tumor. Age and physical, mental, and emotional status are considered in determining treatment.

See also "Medical and Nursing Management" for the patient undergoing cancer surgery, radiation, and chemotherapy under "Cancer" on pages 113–114 for additional information.

Surgical Management

- Transurethral resection (TUR) or fulguration for simple papillomas with intravesical bacille Calmette-Guérin (BCG may be used)
- Life-long monitoring of benign papillomas with cytology and cystoscopy
- Simple or radical cystectomy for invasive or multifocal bladder cancer with urinary diversion
- Urinary diversion redirects urine from the bladder through a surgically created opening (stoma) in the skin. A cutaneous urinary

diversion drains through an opening stoma in the abdominal wall into an external drainage device; a *continent urinary diversion* uses a portion of the intestine to create a new reservoir for urine.

Pharmacologic Therapy

- Chemotherapy with a combination of methotrexate (Rheumatrex), 5-fluorouracil (5-FU), vinblastine (Velban), doxorubicin (Adriamycin), and cisplatin (Platinol) has been effective in producing partial remission of transitional cell carcinoma of the bladder in some patients.
- Topical chemotherapy (intravesical or instillation of antineoplastic agents into the bladder causes contact of the agent with the bladder wall) is considered for patients with high risk of recurrence, for cancer in situ, or for incomplete tumor resection.
- Intravesical BCG (effective with superficial transitional cell carcinoma)

Radiation Therapy

- Radiation of tumor preoperatively to reduce microextension and viability
- Radiation therapy in combination with surgery to control inoperable tumors

Investigational Therapy

Photodynamic techniques in treating superficial bladder cancer are under investigation.

For more information, see Chapter 28 in Pellico, L.H. (2013). *Focus on adult health. Medical-surgical nursing.* Philadelphia: Wolters Kluwer Health | Lippincott Williams & Wilkins.

Cancer of the Breast

Cancer of the breast is a pathologic entity that starts with a genetic alteration in a single cell and may take several years to become palpable.

PATHOPHYSIOLOGY

The most common type of breast cancer is infiltrating ductal carcinoma (80% of cases); tumors arise from the duct system and invade the surrounding tissues. If lymph nodes are unaffected, the prognosis is better. The key to improved cure rates is early diagnosis, before metastasis.

RISK FACTORS

- There is no one specific cause of breast cancer; rather, a combination of genetic, hormonal, and possibly environmental events may contribute to its development.
- Gender (female) and increasing age
- Previous breast cancer: The risk of developing cancer in the same or opposite breast is significantly increased.
- Family history: Having first-degree relative with breast cancer (mother, sister, daughter) increases the risk twofold; having two first-degree relatives increases the risk fivefold.
- Genetic mutations (*BRCA1* or *BRCA2*) account for the majority of inherited breast cancers.
- Hormonal factors: Early menarche (before 12 years of age), nulliparity, first birth after 30 years of age, late menopause (after 55 years of age), and hormone therapy (formerly referred to as hormone replacement therapy).
- Other factors may include exposure to ionizing radiation during adolescence and early adulthood obesity, alcohol intake (beer, wine, or liquor), high-fat diet (controversial, more research needed).

Protective Factors

Protective factors may include regular vigorous exercise (decreased body fat), pregnancy before age 30 years, and breastfeeding.

CLINICAL MANIFESTATIONS AND ASSESSMENT

- Nontender, fixed lesion, hard with irregular borders; most occur in the upper outer quadrant

- May be asymptomatic and discovered on mammogram
- Advanced signs may include skin dimpling, nipple retraction, or skin ulceration

DIAGNOSTIC METHODS

- Breast imaging, including mammography and digital mammography, ultrasound, and MRI
- Biopsy (eg, percutaneous, surgical) and histologic examination of cancer cells
- Tumor staging and analysis of additional prognostic factors are used to determine the prognosis and optimal treatment regimen
- Chest X-rays, CT, PET scan, bone scans, and blood work (complete blood cell count, comprehensive metabolic panel, tumor markers; ie, carcinoembryonic antigen [CEA], CA15-3).

MEDICAL AND NURSING MANAGEMENT

Prevention Strategies

- Chemoprevention with hormonal agents such as tamoxifen (Nolvadex) or raloxifene (Evista)
- Prophylactic mastectomy for *BRCA 1* or *2* gene mutation

Surgical Management

- Lumpectomy: Removal of cancerous tissue with border of normal tissue; typically followed by 5 to 7 weeks of radiation therapy
- Simple or total mastectomy: Removal of the breast and nipple–areola complex but does not include axillary lymph node dissection (ALND)
- Modified radical mastectomy: Removal of the entire breast tissue, including the nipple–areola complex and a portion of the axillary lymph nodes
- Breast-conserving surgery: Lumpectomy, wide excision, partial or segmental mastectomy, quadrantectomy followed by lymph node removal for invasive breast cancer

- Sentinel lymph node biopsy: Used for pathologic axillary staging for patients with breast cancer; involves injecting a radioactive tracer to determine presence of cancer in the axillary lymph nodes. If present, complete ALND is performed.
- Breast reconstruction may be performed at the time of surgery or at a later date.

Radiation Therapy

- External-beam radiation therapy: Typically, whole-breast radiation, but partial-breast radiation (radiation to the lumpectomy site alone) is now being evaluated at some institutions in carefully selected patients.
- Brachytherapy may be used, depending on classification stage and location of the tumor.

Pharmacologic Therapy

- Indication for chemotherapy depends on the size of the tumor, lymph node involvement, the presence or absence of hormone receptors in the tumor, and the amount of HER2/neu present in the breast cancer cells.
- Most common drugs that are recommended for use in early stage breast cancer are cyclophosphamide, docetaxel, doxorubicin, epirubicin, fluorouracil, methotrexate, and paclitaxel.
- Hormonal therapy based on the index of estrogen and progesterone receptors: Tamoxifen (Nolvadex, Soltamox) is the primary hormonal agent used to suppress hormonal-dependent tumors; others are inhibitors anastrazole (Arimidex), letrozole (Femara), and exemestane (Aromasin).
- Targeted therapy: Trastuzumab (Herceptin), bevacizumab (Avastin).

NURSING PROCESS

The Patient Undergoing Surgery for Breast Cancer

See "Nursing Management" under "Cancer" on page 114 for additional information.

(continues on page 130)

Assessment

- Perform a health history.
- Assess coping skills, support systems, knowledge deficit, and presence of discomfort.

Diagnosis

- Deficient knowledge about the planned treatments
- Anxiety related to cancer diagnosis
- Fear related to specific treatments and body image changes
- Risk for ineffective coping (individual or family) related to the diagnosis of breast cancer and treatment options
- Decisional conflict related to treatment options

Postoperative Nursing Diagnoses

- Pain and discomfort related to surgical procedure
- Disturbed sensory perception related to nerve irritation in affected arm, breast, or chest wall
- Disturbed body image related to loss or alteration of the breast
- Risk for impaired adjustment related to the diagnosis of cancer and surgical treatment
- Self-care deficit related to partial immobility of upper extremity on operative side
- Risk for sexual dysfunction related to loss of body part, change in self-image, and fear of partner's responses
- Deficient knowledge: Drain management after breast surgery
- Deficient knowledge: Arm exercises to regain mobility of affected extremity
- Deficient knowledge: Hand and arm care after an ALND

Planning and Goals

The major goals may include increased knowledge about the disease and its treatment; reduction of preoperative and postoperative fear, anxiety, and emotional stress; improvement of decision-making ability; pain management; improvement in coping abilities; improvement in sexual function; and the absence of complications.

Preoperative Nursing Interventions

Providing Education and Preparation About Surgical Treatments

- Review treatment options by reinforcing information provided to the patient and answer any questions.
- Prepare the patient for pre-, intra-, and postoperative care, including need for drains and drain care once home.
- Inform patient that she will often have decreased arm and shoulder mobility after an ALND; demonstrate range-of-motion exercises prior to discharge.
- Reassure patient that appropriate analgesia and comfort measures will be provided.

Reducing Fear and Anxiety and Improving Coping Ability

- Help patient cope with the physical and emotional effects of surgery including fear of pain, mutilation, loss of sexual attractiveness, and coping with an uncertain future.
- Provide patient with realistic expectations about the healing process and expected recovery to help alleviate fears.
- Inform patient about available resources at the treatment facility, as well as in the breast cancer community (eg, social workers, psychiatrists, and support groups); patient may find it helpful to talk to a breast cancer survivor who has undergone similar treatments.

Promoting Decision-Making Ability

- Validate patient's and family's understanding of the risks and benefits of each option.
- Ask patient questions about specific treatment options to help her focus on choosing an appropriate treatment (eg, How would you feel about losing your breast? Are you considering breast reconstruction? If you choose to retain your breast, would you consider undergoing radiation treatments 5 days a week for 5 to 6 weeks?).
- Support the patient's decision.

Postoperative Nursing Interventions

Relieving Pain and Discomfort

- Assess patient for pain; individual pain varies depending on the procedure.

(continues on page 132)

- Encourage patient to use analgesics upon discharge as needed.
- Prepare patient for a possible slight increase in pain after the first few days of surgery as she regains sensation around the surgical site and becomes more active.
- Evaluate patients who report severe pain for complications.
- Suggest alternative methods of pain management (eg, taking warm showers, using distraction methods such as guided imagery).

Managing Postoperative Sensations

- Reassure patients that postoperative sensations such as tenderness, soreness, numbness, tightness, pulling, and twinges or phantom sensations (after mastectomy) are a normal part of healing and not indicative of a problem.
- Reassure patients that sensations may diminish after several months, and they are a normal part of healing.

Promoting Positive Body Image

- Assess the patient's readiness to see the incision for the first time and provide gentle encouragement; ideally, the patient will be with the nurse or another health care provider for support.
- Maintain the patient's privacy.

Promoting Positive Adjustment and Coping

- Provide ongoing assessment of how the patient is coping with her diagnosis and treatment.
- Assist patient in identifying and mobilizing her support systems; the patient's spouse or partner may also need guidance, support, and education.
- Provide resources (eg, Reach to Recovery program of the American Cancer Society [ACS], advocacy groups, or a spiritual advisor).
- Encourage the patient to discuss issues and concerns with other patients who have had breast cancer.
- Provide patient with information about the plan of care after treatment.
- If additional support is required, consultation with a mental health practitioner may be indicated.

Improving Sexual Function

- Explain that, once discharged from the hospital, most patients are permitted to engage in sexual activity.

- Encourage the patient to discuss how she and her partner feel about body image, self-esteem, and sexual function.
- When pertinent, explore reasons for a decrease in libido (eg, fatigue, anxiety, self-consciousness). Suggest varying the time of day for sexual activity, when the patient is less tired, assuming comfortable positions, and expressing affection using alternative measures (eg, hugging, kissing, manual stimulation).
- If sexual issues cannot be resolved, a referral may be helpful.

Evaluation

Expected Patient Outcomes

- Exhibits knowledge about diagnosis and treatment options
- Verbalizes willingness to deal with anxiety and fears related to the diagnosis and the effects of surgery on self-image and sexual functioning.
- Demonstrates ability to cope with diagnosis and treatment
- Makes decisions regarding treatment options in a timely manner
- Reports pain has decreased and states pain management strategies are effective
- Identifies postoperative sensations and recognizes that they are a normal part of healing
- Exhibits clean, dry, and intact surgical incision without signs of inflammation or infection
- Lists signs and symptoms of infection to be reported to the nurse or surgeon
- Verbalizes feelings regarding change in body image
- Participates actively in self-care activities
- Discusses issues of sexuality and resumption of sexual relations
- Demonstrates knowledge of post discharge recommendations and restrictions

COMPLICATIONS

- Lymphedema
- Hematoma
- Infection

For more information, see Chapters 6 and 33 in Pellico, L.H. (2013). *Focus on adult health. Medical-surgical nursing.* Philadelphia: Wolters Kluwer Health | Lippincott Williams & Wilkins.

C Cancer of the Cervix

The most common reproductive cancer among women is cervical cancer; it is the second most common cancer among women. Approximately 11,000 new cases of cervical cancer are diagnosed annually, and approximately 4,000 women will die of cervical cancer each year.

PATHOPHYSIOLOGY

Cervical cancer is predominantly squamous cell cancer and adenocarcinomas.

RISK FACTORS

- Intercourse with an uncircumcised male
- Early age of first coitus
- Multiple sexual partners
- High parity
- Sexually transmitted infections
- Cigarette smoking
- Exposure to human papillomavirus
- Increased risk in lesbian women due to misinformation

CLINICAL MANIFESTATIONS AND ASSESSMENT

- Routine screening for cervical cancer increases a woman's chances of being diagnosed at an earlier stage.

- Often asymptomatic; advanced disease may include irregular vaginal bleeding, or pelvic pain and pressure, dyspareunia, and rectal pressure.
- Malodorous vaginal discharge gradually increases in amount, becomes watery, and finally dark and foul-smelling; occurs as a result of tumor.

DIAGNOSTIC METHODS

- Pap smear and biopsy results show precancerous or cancerous changes.
- Other tests may include pelvic ultrasound, colposcopy, and cervical biopsy.
- Chest X-ray and abdominal/pelvic imagining such as CT scan or MRI are performed to rule out metastasis.

MEDICAL AND NURSING MANAGEMENT

Staging is performed (usually TNM system) to determine the extent of the disease and to plan for treatment.

- Abnormal Pap smears demonstrating precancerous lesions are followed up with colposcopy and cervical biopsy; once diagnosis is established, conization, cold knife conization, or LEEP procedures may be performed.
- Patients diagnosed with a stage 1B or IIA undergo a radical hysterectomy: Removal of the uterus and upper one-third of the vagina and cervix; ovaries remain. Bilateral pelvic lymph node sampling is also done.
- Pelvic radiation and chemotherapy may follow but is dependent upon the size and extent of the tumor.
- Neoadjuvant chemotherapy may decrease tumor size and increase survival when used prior to a radical hysterectomy

Patient Education

- Nurses working in a variety of settings have the opportunity to educate women on cervical cancer screenings.

- Assist patient with access to screening: Federally funded cervical cancer screening programs through public health departments, hospital-based primary care centers, and community health care clinics are available.
- Educate parents and young women about human papilloma virus (HPV) vaccination, which is 94% to 98% effective against cervical intraepithelial neoplasia (CIN) lesions caused by HPV.
- Post cervical biopsy, instruct the patient about importance of pelvic rest and contacting the provider for fever, increased bleeding, pelvic pain, or malodorous vaginal discharge.

For more information, see Chapter 33 in Pellico, L.H. (2013). *Focus on adult health. Medical-surgical nursing.* Philadelphia: Wolters Kluwer Health | Lippincott Williams & Wilkins.

Cancer of the Colon and Rectum (Colorectal Cancer)

Tumors of the colon and rectum are relatively common; the colorectal area is now the third most common site of new cancer cases and deaths in the United States.

PATHOPHYSIOLOGY

Cancer of the colon and rectum is predominantly (95%) adenocarcinoma (ie, arising from the epithelial lining of the intestine). It may start as a benign polyp but may become malignant, invade and destroy normal tissues, and extend into surrounding structures. Cancer cells may migrate away from the primary tumor and spread to other parts of the body (most often to the liver). Most people are asymptomatic for long periods and seek health care only when they notice a change in bowel habits or rectal bleeding. Prevention and early screening are the keys to detection and reduction of mortality rates.

RISK FACTORS

- Western cultures
- Increasing age
- Family history of colon cancer
- Irritable bowel disease (IBD) or polyps
- Dietary carcinogens
- Lack of fiber
- Excess dietary fat
- High alcohol consumption
- Smoking

CLINICAL MANIFESTATIONS AND ASSESSMENT

- Symptoms are often insidious and determined by location of the cancer, stage of disease, and function of the area where it is located.
- The most common presenting symptom is a change in bowel habits; second most common symptom is blood in the stools.
- Symptoms may also include unexplained anemia, anorexia, weight loss, and fatigue.
- The later symptoms most commonly reported by the elderly are abdominal pain, obstruction, tenesmus, and rectal bleeding.
- Right-sided lesions are possibly accompanied by dull abdominal pain and melena (black tarry stools).
- Left-sided lesions are associated with obstruction (abdominal pain and cramping, narrowing stools, constipation, and distention) and bright red blood in stool.
- Rectal lesions are associated with tenesmus (ineffective painful straining at stool), rectal pain, feeling of incomplete evacuation after a bowel movement, alternating constipation and diarrhea, and bloody stool.

DIAGNOSTIC METHODS

- Abdominal and rectal examination; fecal occult blood testing; barium enema; proctosigmoidoscopy; and colonoscopy, biopsy, or cytology smears

- CEA studies may be performed; they are reliable prognostic indicators and should return to normal within 48 hours of tumor excision. Later elevations suggest recurrence.

MEDICAL AND NURSING MANAGEMENT

- Intravenous fluids and nasogastric (NG) suction are used for symptoms of intestinal obstruction. Blood component therapy may be required for excessive bleeding.
- Treatment depends on the stage of the disease; surgery to remove the tumor, supportive therapy, and adjuvant therapy including chemotherapy, radiation therapy, immunotherapy, or multimodality therapy to delay tumor recurrence and increase survival time are performed.
- Radiation therapy is used before, during, and after surgery to shrink the tumor, to achieve better results from surgery, and to reduce the risk of recurrence or for palliation.
- The type of surgery recommended depends on the location and size of the tumor.
- Segmental resection with anastomosis involves removal of the tumor and portions of the bowel on either side of the growth, as well as the blood vessels and lymphatic nodes.
- Abdominoperineal resection with permanent sigmoid colostomy involves removal of the tumor and a portion of the sigmoid and all of the rectum and anal sphincter.
- Temporary colostomy is followed by segmental resection and anastomosis and subsequent reanastomosis of the colostomy, allowing initial bowel decompression and bowel preparation before resection.
- Permanent colostomy or ileostomy is used for palliation of unresectable obstructing lesions.
- Construction of a coloanal reservoir called a colonic J pouch, is performed in two steps. A temporary loop ileostomy is constructed to divert intestinal flow, and the newly constructed J pouch (made from 6 to 10 cm of colon) is reattached to the anal stump. After 3 months, the ileostomy is reversed and intestinal continuity is restored, preserving the anal sphincter and continence.

- With improved surgical techniques, colostomies are performed in less than one-third of patients with colorectal cancer.

Gerontologic Considerations

The elderly are at increased risk of complications after surgery and may have difficulty managing colostomy care due to decreased vision, impaired hearing, and difficulty with fine motor coordination.

- Allow patients to handle ostomy equipment and simulate cleaning the peristomal skin and irrigating the stoma before surgery.
- Skin care is a major concern in older patients with a colostomy because of changes that occur with aging—the epithelial and subcutaneous fatty layers become thin, and the skin is irritated easily. To prevent skin breakdown, special attention is paid to skin cleansing and the proper fit of an appliance.
- Recognize atherosclerosis because it may cause decreased blood flow to the wound and stoma site, prolonging wound healing
- Some patients have delayed elimination after irrigation because of decreased peristalsis and mucus production.
- Explain to the patient that many patients require 6 months before they feel comfortable with their ostomy care.

COMPLICATIONS

- Partial or complete bowel obstruction
- Perforation
- Abscess formation
- Peritonitis
- Sepsis
- Shock

For more information, see Chapter 24 in Pellico, L.H. (2013). *Focus on adult health. Medical-surgical nursing.* Philadelphia: Wolters Kluwer Health | Lippincott Williams & Wilkins.

Cancer of the Endometrium

Cancer of the endometrium or uterus is the most commonly reported female reproductive cancer and comprises approximately 6% of all reproductive cancers in the United States.

PATHOPHYSIOLOGY

Most endometrial cancers are considered endometrioid. Less common are nonendometrioid, including serous, clear cell, and carcinosarcomas. Nonendometrioid cancers are more aggressive, with an increased mortality rate. Unopposed estrogen causes endometrial hyperplasia or an overgrowth of the uterine lining. Simple hyperplasia often spontaneously regresses but complex hyperplasia and atypical hyperplasia are more likely to progress to cancer. Patients can be treated with progesterone prior to considering surgical hysterectomy.

RISK FACTORS

- Unopposed estrogen
- Early onset of menarche (before age 12) or late menopause (after age 50)
- Nulliparous
- Polycystic ovarian syndrome (PCOS)
- Use of tamoxifen
- Obesity
- Diabetes
- Prior pelvic radiation
- Personal or family history of breast, uterine, ovarian, or colon cancer
- Previous history of atypical hyperplasia

CLINICAL MANIFESTATIONS AND ASSESSMENT

- Abnormal vaginal bleeding is the most common early symptom of endometrial cancer; may be present in postmenopausal women.

- Any unexplained vaginal bleeding or an irregularity in menstrual cycle should be evaluated by a health care professional.

DIAGNOSTIC METHODS

- Endometrial biopsy is the preferred method as it does not require anesthesia.
- Dilation and curettage (D & C) is gold standard when biopsy is indicative of endometrial cancer.
- Hysteroscopic-directed biopsy or transvaginal ultrasound may be performed.

MEDICAL AND NURSING MANAGEMENT

See also "Medical and Nursing Management" under "Cancer of the Cervix" on pages 135–136 for additional information.

- Total abdominal hysterectomy and bilateral salpingo-oophorectomy; node sampling with pelvic lymph node removal is of questionable value.
- Laparoscopic vaginal hysterectomy decreases morbidity in morbidly obese women or those with severe comorbid conditions.
- Vaginal brachytherapy is preferred over external beam radiation, due to lessened side effect: Patient is in isolation, on strict bed rest, and given a low-residue diet. Nurses wear dosimeter and stand behind a lead shield to deliver care.
- Educate women who have high risk factors, including decreasing obesity and controlling diabetes.
- Monitor CA125 levels; elevated levels are a significant predictor of extrauterine disease or metastasis.

For more information, see Chapter 33 in Pellico, L.H. (2013). *Focus on adult health. Medical-surgical nursing.* Philadelphia: Wolters Kluwer Health | Lippincott Williams & Wilkins.

Cancer of the Esophagus

The rate of adenocarcinoma is rapidly increasing in the United States, as well as in other Western countries.

PATHOPHYSIOLOGY

Esophageal cancer can be of two cell types: Adenocarcinoma and squamous cell carcinoma. Adenocarcinoma is found in gland cells not common to the esophagus, except in patient's having Barrett's esophagus (typically secondary to gastroesophageal reflux disease [GERD]), which places them at greater risk developing esophageal cancer.

Tumor cells of adenocarcinoma and of squamous cell carcinoma may spread beneath the esophageal mucosa or directly into, through, and beyond the muscle layers into the lymphatics. In the latter stages, obstruction of the esophagus is noted, with possible perforation into the mediastinum and erosion into the great vessels.

RISK FACTORS

- Male
- Chronic esophageal irritation such as GERD, alcohol, tobacco
- Chronic ingestion of hot liquids or foods
- Nutritional deficiencies
- Poor oral hygiene
- Exposure to nitrosamines in the environment or food

CLINICAL MANIFESTATIONS AND ASSESSMENT

- Many patients have advanced ulcerated lesion of the esophagus before symptoms are manifested.
- Dysphagia, first with solid foods and eventually liquids

- Feeling of a mass in the throat; painful swallowing.
- Intermittent and increasing dysphagia
- Later, regurgitation of undigested food and saliva, foul breath, hiccups, substernal pain or fullness
- Hemorrhage; progressive loss of weight and strength from starvation
- The delay between the onset of early symptoms and the time when the patient seeks medical advice is often 12 to 18 months.

DIAGNOSTIC METHODS

- Esophagogastroduodenoscopy (EGD) with biopsy and brushings
- CT, MRI, PET, endoscopic ultrasound (EUS)

MEDICAL AND NURSING MANAGEMENT

Treatment of esophageal cancer is directed toward cure if cancer is in early stage; in late stages, palliation is the goal of therapy.

- Surgery (eg, esophagectomy), radiation, chemotherapy, or a combination of these modalities, depending on extent of disease and patient condition
- Standard surgical management is total resection of the esophagus (esophagectomy) with removal of the tumor plus a wide tumor-free margin of the esophagus and the lymph nodes in the area. Thoracic or abdominal approach may be used based on location of the tumor.
- Palliative treatment to maintain esophageal patency: Dilation of the esophagus, laser therapy, placement of an endoprosthesis (stent), radiation, and chemotherapy

Nursing Management

See "Nursing Management for the Patient With Cancer" under "Cancer" on pages 120–123 for additional information on preparation for surgery, radiation therapy, or chemotherapy.

- Implement program to promote weight gain based on a high-calorie and high-protein diet, in liquid or soft form, if adequate food can be taken by mouth. If this is not possible, initiate parenteral or enteral nutrition.
- Monitor nutritional status throughout treatment.
- Inform patient about the nature of the postoperative equipment that will be used, including that required for closed chest drainage, NG suction, parenteral fluid therapy, and gastric intubation.
- Postoperatively, the NG tube should not be manipulated; patient is NPO until anastomosis is free from leakage, there is no obstruction and no evidence of pulmonary aspiration.

☼ N U R S I N G   A L E R T

The NG tube is not manipulated; if displacement occurs, it is not likely to be replaced unless by the surgeon because damage to the anastomosis may occur.

- Immediate postoperative care is similar to that provided for patients undergoing thoracic surgery: Place patient in a low Fowler's position after recovery from anesthesia and later in a Fowler's position to prevent reflux of gastric secretions.
- Observe patient carefully for regurgitation, dyspnea, and aspiration pneumonia.
- Implement vigorous pulmonary plan of care that includes incentive spirometry, sitting up in a chair, and, if necessary, nebulizer treatments; avoid chest physiotherapy due to the risk of aspiration.
- Monitor the patient's temperature to detect any elevation that may indicate an esophageal leak (drainage from the cervical neck wound, usually saliva).
- Monitor for and treat cardiac complications, including atrial fibrillation.
- Arrange for speech therapist to evaluate patient's ability to swallow and rule out aspiration after NG tube removed (5 to 7 days postoperatively).
- Small, frequent feedings (six to eight per day) are recommended because large quantities of food overload the stomach and promote gastric reflux.

- Encourage the patient to eat, because the appetite is usually poor. Family involvement and home-cooked favorite foods may be helpful. Antacids may decrease gastric distress. Metoclopramide (Reglan) is useful in promoting gastric motility.
- Avoid supplements such as Boost and Ensure because they promote dumping syndrome.
- Perform daily assessment of weight and nutritional intake.
- When the patient is ready to go home, instruct the family about how to promote nutrition, what observations to make, what measures to take if complications occur, how to keep the patient comfortable, and how to obtain needed physical and emotional support.

C

For more information, see Chapter 22 in Pellico, L.H. (2013). *Focus on adult health. Medical-surgical nursing.* Philadelphia: Wolters Kluwer Health | Lippincott Williams & Wilkins.

Cancer of the Larynx

Cancer of the larynx is a malignant tumor in and around the larynx (voice box).

PATHOPHYSIOLOGY

Squamous cell carcinoma is the most common form of cancer of the larynx (95%). Approximately 55% of patients with laryngeal cancer present with involved lymph nodes at time of diagnosis.

Metastatic disease from the true vocal cords is very rare, because they are devoid of lymph nodes. The survival for patients who have small laryngeal cancers without evidence of spread to the lymph nodes is about 75% to 95%. Recurrence occurs usually within the first 2 to 3 years after diagnosis. The presence of disease after 5 years is very often secondary to a new primary malignancy. The incidence of laryngeal cancer continues to decline, but the incidence in women versus men continues to increase.

C

RISK FACTORS

- Male
- Aged 60 to 70 years
- African Americans twice as likely as Caucasians
- Exposure to carcinogens: Tobacco (smoke, smokeless) and alcohol and their combined effects
- Occupational or environmental exposure: Asbestos, wood dust, coal dust, steel dust, cement dust, tar products, leather, formaldehyde, and iron compounds and fumes have also been implicated.
- Other contributing factors include straining the voice, chronic laryngitis, nutritional deficiencies (riboflavin), family predisposition, and a weakened immune system.

CLINICAL MANIFESTATIONS AND ASSESSMENT

- Hoarseness, noted early with cancer in glottic area; harsh, raspy, low-pitched voice
- Persistent cough; pain and burning in the throat when drinking hot liquids and citrus juices
- Palpable lump in the neck
- Later symptoms: Dysphagia, dyspnea, unilateral nasal obstruction or discharge, persistent hoarseness or ulceration, foul breath
- Enlarged cervical nodes, weight loss, general debility, and pain radiating to the ear may occur with metastasis.

DIAGNOSTIC METHODS

- Indirect laryngoscopy
- Endoscopy, virtual endoscopy, optical imaging, CT, MRI, and PET scanning (to detect recurrence of tumor after treatment)
- Direct laryngoscopic examination under local or general anesthesia
- Biopsy of suspicious tissue

MEDICAL AND NURSING MANAGEMENT

- The goals of treatment of laryngeal cancer include cure; preservation of safe, effective swallowing; preservation of useful voice; and avoidance of permanent tracheostoma.
- Treatment options include surgery, radiation therapy, and chemotherapy, depending on whether initial diagnosis or recurrence.
- Chemotherapy traditionally has been used for recurrence or metastatic disease. It has also been used more recently in conjunction with radiation therapy, to avoid a total laryngectomy, or preoperatively, to shrink a tumor before surgery.

Surgical Management

Surgical management depends largely on the stage of the disease.

- Total laryngectomy, removal of the larynx, including the hyoid bone, epiglottis, cricoid cartilage, and two or three rings of the trachea, can provide the desired cure, but leaves the patient with significant loss of the natural voice and need to breathe through a stoma; often used as salvage therapy.
- Voice-sparing surgeries, which achieve a positive cure rate for the patient who has an early laryngeal carcinoma, include:
  - Vocal cord stripping, which involves removal of the mucosa of the edge of the cord
  - Cordectomy, using a transoral laser (for lesions in middle one-third of vocal cords)
  - Partial laryngectomy (laryngofissure–thyrotomy), which involves removal of a portion of the larynx and one vocal cord with tumor
  - Supraglottic laryngectomy, in which the hyoid bone, glottis, and false cords are removed
  - Hemilaryngectomy, in which the thyroid cartilage is split in the midline, and one true cord and one false cord is removed with the tumor
- Wound drains may be placed; observe measure and record drainage. Drains are removed when drainage is less than 30 mL for 2 consecutive days.

- Complications may include salivary leak, wound infection from development of pharyngocutaneous fistula, stomal stenosis, and dysphagia secondary to pharyngeal and cervical esophageal stricture.

Radiation Therapy

- The goal of radiation therapy is to eradicate the cancer and preserve the function of the larynx.
- Decision to use radiation therapy is based on several factors, including the staging of the tumor and the patient's overall health status, lifestyle (including occupation), and personal preference.
- Early-stage vocal cord tumors are initially treated with irradiation.
- Radiation therapy may also be used preoperatively to reduce the tumor size. Radiation therapy is combined with surgery in advanced laryngeal cancer as adjunctive therapy to surgery or chemotherapy and as a palliative measure.
- Complications from radiation therapy are a result of external radiation to the head and neck area, which may also include the parotid gland, which is responsible for mucus production. Symptoms may include acute mucositis, ulceration of the mucous membranes, pain, xerostomia (dry mouth), and loss of taste, dysphasia, fatigue, and skin reactions. Complications occurring late may include laryngeal necrosis, edema, and fibrosis

Speech Therapy

- The patient who undergoes a laryngectomy faces potentially complex and frustrating communication problems.
- Loss or alteration of speech is discussed with the patient and family before surgery; the speech therapist conducts a preoperative evaluation.
- Plan with the patient and family those methods of communication available in the immediate postoperative period. Writing, lip speaking, and communication or word boards are options that can be utilized by patient, family, nurse, and physician consistently after surgery.

- Postoperatively, alaryngeal communication is used: The three most common techniques of alaryngeal communication are esophageal speech, artificial larynx (electrolarynx), and tracheoesophageal puncture using a voice prosthesis.

Nursing Management

Teaching the Patient Preoperatively

- Teach the patient undergoing complete laryngectomy that the natural voice and ability to sing, laugh, and whistle will be lost, but that special training can provide a means for communicating.
- Review equipment and teach importance of coughing and deep-breathing exercises.

Reducing Anxiety and Depression

- Provide the patient and family with opportunities to ask questions, verbalize feelings, and discuss perceptions, fears related to cancer diagnosis, and possibility of loss of voice and disfigurement.
- A visit from someone who has had a laryngectomy may reassure the patient that people are available to assist with rehabilitation; such visits may be planned pre- or postoperatively.
- In immediate postoperative period, the nurse spends time with the patient, focusing on building trust and reducing the patient's anxiety.
- Seek to learn from the patient what activities promote feelings of comfort; assist the patient in such activities (eg, listening to music, reading). Relaxation techniques such as guided imagery and meditation are often helpful.

Maintaining a Patent Airway

- Promote a patent airway by positioning the patient in semi-Fowler's or Fowler's position after recovery from anesthesia. This decreases surgical edema and promotes lung expansion.
- Observe the patient for restlessness, labored breathing, apprehension, and increased pulse rate, which helps to identify possible respiratory or circulatory problems.
- Use opioids cautiously, providing adequate analgesia for turning, coughing, and deep breathing.

- Provide suctioning to remove secretions, avoiding disruption of the suture line.
- Monitor pulse oximetry.
- Encourage and assist the patient with early ambulation to prevent atelectasis, pneumonia, and deep vein thrombosis (DVT).
- Recognize that the laryngectomy tube (shorter than a tracheostomy tube but has a larger diameter) is the patient's only airway; humidification is required if no inner cannula is present. (Care is the same as for tracheostomy tube). Reassure the patient that excess mucus will diminish over time.

Promoting Alternative Communication Methods

- Establishing an effective means of communication is the primary goal in the rehabilitation of the laryngectomy patient.
- A call bell or hand bell must be placed within easy reach of the patient; the patient is unable to use an intercom system.
- Provide a magic slate; place IV in nondominant arm for ease of writing.
- Picture-word-phrase board or hand signals may be used for those who cannot write.
- Give patient adequate time to communicate as writing or gesturing is time-consuming and frustrating; patient may become impatient and angry when not understood.

Promoting Adequate Nutrition and Hydration

- Patient may be NPO for several days after surgery; plan for alternative methods of nutritional and hydration via IV, NG, or gastrostomy or parenteral nutrition.
- When able to start oral feedings, a swallowing study to evaluate risk for aspiration is performed.
- Initiate diet with thick liquids for ease of swallowing.
- Remain with patient during initial oral feedings; keep suction setup at bedside if needed. Solid foods are introduced as tolerated.
- The nurse instructs the patient to avoid sweet foods, which increase salivation and suppress the appetite.
- The patient is instructed to rinse the mouth with warm water or mouthwash after oral feedings and to brush the teeth frequently.

- Changes in taste and olfactory sensation adapt, often with return of interest in eating. Monitor weight and laboratory data to ensure that nutritional and fluid intake are adequate. Skin turgor and vital signs are assessed for signs of decreased fluid volume.

Promoting Positive Body Image and Self-Esteem

- Disfiguring surgery and an altered communication pattern are a threat to a patient's body image and self-esteem. The reaction of family members and friends is a major concern for the patient.
- Encourage the patient to express feelings about the changes brought about by surgery, particularly feelings related to fear, anger, depression, and isolation.
- Encouraging use of previous effective coping strategies may be helpful.
- Support groups, such as the International Association of Laryngectomees ([IAL) and I Can Cope (the American Cancer Society), may help the patient and family deal with the changes in their lives.

Promoting Self-Care

- Maintaining a positive approach is important when caring for the patient and includes promotion of self-care activities.
- Patient and family should begin participating in self-care activities as soon as possible.
- Support the patient and the family, especially when explaining the tubes, dressings, and drains that are in place postoperatively.

COMPLICATIONS

- Respiratory distress and hypoxia
- Hemorrhage
- Infection
- Wound breakdown
- Aspiration
- Tracheostomal stenosis

For more information, see Chapter 9 in Pellico, L.H. (2013). *Focus on adult health. Medical-surgical nursing.* Philadelphia: Wolters Kluwer Health | Lippincott Williams & Wilkins.

Cancer of the Liver (Hepatocellular Carcinoma)

Hepatocellular carcinoma (HCC) has a high mortality rate and is the fifth leading cause of cancer.

PATHOPHYSIOLOGY

The clinical manifestations of hepatocellular carcinoma (HCC) are usually found within the context of the patient with known cirrhosis.

RISK FACTORS

- Cirrhosis
- Hepatitis B and C
- Alcoholic liver disease
- Nonalcoholic steatohepatitis (inflammation and fat accumulation of the liver)
- Primary biliary cirrhosis
- Hemochromatosis
- Age older than 50 years
- Male gender

CLINICAL MANIFESTATIONS AND ASSESSMENTS

- Symptoms of cirrhosis include jaundice, ascites, varices, and the stigmata of chronic liver disease are common features.
- Unintentional weight loss, anorexia, and right upper quadrant pain are noted.
- In late cases, the patient may present with intra-abdominal bleeding from tumor rupture.

DIAGNOSTIC METHODS

The diagnosis of liver cancer is based on clinical signs and symptoms, the history and physical examination, and the results of laboratory and imaging studies.

- For patients deemed at high risk, routine screening with abdominal ultrasound and measurement of alpha fetoprotein levels improves detection.
- Increased serum levels of bilirubin, alkaline phosphatase, GGT, and alpha-fetoprotein levels may occur.
- Anemia and leukocytosis are common.
- Hypercalcemia, hypoglycemia, and hypocholesterolemia may also be seen.
- Confirmation is made radiologically with use of CT scan imaging or MRI to determine the number, size, and location of tumors and if vascular invasion has occurred.
- Liver biopsy may be used to obtain tissue samples of the lesion to determine malignancy.

MEDICAL AND NURSING MANAGEMENT

Surgical Management

Surgical resection is the preferred treatment for patients without cirrhosis and with adequate hepatic reserve.

- In HCC and cirrhosis, liver transplantation is the treatment of choice.
- Other treatments for HCC are percutaneous ethanol injection (PEI) and radiofrequency ablation (RFA), which induce tumor necrosis.
- Transarterial chemoembolization (TACE) blocks hepatic blood flow to the tumor and is used in combination with chemotherapeutic agents.
- Systemic chemotherapy includes sorafenib and other agents; clinical trials are under way to study effectiveness of chemotherapeutics for HCC.

Liver Transplantation

With recent advances in surgical techniques, immunosuppressant medications, and increased knowledge of immunology, liver transplantation has become the treatment of choice for patients with end-stage liver disease and acute liver failure.

- Procedure involves surgical removal of the diseased liver and replacement with a healthy donor organ in the same anatomic location (orthotopic liver transplantation).
- The benefit of this option is limited by the shortage of cadaveric donor organs.
- Contraindications include uncontrolled infection, extrahepatic malignancy or advanced hepatobiliary metastatic disease, irreversible brain damage, anatomic difficulties, and multiorgan failure.
- Psychosocial contraindications include active substance use, medical nonadherence, and severe psychiatric instability.
- Other obstacles to successful transplant are comorbidities such as advanced cardiac or pulmonary disease and poor psychosocial support.
- Postoperatively, the nurse maintains asepsis and observes for infection and rejection.
- Life-long immunosuppressant therapy is required; side effects include renal dysfunction, hypertension, hyperlipidemia, and hyperkalemia.

For more information, see Chapter 25 in Pellico, L.H. (2013). *Focus on adult health. Medical-surgical nursing.* Philadelphia: Wolters Kluwer Health | Lippincott Williams & Wilkins.

Cancer of the Lung (Bronchogenic Carcinoma)

Lung cancer is the leading cancer killer among men and women in the United States. The incidence of lung cancer in men has remained relatively constant, but an increased incidence in women has occurred since 1991.

PATHOPHYSIOLOGY

Eighty percent of lung cancer in women and 90% in men is caused by cigarette smoking, with the remainder being attributed to other carcinogens, including radon gas and occupational and environmental agents. In approximately 70% of patients with lung cancer, the disease has spread to regional lymphatics and other sites by the time of diagnosis. As a result, the long-term survival rate is low.

Classification and Staging

- For purposes of staging and treatment, most lung cancers are classified into one of two major categories: Small cell lung cancer (25% of lung cancers) and non–small cell lung cancer (NSCLC) (75% of lung cancers), which includes squamous cell carcinoma (20% to 30%), large cell carcinoma (10%), and adenocarcinoma (30% to 40%), including bronchoalveolar carcinoma. Most small cell carcinomas arise in the major bronchi and spread by infiltration along the bronchial wall.
- Tumors are staged by lymph node involvement and spread of the cancer. NSCLC is staged as I to IV. Stage I is the earliest stage and has the highest cure rates, whereas stage IV designates metastatic spread. Small cell lung cancers are classified as limited or extensive

RISK FACTORS

- Tobacco smoke, passive smoking/second-hand smoke
- Occupational and environmental agents (vehicle emissions, pollutants, urban areas, radon gas, arsenic, asbestos, chromates, coal fumes, radiation)
- Male
- Genetic predisposition
- Underlying diseases (chronic obstructive pulmonary disease [COPD], tuberculosis [TB])
- Family history (close relative with lung cancer)
- Low intake of fruits and vegetables

CLINICAL MANIFESTATIONS AND ASSESSMENT

- Lung cancer develops insidiously and is asymptomatic until late in its course.
- Cough or change in a chronic cough is the most common symptom.
- Cough starts as a dry, persistent cough, without sputum production. When obstruction of airways occurs, the cough may become productive due to infection.
- Dyspnea occurs frequently.
- Hemoptysis or blood-tinged sputum may be expectorated.
- Chest or shoulder pain may indicate chest wall or pleural involvement by a tumor.
- Pain is a late manifestation, and may be related to metastasis to the bone.
- Recurring fever is an early symptom in response to a persistent infection distal to the tumor.
- Suspect lung cancer in people with repeated unresolved upper respiratory tract infections.
- If the tumor spreads to adjacent structures and regional lymph nodes, chest pain and tightness, hoarseness (involving the recurrent laryngeal nerve), dysphagia, head and neck edema, and symptoms of pleural or pericardial effusion may occur.
- The most common sites of metastases are lymph nodes, bone, brain, contralateral lung, adrenal glands, and liver.
- Nonspecific symptoms of weakness, anorexia, and weight loss also may be present.
- As pulmonary symptoms occur in smokers, cancer of the lung should always be considered.

DIAGNOSTIC METHODS

- Chest X-ray, CT scans, fiberoptic bronchoscopy for brushings, washings and biopsies of suspicious areas
- Transthoracic fine needle aspiration may be performed under CT guidance to aspirate cells from a suspicious area.
- Endoscopy with transesophageal ultrasound and biopsy

- PET scan, ultrasound of liver, CT of brain, MRI, and mediastinoscopy or mediastinotomy for biopsy
- Pulmonary function tests, arterial blood gas analysis, ventilation/perfusion scans, and exercise testing may all be used as part of the preoperative assessment.
- Staging of the tumor is performed. (See "Tumor Staging and Grading" under "Cancer Care" on page 112 for additional information.)

MEDICAL AND NURSING MANAGEMENT

See also "Medical and Nursing Management" under "Cancer" on pages 113–123 for additional information.

- The objective of management is to provide a cure if possible. Treatment depends on cell type, stage of the disease, and physiologic status.
- Treatment may involve surgery, radiation therapy, or chemotherapy. Therapies to modulate the immune system (gene therapy, therapy with defined tumor antigens) are under study and show promise.

Surgical Management

- Surgical resection is the preferred method for localized non–small cell tumors with no evidence of metastatic spread and adequate cardiopulmonary function. Lesions of many patients with bronchogenic cancer are inoperable at the time of diagnosis.
- The most common surgical procedure for a small, apparently curable tumor of the lung is lobectomy. In some cases, an entire lung may be removed (pneumonectomy).

Radiation Therapy

- Radiation therapy (XRT) is useful in controlling neoplasms that cannot be surgically resected but are responsive to radiation.
- Irradiation may be used to reduce tumor mass, to make an inoperable tumor operable, or to relieve the pressure on vital

structures. It can reduce symptoms of spinal cord metastasis and superior vena cava compression and treat metastases to the brain.

- Radiation therapy may help relieve cough, chest pain, dyspnea, hemoptysis, and bone and liver pain, and it improves the quality of life.
- Radiofrequency ablation and cryoablation are two types of non-surgical therapies that have been used to treat lung tumors.

Chemotherapy

- Chemotherapy is used to alter tumor growth patterns, to treat distant metastases or small cell cancer of the lung, and as an adjunct to surgery or radiation therapy. Chemotherapy may provide relief, especially of pain, pressure symptoms in brain, spinal cord, and pericardial metastasis, but it does not usually cure the disease or prolong life.
- The choice of agent depends on the growth of the tumor cell and the specific phase of the cell cycle that the medication affects. Combinations of two or more medications may be more beneficial than single-dose regimens.

Palliative Therapy

- Palliative therapy may include radiation therapy or chemo-therapy to shrink the tumor to provide pain relief, a variety of bronchoscopic interventions to open a narrowed bronchus or airway, and pain management and other comfort measures.
- Evaluation and referral for hospice care are important in planning for comfortable and dignified end-of-life care for the patient and family.

Treatment-Related Complications

A variety of complications may occur as a result of treatment for lung cancer.

- Surgical resection may result in respiratory failure, particularly if the cardiopulmonary system is compromised before surgery. Surgical complications and prolonged mechanical ventilation are potential outcomes.

- Radiation therapy may result in diminished cardiopulmonary function and other complications, such as pulmonary fibrosis, pericarditis, myelitis, and cor pulmonale.
- Chemotherapy, particularly in combination with radiation therapy, can cause pneumonitis and pulmonary toxicity.

Nursing Management

Nursing care of patients with lung cancer is similar to that for other patients with cancer and addresses the physiologic and psychological needs of the patient.

- The physiologic problems are primarily due to the respiratory manifestations of the disease.
- Nursing care includes strategies to ensure relief of pain and discomfort and to prevent complications.

Managing Symptoms

- Instruct patient and family about side effects of the specific treatment and strategies, such as dyspnea, fatigue, nausea and vomiting, anorexia, and fatigue.
- Help the patient and family cope with therapeutic measures.

Relieving Breathing Problems

- Maintain patent airway through the removal of excess secretions; deep-breathing exercises, chest PT, directed cough, suctioning, and in some instances bronchoscopy are performed.
- Administer bronchodilators as prescribed to promote bronchial dilation.
- Provide supplemental oxygen as needed; as the tumor enlarges or spreads, it may compress a bronchus or involve a large area of lung tissue, resulting in an impaired breathing pattern and poor gas exchange.
- Encourage the patient to assume positions that promote lung expansion and to perform breathing exercises for lung expansion and relaxation.
- Provide patient education about energy conservation and airway clearance. A referral to a pulmonary rehabilitation program may be helpful in managing respiratory symptoms.

Providing Psychological Support

Provide psychological support and identify potential resources for the patient and family.

Gerontologic Considerations

- At the time of diagnosis of lung cancer, most patients are older than 65 years of age and have stage III or IV disease.
- Age is not a significant prognostic factor for overall survival and response to treatment.
- Depending on the comorbidities and functional status of elderly patients, chemotherapy agents, doses, and cycles may need to be adjusted to maintain quality of life.
- Issues that must be considered in care of elderly patients with lung cancer include functional status, comorbid conditions, nutritional status, cognition, concomitant medications, and psychological and social support.

For more information, see Chapter 10 in Pellico, L.H. (2013). *Focus on adult health. Medical-surgical nursing.* Philadelphia: Wolters Kluwer Health | Lippincott Williams & Wilkins.

Cancer of the Oral Cavity and Pharynx

Cancer of the oral cavity and throat can occur in any part of the mouth (lips, lateral tongue, floor of mouth most common) or throat.

PATHOPHYSIOLOGY

Malignancies of the oral cavity are usually squamous cell cancers and are considered highly curable if discovered early.

RISK FACTORS

- Alcohol
- Tobacco product

- Dietary deficiency
- Smoked meat
- Prolonged exposure to sun and wind (cancer of the lip)
- African Americans are more at risk than Caucasians.

CLINICAL MANIFESTATIONS AND ASSESSMENTS

- Few or no symptoms in early phase
- Later, most frequent symptom is a painless sore or mass that will not heal.
- Typical lesion is a painless indurated ulcer with raised edges.
- As the cancer progresses, patient may complain of tenderness; difficulty in chewing, swallowing, or speaking; coughing of blood-tinged sputum; or enlarged cervical lymph nodes.
- High-risk areas include the buccal mucosa and gingiva in people who use snuff or smoke cigars or pipes.
- In cigarettes smokers and those who drink alcohol, high-risk areas include the floor of the mouth, the ventrolateral tongue, and the soft palate complex (soft palate, anterior and posterior tonsillar area, uvula, and the area behind the molar and tongue junction).

MEDICAL AND NURSING MANAGEMENT

Management varies with the nature of the lesion, preference of the physician, and patient choice. Resectional surgery, radiation therapy, chemotherapy, or a combination may be effective.

- Tissue from any ulcer of the oral cavity that does not heal in 2 weeks should be examined through biopsy.
- Lip cancer: Small lesions are excised liberally; larger lesions may be treated by radiation therapy for cosmetic reasons.
- Tongue cancer: Radiation with chemotherapy may preserve organ function and quality of life. Surgeries may include hemi-glossectomy (removal of half the tongue) or total glossectomy (removal of the tongue).

- Radical neck dissection or radical neck dissection with reconstruction for metastasis of oral cancer to lymphatic channel in the neck region with reconstructive surgery may be performed.

Nursing Management

- Preoperatively assess the patient's nutritional status; a dietary consultation may be necessary. Enteral or IV feedings may be needed
- If a radial graft is to be performed, an Allen test on the donor arm must be performed to ensure that the ulnar artery is patent.
- Postoperatively, monitor ability for patient to protect his or her airway by assessing ability to swallow and management of oral secretions. Suction oral secretions and instruct patient on use of Yankauer suction (tonsil tip suction).
- Assess the patient's ability to communicate in writing; verbal communication may be impaired by radical surgery. (Provide a pen and paper after surgery to patients who can use them to communicate.)
- Perform suction carefully if a graft is present, to prevent damage. Assess graft for viability; white color may indicate arterial occlusion, and blue mottling may indicate venous congestion.
- Perform an Allen test, if a radial graft is anticipated, to ensure patency of the ulnar artery, which will provide blood flow to the hand.
- Monitor for xerostomia (dry mouth), a frequent sequela of oral cancer, particularly after radiation or major surgery. Encourage patient to increase fluid intake (when not contraindicated) and to use a humidifier during sleep. The use of synthetic saliva, a moisturizing antibacterial gel such as Oral Balance, or a saliva production stimulant such as Salagen may be helpful.
- Advise patient to avoid dry, bulky, and irritating foods and fluids, as well as alcohol and tobacco.
- Observe for stomatitis or mucositis (inflammation and breakdown of the oral mucosa), a side effect of chemotherapy or radiation therapy.
- Observe for alcohol and nicotine use as individuals with cancers of the head and neck frequently have used alcohol or tobacco.
- Monitor for depression, especially at diagnosis and during treatment.

NURSING PROCESS

The Patient Undergoing a Neck Dissection

Assessment

- Assess the patient's physical and psychological preparation for surgery, along with knowledge of the preoperative and postoperative procedures.
- Postoperatively, assess the patient for complications such as altered respiratory status, wound infection, and hemorrhage.

Diagnosis

- Deficient knowledge about preoperative and postoperative procedures
- Ineffective airway clearance related to obstruction by mucus, hemorrhage, or edema
- Acute pain related to surgical incision
- Risk for infection related to surgical intervention secondary to decreased nutritional status, or immunosuppression from chemotherapy or radiation therapy
- Impaired tissue integrity secondary to surgery and grafting
- Imbalanced nutrition, less than body requirements, related to disease process or treatment
- Situational low self-esteem related to diagnosis or prognosis
- Impaired verbal communication secondary to surgical resection
- Impaired physical mobility secondary to nerve injury

Potential Postoperative Complications

- Hemorrhage
- Chyle fistula
- Nerve injury

Planning

The major goals for the patient include participation in the treatment plan, maintenance of respiratory status, attainment of comfort, absence of infection, viability of the graft, maintenance

(continues on page 164)

of adequate intake of food and fluids, effective coping strategies, effective communication, maintenance of shoulder and neck
motion, and absence of complications.

Nursing Interventions

- Preoperatively, inform patient about the nature and extent of
  the surgery and what the postoperative period will be like.
- To maintain the airway post extubation, place patient in
  Fowler's position. Assess for stridor, indicative of airway
  obstruction:
  - Observe for respiratory distress including dyspnea, cyanosis,
    changes in mental status, and changes in vital signs; these
    may suggest edema, hemorrhage, inadequate oxygenation,
    or inadequate drainage.
  - Prevent pneumonia with suction, coughing, and deep
    breathing.
- Relieve pain; administer analgesics as prescribed based on
  individual's pain experience. Patients with head and neck
  cancer often report less pain than do patients with other types
  of cancer.
- Provide wound care; observe wound drainage tubes, anticipating 80 to 120 mL of serosanguineous material over the first
  24 hours. Excessive drainage may indicate fistula or hemorrhage. Assess graft for pink color and warmth and incision for
  signs of infection. Prophylactic antibiotics may be prescribed.

Maintaining Adequate Nutrition

- Provide early intervention to correct nutritional deficiencies,
  using enteral or parenteral nutrition to maintain positive
  nitrogen balance.
- Ability to chew will direct whether diet modifications for soft,
  pureed, or liquid food is needed.
- Oral care before eating may enhance the patient's appetite;
  after eating it is important to prevent infection and dental
  caries.

Supporting Coping Measures

- Preoperatively, information about the planned surgery is given
  to the patient and family.

- Postoperatively, psychological nursing interventions are aimed at supporting the patient, who has had a change in body image or who has major concerns regarding the prognosis.
- The patient may have difficulty communicating and may be concerned about his or her ability to breathe and swallow normally.
- Support the patient's family and friends in encouraging and reassuring the patient that adjusting to the results of this surgery will take time.
- The person who has had extensive neck surgery often is sensitive about his or her appearance; the nurse accepts the patient's appearance and expresses a positive, optimistic attitude to encourage the patient.

Promoting Effective Communication

- Post laryngectomy, the nurse explores other methods of communicating with the patient. Use of a pencil and paper or pointing to needed items on a picture pad may be used.
- Obtain a consultation with a speech/language therapist.
- Alternative speech techniques, such as an electrolarynx (a mechanical device held against the neck) or esophageal speech, may be taught by a speech/language therapist.

Maintaining Physical Mobility

- Excision of muscles and nerves results in weakness at the shoulder that can cause shoulder drop, a forward curvature of the shoulder.
- Begin an exercise program, usually after drains have been removed and the neck incision is sufficiently healed. Physical therapists and occupational therapists can assist patients in performing these exercises.

Monitoring and Managing Potential Complications

Hemorrhage

- Observe for hemorrhage secondary to carotid artery rupture; this results from necrosis of the graft or damage to the artery itself from tumor or infection.
- Assess vital signs. Tachycardia, tachypnea, and hypotension may indicate hemorrhage and impending hypovolemic shock.

(continues on page 166)

- Instruct the patient to avoid the Valsalva maneuver (bearing down, such as when having a bowel movement) to prevent stress on the graft and carotid artery.
- Observe for signs of impending rupture, such as high epigastric pain or discomfort.
- Monitor dressings and wound drainage for excessive bleeding.
- If hemorrhage occurs, call for immediate assistance and apply continuous pressure to the bleeding site or major associated vessel.
- Recognize that some advocate placing the patient in a supine position and elevating the legs to maintain blood pressure, others recommend elevating the head of bed to maintain airway patency and prevent aspiration.
- A controlled, calm manner allays the patient's anxiety.
- The surgeon is notified immediately, because a vascular or ligature tear requires surgical intervention.

Chyle Fistula
- A chyle fistula (milk-like drainage from the thoracic duct into the thoracic cavity) may develop as a result of damage to the thoracic duct during surgery.
- The diagnosis is made if there is excess drainage that has a 3% fat content and a specific gravity of 1.012 or greater.
- Treatment of a small leak (≤500 mL) includes application of a pressure dressing and a diet of medium-chain fatty acids or parenteral nutrition. Surgical intervention to repair the damaged duct is necessary for larger leaks.

Nerve Injury
- Nerve injury can occur if the cervical plexus or spinal accessory nerves are severed during surgery.
- Observe for lower facial paralysis as a result of injury to the facial nerve
- Monitor for damage to the superior laryngeal nerve; difficulty swallowing liquids and food because of the partial lack of sensation of the glottis will develop
- Speech therapy may be indicated to assist with problems related to nerve injury.

Teaching Patients Self-Care

- Teach the patient and caregiver about wound management, the dressing, and any drains.
- Encourage the caregiver to demonstrate his or her ability to provide suction and tracheostomy care.
- Instruct the patient and caregiver about possible complications, such as bleeding and respiratory distress and when to notify the health care provider of signs and symptoms of these complications.
- Provide detailed instructions and demonstration of enteral or parenteral feedings if the patient cannot take food by mouth. Education in techniques of effective oral hygiene is also important.
- Obtain a referral for home care nursing. The nurse assesses healing, the patient's adjustment to changes in physical appearance and status, and ability to communicate and to eat normally; ensures that feedings are being administered properly; and monitors for any complications.
- Physical and speech therapy also may be continued at home.
- The patient is given information regarding local support groups such as "I Can Cope" or "New Voice Club," if indicated. The local chapter of the American Cancer Society may be contacted for information and equipment needed for the patient.

Evaluation

Expected patient outcomes may include:

- Discusses expected course of treatment
- Demonstrates good respiratory exchange
- Remains free of infection
- Graft is pink and warm to touch
- Maintains adequate intake of foods and fluids
- Demonstrates ability to cope
- Verbalizes comfort
- Attains maximal mobility
- Exhibits no complications

For more information, see Chapter 22 in Pellico, L.H. (2013). *Focus on adult health. Medical-surgical nursing.* Philadelphia: Wolters Kluwer Health | Lippincott Williams & Wilkins.

Cancer of the Ovary

Ovarian cancer is referred to as a cancer that "whispers" because its clinical manifestations are not apparent until the tumor has invaded surrounding structures and causes symptoms.

PATHOPHYSIOLOGY

Ovarian cancer is highly fatal due to the aggressiveness of the malignancy. Five-year survivorship rate is not unforeseeable if the cancer is diagnosed at an early stage, but only 20% of women with ovarian cancer are diagnosed at that stage. Eighty-five percent of women diagnosed are over age 50; 15% have genetic links; 10% have *BRCA 1* and *2* mutations, and 5% have HNPCC risk factors. Use of oral contraceptives has been proven to decrease the risk of developing ovarian cancer by 50%, with long-term protection benefits.

Cancers of the ovary occur as a result of cancerous epithelial cells from the lining of the ovary. Shedding of malignant ovarian cells from the ovary implant onto the surfaces of the peritoneal cavity. These cancerous cells then undergo transformation of ovarian surface epithelium

RISK FACTORS

- *BRCA 1* and *2* mutations
- Age over 40 or postmenopausal
- Nulliparous
- Northern American or Northern European descent
- Personal history of breast, colon, or endometrial cancer
- Obesity; BMI greater than 30
- Use of fertility drugs

- Long-term use of hormone replacement therapy
- Genetic predisposition; positive family history of ovarian cancer

CLINICAL MANIFESTATIONS AND ASSESSMENTS

- Symptoms of ovarian cancer are subtle and start with persistent bloating, early satiety, or a change in bowel or bladder habits.
- Women will typically complain of weight gain confined to their abdominal area.
- Early symptoms include early satiety, feeling of abdominal fullness.
- Ascites (fluid accumulation in the peritoneal cavity) is considered a late-stage symptom, and prognosis is poor.
- Ovarian cancer carries a high rate of misdiagnosis, with patients commonly receiving treatment for a variety of disorders including IBS, GERD, menopause, or urinary tract infections.

DIAGNOSTIC METHODS

No reliable screening tools are available for this disease. Treatment is hindered by late diagnosis, when the disease has already invaded peritoneal tissues and surrounding structures.

- Bimanual examinations diagnose approximately one-third of ovarian masses.
- Pelvic ultrasounds and CA 125, a tumor marker are the first diagnostics performed when ruling out an ovarian mass.
- If either of these tests is suggestive of a tumor, an abdominal and pelvic CT scan is performed. Patients are always referred to a gynecologic/oncologist for management.

MEDICAL AND NURSING MANAGEMENT

- Surgical staging allows for identification of treatment options and determines the prognosis based on tumor type.

- Frozen section of suspicious tissue removed during surgery is sent for immediate evaluation. If positive, the surgeon then performs extensive cytoreduction surgery or debulking to obtain clean tissue margins. Total abdominal hysterectomy (TAH) with bilateral salpingo-oophorectomy (BSO), removal of the omentum, peritoneal washings, and partial colectomy in the case of colon involvement are performed.
- Chemotherapy treats residual tumor and controls metastatic disease. For advanced tumors, chemotherapy is given first to decrease the size of the tumor, then surgical debulking is performed.
- First-line chemotherapy consists of platinum and paclitaxel. Patients undergo two to three cycles to evaluate the response and toxicity before proceeding with further treatment.
- Patients whose tumors are resistant to platinum receive single-agent therapy. CA 125 is a sensitive indicator of disease relapse.

Nursing Management

- Education and support begin preoperatively and continue through discharge; support is individualized based on the patient's psychological and physical status, stage of illness, and treatment plan.
- Postoperatively, monitor for signs and symptoms of infection, ileus, DVT, pulmonary embolus (PE) and bleeding. Encourage regular use of incentive spirometry and ambulation to decrease development of DVTs and atelectasis.
- Provide anticipatory guidance with the patient and her support system regarding diagnosis of cancer and side effect of chemotherapy.
- Hair loss, nutrition, neuropathies, nausea, and vomiting, as well as self-image alterations should be addressed regularly postoperatively and during treatment

For more information, see Chapter 33 in Pellico, L.H. (2013). *Focus on adult health. Medical-surgical nursing.* Philadelphia: Wolters Kluwer Health | Lippincott Williams & Wilkins.

Cancer of the Pancreas

Pancreatic cancer is the fourth leading cause of cancer death in the United States. Cancer may develop in the head, body, or tail of the pancreas; most pancreatic cancers originate in the head of the pancreas.

PATHOPHYSIOLOGY

Patients usually do not seek medical attention until late in the disease; most patients have advanced, unresectable tumor when first detected. A 5% survival rate at 5 years regardless of the stage of disease at diagnosis or treatment exists.

RISK FACTORS

- 65 to 84 years
- Tobacco
- Obesity
- Nonhereditary pancreatitis
- Genetic predisposition; first-degree relative with pancreatic cancer

CLINICAL MANIFESTATIONS AND ASSESSMENT

- Pain, jaundice, and weight loss are classic signs but often do not appear until the disease is advanced.
- Weight loss is rapid, profound, and progressive.
- Vague upper- or mid-abdominal pain or discomfort often unrelated to GI function and difficult to describe.
- Radiating, boring pain in the mid-back, unrelated to posture or activity; more severe at night.
- Meals aggravate epigastric pain; pain occurs before jaundice and pruritus.
- Diarrhea and steatorrhea is present.

- Ascites is common.
- Symptoms of insulin deficiency (diabetes: glycosuria, hyperglycemia, and abnormal glucose tolerance) may be an in early sign of carcinoma.

DIAGNOSTIC METHODS

- Spiral (helical) CT has a greater than 90% accuracy in the diagnosis and staging; CT can accurately image pancreatic masses, dilatation of pancreatic duct, and metastases to the liver or peritoneum.
- ERCP and magnetic resonance cholangiopancreatography (MRCP) are also used to diagnosis pancreatic cancer.
- Cells obtained during ERCP are sent to the laboratory for histologic analysis.
- Although CA 19-9 (cancer-associated antigen) serum levels may be elevated, this tumor marker is used primarily to monitor disease progression and treatment efficacy.

MEDICAL AND NURSING MANAGEMENT

- Only 10% to 15% of patients with pancreatic cancer benefit from surgical resection; the majority of patients present at a late stage, frequently with metastatic spread to other organs or vascular invasion.
- Whipple procedure (pancreaticoduodenectomy) is used in early stages.
- Use of adjuvant therapy (ie, chemotherapy) continues to be controversial and nonstandard in this small group of surgical patients with ongoing clinical trials to evaluate potential benefits of treatment.
- Gemcitabine alone or in combination with other chemotherapeutic agents remains the treatment of choice for most patients with pancreatic cancer.
- Palliative measures to address symptoms of pancreatic cancer include nutritional support and pain management.

Nursing Management

See also "Preoperative and Postoperative Nursing Management" in Chapter P on pages 531–554 for additional information.

- Provide skin care and nursing measures to relieve pain and discomfort associated with jaundice, anorexia, and profound weight loss.
- Specialty mattresses protect bony prominences from pressure.
- Pain may be severe and may require liberal use of opioids; patient-controlled analgesia should be considered for the patient with severe, escalating pain.
- Discuss and honor end-of-life referral to hospice care as indicated.
- The postoperative management of patients who have undergone a pancreaticoduodenectomy is similar to the management of patients after extensive GI or biliary surgery.
- Monitor for complications: hemorrhage, vascular collapse, and hepatorenal failure; ongoing monitoring incudes vital signs, ABGs, pulse oximetry, laboratory values, and urine output.
- Plan for NG tube with suction, NPO status, and nutrition that allows the GI tract to rest while promoting adequate nutrition.
- The patient may require intensive care after surgery; IV and arterial lines are used for fluid and blood replacement and hemodynamic monitoring, and a mechanical ventilator is used.
- Monitor for malabsorption syndrome and diabetes mellitus, acutely and long term.
- Provide psychological and emotional state support and understanding for patient and family; after major and high-risk surgery, anxiety and depression may affect recovery.

Promoting Home and Community-Based Care

- Provide careful and thorough preparation for self-care at home, including modifications in the diet because of malabsorption and hyperglycemia resulting from the surgery.
- Teach about the continuing need for pancreatic enzyme replacement, a low-fat diet, and vitamin supplementation.
- Discuss strategies to relieve pain and discomfort, along with strategies to manage drains, if present, and to care for the

surgical incision, wound care, skin care, and management of drainage.

- Describe, verbally and in writing, the signs and symptoms of complications, and teach the patient and family about indicators of complications that should be reported promptly.
- Discharge of the patient to a long-term care or rehabilitation facility may be warranted after the extensive surgery, particularly if the patient's preoperative status was not optimal.
- If the patient elects to receive chemotherapy, the nurse focuses teaching on prevention of side effects and complications of the agents used.
- A referral for home care may be indicated to assess physical status, fluid and nutritional status, skin integrity, and the adequacy of pain management.
- Teach the patient and family strategies to prevent skin breakdown and relieve pain, pruritus, and anorexia.
- Discuss hospice services with the patient and family, and make a referral if indicated.

For more information, see Chapter 25 in Pellico, L.H. (2013). *Focus on adult health. Medical-surgical nursing.* Philadelphia: Wolters Kluwer Health | Lippincott Williams & Wilkins.

Cancer of the Prostate and Prostatectomy

Cancer of the prostate is the most common cancer in men (other than nonmelanoma skin cancer) and is the second most common cause of cancer deaths in American men.

PATHOPHYSIOLOGY

Among men diagnosed with prostate cancer, 5-year survival is nearly 100%, 93% survive at least 10 years, and 79% survive 15 years.

RISK FACTORS

- Common in the United States and northwestern Europe but rare in Asia, Africa, Central America, and South America.
- Highest in African American men worldwide
- Increasing age
- Familial
- Diet high in red meat or high fat dairy products

CLINICAL MANIFESTATIONS AND ASSESSMENT

- Usually asymptomatic in early stage
- Difficulty with urination, urinary retention, decreased size and force of urinary stream
- Hematuria may result if the cancer invades the urethra or bladder, or both.
- Symptoms of metastases include backache, hip pain, perineal and rectal discomfort, anemia, weight loss, weakness, nausea, and oliguria (<400 mL/day). These symptoms may be the first indications of prostate cancer.
- The American Urological Association (AUA) recommends that men who elect screening should have both a prostate-specific antigen (PSA) test, digital rectal exam (DRE), and counseling. The American Cancer Society does not support routine PSA screening, but recommends that providers offer PSA testing and DRE yearly, beginning at age 50, to men who are at average risk of prostate cancer and have at least a 10-year life expectancy.

DIAGNOSTIC METHODS

- PSA level in the blood is proportional to the total prostatic mass and does not necessarily indicate malignancy.
- Digital rectal examination (preferably by the same examiner) reveals nodule within the substance of the gland or extensive hardening in the posterior lobe; later lesion is stony hard and fixed.

- Gleason score is the system used most often to grade prostate cancer and to guide the physician in determining the most appropriate treatment.
- Diagnosis of prostate cancer is confirmed by a histologic examination of tissue.
- Cancer detected when transurethral resection of the prostate (TURP) is performed for benign prostatic enlargement and lower urinary tract symptoms occurs in about 1 out of 10 cases.
- Needle biopsies of the prostate are guided by transrectal ultrasound (TRUS) and may be indicated for men who have elevated PSA levels and abnormal DRE findings.
- Other tests that may be used to establish the extent of disease include bone scans to detect metastasis to the bones and CT scan to identify metastases in the pelvic lymph nodes.
- Symptoms of metastases include backache, hip pain, perineal and rectal discomfort, anemia, weight loss, weakness, nausea, oliguria, and spontaneous pathologic fractures; hematuria may result from urethral or bladder invasion.

MEDICAL AND NURSING MANAGEMENT

Treatment is based on the stage of the disease and the patient's age and symptoms. Review of data from clinical assessment, laboratory and radiology tests, transrectal ultrasound (TRUS), and/or biopsy results assists in the treatment decision process.

Surgical Management

Radical prostatectomy is the complete surgical removal of the prostate, seminal vesicles, and often the surrounding fat, nerves, lymph nodes and blood vessels; erectile dysfunction (ED) typically results.

Radiation Therapy

- Teletherapy (external) or brachytherapy (internal) may be employed:
- Teletherapy (external-beam radiation therapy) for 6 to 7 weeks.

- Brachytherapy involves the implantation of interstitial radioactive seeds under anesthesia, via the perineum, into the prostate. Patient should avoid close contact with pregnant women and infants for up to 2 months.
- Side effects of teletherapy and brachytherapy include inflammation of the rectum, bowel, and bladder due to their proximity to the prostate.
- Combination therapy (radiation therapy followed by hormonal therapy) may improve overall survival.

Hormonal Therapy

- Hormonal therapy includes surgical castration (orchiectomy), medications to reduce androgens. Orchiectomy is associated with considerable emotional impact.
- Effective hormonal alternatives to orchiectomy include the nonsteroidal antiandrogen bicalutamide, luteinizing hormone-releasing hormone (LHRH) agonists (leuprolide and goserelin), and antiandrogen agents, such as flutamide. Hot flashes can occur with orchiectomy or LHRH agonist therapy.

Second-Line Medical Treatment

- Ketoconazole lowers testosterone by decreasing both testicular and endocrine production of androgens.
- Survival may be increased with chemotherapy (paclitaxel and docetaxel) for non–androgen-dependent prostate cancer.

Other Therapies

- Ablation with cryosurgery may be used in patients who cannot tolerate surgery or those with recurrent prostate cancer; a transperineal probe freezes the tissue.
- Repeated TURs may be required to keep ureteral passage open. Alternatives include suprapubic catheter drainage or transurethral catheters.
- For advanced prostate cancer, palliative measures such as pain management, complementary and alternative medicine (CAM), and androgen deprivation can be options. Many men survive for a long period, apparently free of metastatic disease.

- Pain management using opioid and nonopioid medications, external-beam radiation therapy, and radiopharmaceuticals may be used; metastatic lesions may be very painful.
- More than one-third of men with a diagnosis of prostate cancer elect to use some form of CAM.

Complications Associated With Therapies

- Each treatment for prostate cancer has some incidence of sexual dysfunction. With nerve-sparing radical prostatectomy, ability to have erections is better for men who are younger and in whom both neurovascular bundles are spared.
- Hormonal therapy also affects sexual desire and arousability. PDE-5 inhibitors may improve erectile function in men with partial or moderate ED after radiation therapy for localized prostate cancer.

Prostate Surgery

Prostate surgery may be indicated for the patient with benign prostatic hyperplasia (BPH) or prostate cancer. Surgery should be performed before acute urinary retention and damage to the upper urinary tract and collecting system occurs, or before cancer progresses.

Procedures

Transurethral Resection of the Prostate

TURP is carried out through the urethra to the prostate, which is removed in small chips with an electrical cutting loop.

- Urethral strictures occur more frequently than with non-transurethral procedures.
- Retrograde ejaculation may occur due to removal of prostatic tissue at the bladder neck, which causes the seminal fluid to flow backward into the bladder.

Suprapubic Prostatectomy

Suprapubic prostatectomy removes the gland through an abdominal incision and bladder; the prostate gland is removed from above.

Perineal Prostatectomy

Perineal prostatectomy involves removal of the gland through an incision in the perineum.

- Postoperatively, the wound may easily become contaminated because the incision is near the rectum, and incontinence is common.
- Erectile dysfunction and rectal injury are more likely.

Retropubic Prostatectomy

A low abdominal incision is made, and the prostate gland can be reached between the pubic arch and the bladder without entering the bladder; allows better control of blood loss and better visualization of the surgical site.

Transurethral Incision of the Prostate

TUIP is indicated when the prostate gland is small (≤30 g). An instrument is passed through the urethra, incisions are made in the prostate and prostate capsule to reduce the prostate's pressure on the urethra and to reduce urethral constriction. It is performed on an outpatient basis and has a low complication rate.

Robotic or Laparoscopic Prostatectomy

Laparoscopic prostatectomy provides better visualization of the surgical site and surrounding areas. Less bleeding, shorter hospital stays, less postoperative pain, and more rapid return to normal activity typically result.

Complications

Postoperative complications depend on the type of prostatectomy performed:

- Hemorrhage
- Clot formation
- Catheter obstruction
- Sexual dysfunction; options to produce erections sufficient for sexual intercourse include prosthetic penile implants, vacuum devices, and pharmacologic interventions.

C

NURSING PROCESS

Patient Undergoing Prostatectomy

Assessment

- Assess impact of underlying disorder on patient's lifestyle.
- Question patient about family history of cancer and heart or kidney disease, including hypertension.
- Observe for weight loss, pallor, ability to get in and out of bed without assistance, and ability to perform activities of daily living (ADL) to help plan resumption of postoperative activity.

Diagnosis

Preoperative Nursing Diagnoses

- Anxiety related to surgery and its outcome
- Acute pain related to bladder distention
- Deficient knowledge about factors related to the disorder and the treatment protocol

Postoperative Nursing Diagnoses

- Acute pain related to the surgical incision, catheter placement, and bladder spasms
- Deficient knowledge about postoperative care and management

Planning

The major preoperative goals for the patient may include reduced anxiety and learning about the prostate disorder and the perioperative experience. The major postoperative goals may include maintenance of fluid volume balance, relief of pain and discomfort, ability to perform self-care activities, and absence of complications.

Preoperative Nursing Interventions

Reducing Anxiety

- Assess patient's understanding of the diagnosis and of the planned surgical procedure.

- Clarify the nature of the surgery and expected postoperative outcomes; familiarize the patient with the pre- and postoperative routines.
- Provide privacy and establish a trusting and professional relationship. Encourage patient to verbalize his feelings and concerns.

Relieving Discomfort

- If the patient experiences discomfort before surgery, provide analgesics and bed rest.
- Monitor voiding patterns for bladder distention, and assist with catheterization if indicated.

Providing Instruction

- Preoperatively, review the anatomy of the affected structures and their function in relation to the urinary and reproductive systems, using diagrams and other teaching aids if indicated.
- Describe the type of incision, which varies with the surgery, and inform the patient about the likely type of urinary drainage system and the recovery room procedure.
- Base the amount of information given on the patient's needs and questions.

Postoperative Nursing Interventions

Maintaining Fluid Balance

- Postoperatively, the patient is at risk for fluid imbalance due to irrigation of the surgical site during and after surgery.
- Observe for signs of fluid volume excess such as jugular vein distention (JVD), the development of an S_3 gallop, and pulmonary crackles.
- Monitor inputs and outputs (I & O), the amount of irrigating fluid used, and for adequate urine output.
- Monitor for hyponatremia, increasing blood pressure, confusion, and respiratory distress.
- Observe for signs and symptoms of hemorrhage, including hypotension, tachycardia, tachypnea, gross hematuria, restlessness, pallor, and decreasing hemoglobin and hematocrit. Notify the surgeon immediately and plan for fluid resuscitation with IV fluids and blood products.

(continues on page 182)

⚡*N u r s i n g   A l e r t*

In assessing urinary output, the nurse anticipates a minimum of 0.5 mL/kg/hr; thus, if the patient weighs 70 kg, 35 mL of urine is expected hourly. To calculate the actual urine output, the nurse must consider all irrigating fluids instilled against total urine collection bag drainage. If large amounts of irrigating solutions are required postoperatively, the nurse empties the collection bag frequently to prevent overfilling of collection bag and creating back pressure within the bladder. Meticulous I & O is required.

Relieving Pain

- Assess for pain, which may be incisional, referred to the flank area, or caused by bladder spasms. If present, determine cause, location, and severity using a pain scale.
- Bladder spasms are typically described as severe, cramping, spasmodic, and located in the suprapubic region.

⚡*N u r s i n g   A l e r t*

Bladder spasms are associated with irritation to the detrusor muscle causing spasm of the muscle. If spasms are present, ensure the urinary drainage system is patent; obstruction is associated with spasms. Administers antispasmodic medication as ordered.

- If clots impede urinary drainage, irrigate with 50 to 60 mL of irrigating fluid at a time; ensure that the same amount is recovered after irrigation.
- Secure the catheter drainage tubing to the leg or the lower abdomen to decrease tension on the catheter and prevent bladder irritation.
- After the patient is ambulatory, he is encouraged to walk; sitting for prolonged periods is avoided, as this increases intra-abdominal pressure, discomfort, and bleeding.

Monitoring and Managing Potential Complications

Hemorrhage
- Monitor for bleeding and hemorrhagic shock. The drainage normally begins as reddish-pink and then clears to a light pink within 24 hours after surgery.

- Bright red bleeding with increased viscosity and numerous clots usually indicates arterial bleeding and requires surgical intervention. Venous bleeding, which is dark red in color, may be controlled by the provider via "over-inflating" the catheter balloon and applying traction so that the balloon applies pressure to the prostatic fossa.
- Surgical exploration may be considered if bleeding is not controlled.

Infection
- After perineal prostatectomy, the surgeon usually changes the dressing on the first postoperative day with careful aseptic technique.
- Avoid rectal thermometers, rectal tubes, and enemas due to risk of injury and bleeding in the prostatic fossa.
- Sitz baths are used to promote healing.
- Urinary tract infections may occur; the patient and family are instructed to monitor for signs and symptoms of infection (fever, chills, sweating, myalgia, dysuria, urinary frequency, and urgency).

Deep Vein Thrombosis
- Administer prophylactic, low dose heparin, to prevent DVT and PE; patients undergoing prostatectomy have a high incidence of these complications.
- Assess for manifestations of DVT; apply elastic compression stockings.

Obstructed Catheter
- Maintain free flow through catheter; obstruction produces distention of the prostatic capsule and may cause hemorrhage.
- Administer diuretic as prescribed to promote urination and initiate postoperative diuresis, which helps keep the catheter patent.
- Observe the lower abdomen for increasing distention or dullness to percussion to ensure that the catheter has not become blocked.
- A three-way drainage system with continuous bladder irrigation (CBI) is used after a TURP to maintain the drainage of the

(continues on page 184)

urinary catheter, remove blood clots from the bladder that are the result of the procedure, and cleanse the surgical area to promote healing, as well as to prevent potentially obstruction clots.

Sexual Dysfunction
The patient may experience sexual dysfunction related to ED, decreased libido, and fatigue.

- Discuss options to restore erectile function including medications, surgically placed implants, or vacuum devices.
- Explain that the patient may experience fatigue during rehabilitation postoperatively, which may decrease libido and alter enjoyment of usual activities.
- Explore the emotional challenges of prostate surgery and its implications with the patient and his partner.

Teaching Patients Self-Care

- Instruct the patient and family how to manage the urinary drainage system, how to assess for complications, and how to promote recovery.
- Give verbal and written instructions, including signs and symptoms that should be reported to the physician; these include blood in urine, decreased urine output, fever, change in wound drainage, calf tenderness.
- Tell the patient some urinary incontinence may occur after catheter removal, and that this is likely to subside over time.

Continuing Care

- Referral for home care may be indicated if the patient is elderly or has other health problems, if the patient and family cannot provide care in the home, or if the patient lives alone without available supports.
- The home care nurse assesses the patient's physical status, provides catheter and wound care, and encourages the patient to ambulate and to carry out perineal exercises as prescribed.
- If the prostatectomy was performed to treat prostate cancer, the patient and family are also instructed about the importance of follow-up and monitoring with the urologist.

Evaluation

Expected postoperative patient outcomes may include the following:

- Reports relief of discomfort
- Exhibits fluid and electrolyte balance
- Participates in self-care measures
- Performs perineal exercises and interrupts urinary stream to promote bladder control
- Avoids straining and lifting heavy objects
- Is free of complications

For more information, see Chapter 34 in Pellico, L.H. (2013). *Focus on adult health. Medical-surgical nursing.* Philadelphia: Wolters Kluwer Health | Lippincott Williams & Wilkins.

Cancer of the Skin (Malignant Melanoma)

Malignant melanoma is a cancerous neoplasm in which atypical melanocytes are present in both the epidermis and the dermis (at times in subcutaneous cells).

PATHOPHYSIOLOGY

The most lethal of all skin cancers, malignant melanoma is responsible for about 3% of all cancer deaths. It can occur in one of several forms: Superficial spreading melanoma, lentigo-maligna melanoma, nodular melanoma, and acral-lentiginous melanoma.

Most melanomas arise from cutaneous epidermal melanocytes, but some appear in preexisting nevi (ie, moles) in the skin or develop in the uveal tract of the eye. Melanomas occasionally appear simultaneously with cancer of other organs.

The worldwide incidence of melanoma doubles every 10 years, an increase probably related to increased recreational sun exposure, changes in the ozone layer, and improved methods of early detection.

RISK FACTORS

The cause of malignant melanoma is unknown, but ultraviolet rays are strongly suspected.

- Peak incidence 20 to 45 years
- Living near equator or using tanning bed more than 10 times a year
- Caucasian
- Melanoma-prone families with dysplastic nevi

CLINICAL MANIFESTATIONS AND ASSESSMENT

Superficial Spreading Melanoma

- Most common form; usually affects middle-aged people, occurs most frequently on trunk and lower extremities
- Circular lesions with irregular outer portions
- Margins of lesion flat or elevated and palpable
- May appear in combination of colors, with hues of tan, brown, and black mixed with gray, bluish black, or white; sometimes a dull, pink-rose color is noted in a small area within the lesion

Lentigo-Maligna Melanoma

- Slowly evolving pigmented lesion
- Occurs on exposed skin areas; hand, head, and neck in elderly people
- First appears as tan, flat lesion, which in time undergoes changes in size and color

Nodular Melanoma

- Spherical, blueberry-like nodule with relatively smooth surface and uniform blue-black color
- May be dome-shaped with a smooth surface or have other shadings of red, gray, or purple
- May appear as irregularly shaped plaques, described as a blood blister that fails to resolve
- Invades directly into adjacent dermis (vertical growth); poor prognosis

Acral-Lentiginous Melanoma

- Occurs in areas not excessively exposed to sunlight and where hair follicles are absent
- Found on the palms of the hands, soles, in nail beds, and mucous membranes in dark-skinned people
- Appears as an irregular pigmented macule that develops nodules
- Becomes invasive early

DIAGNOSTIC METHODS

Biopsy confirms the diagnosis of melanoma:

- Excisional biopsy specimen including a 1 cm margin of normal tissue and a portion of underlying subcutaneous fatty tissue is sufficient for staging a melanoma in situ or an early, noninvasive melanoma.
- Incisional biopsy is performed when the suspicious lesion is too large to be removed safely without extensive scarring.
- Meticulous skin examination and palpation of regional lymph nodes that drain the lesional area is essential.
- Investigate for positive family history of melanoma; arrange for first-degree relatives, who may be at high risk, to be evaluated for atypical lesions.
- After diagnosis confirmed, chest X-ray, complete blood cell count, liver function tests, and radionuclide or CT scans are performed to stage extent of disease.

MEDICAL AND NURSING MANAGEMENT

Treatment depends on the level of invasion and the depth of the lesion.

Surgical Management

- Surgical excision is the treatment of choice for small superficial lesions.
- Deeper lesions require wide local excision and possible skin grafting.
- Regional lymph node dissection may be performed to rule out metastasis, although newer approaches call for sentinel node biopsy to avoid problems from extensive lymph node removal.
- Surgical debulking is undertaken to remove the tumor or to remove part of the organ involved (eg, lung, liver, or colon). However, the rationale for more extensive surgery is for relief of symptoms, not for cure.

Pharmacologic Management

- Immunotherapy to modify immune function and other biologic responses to cancer:
  - Bacillus Calmette-Guérin vaccine, *Corynebacterium parvum,* levamisole offer encouraging results.
  - Investigational therapies include biologic response modifiers (eg, interferon-alpha, interleukin-2), adaptive immunotherapy (ie, lymphokine-activated killer cells), and aldesleukin (Proleukin), a monoclonal antibody that may prevent recurrence of melanoma.
- Autologous immunization against tumor cells in the form of a vaccine is in the experimental stage.
- Chemotherapy for metastatic melanoma may be used; however, only a few agents (eg, dacarbazine, nitrosoureas, cisplatin) have been effective in controlling the disease.
- For melanoma in an extremity, inducing hyperthermia to enhance the effects of chemotherapy is performed to control metastasis, along with surgical excision of the primary lesion.

Nursing Management

See "Cancer" overview on pages 113–123 for nursing care measures

For more information see Chapter 52 in Pellico, L.H. (2013). *Focus on adult health. Medical-surgical nursing.* Philadelphia: Wolters Kluwer Health | Lippincott Williams & Wilkins.

Cancer of the Stomach (Gastric Cancer)

The incidence of gastric or stomach cancer continues to decrease in the United States; however, it still accounts for almost 11,000 deaths annually.

PATHOPHYSIOLOGY

Most gastric cancers are adenocarcinomas and occur anywhere in the stomach. The tumor infiltrates the surrounding mucosa, penetrating the wall of the stomach and adjacent organs and structures. The liver, pancreas, esophagus, and duodenum are often affected at the time of diagnosis. Metastasis through lymph to the peritoneal cavity occurs later in the disease. Prognosis is generally poor. The diagnosis is usually made late because most patients are asymptomatic during the early stages of the disease. Most cases of gastric cancer are discovered only after local invasion has advanced or metastases are present.

RISK FACTORS

- 40 to 70 years
- Men more so than women
- Native Americans, Hispanic Americans, and African Americans twice as likely as Caucasian

- High incidence in Japan
- Diets high in smoked, salted, or pickled foods
- Diets low in fruits and vegetables
- Chronic inflammation of the stomach
- *Helicobacter pylori* infection
- Pernicious anemia
- Smoking
- Achlorhydria
- Gastric ulcers
- Previous subtotal gastrectomy (>20 years ago)
- Genetics

CLINICAL MANIFESTATIONS AND ASSESSMENT

- Early stages: Symptoms may resemble those of patients with benign ulcers (eg, pain relieved with antacids).
- Progressive disease: Symptoms include dyspepsia (indigestion), early satiety, weight loss, abdominal pain just above the umbilicus, loss or decrease in appetite, bloating after meals, nausea and vomiting, and symptoms similar to those of peptic ulcer disease.
- Advanced gastric cancer may be palpable as a mass.
- Ascites and hepatomegaly (enlarged liver) are present with liver metastasis.
- Palpable nodules around the umbilicus, Sister Mary Joseph's nodules, are a sign of a GI malignancy, usually a gastric cancer.

DIAGNOSTIC METHODS

- EGD for biopsy and cytologic washings is the diagnostic study of choice.
- Barium X-ray examination of the upper GI tract
- Endoscopic ultrasound for tumor depth and lymph node involvement
- CT to assess for surgical resectability and to assess chest, abdomen, and pelvis in staging

MEDICAL AND NURSING MANAGEMENT

- Removal of gastric carcinoma; if tumor can be removed while still localized to the stomach, cure may be possible.
- Palliation to prevent obstruction or dysphagia may be accomplished by resection of the tumor.
- Diagnostic laparoscopy may be the initial surgical approach to evaluate the tumor, obtain tissue for pathologic diagnosis, and detect metastasis.
- Total gastrectomy, radical subtotal gastrectomy, proximal subtotal gastrectomy, or esophagogastrectomy may be performed.
- Palliative procedures such as gastric or esophageal bypass, gastrostomy, or jejunostomy may temporarily alleviate nausea and vomiting.
- Chemotherapy may be used for further disease control or for palliation (5-fluorouracil, cisplatin, doxorubicin, etoposide, and mitomycin-C).
- Radiation may be used for palliation in patients with obstruction.
- Tumor marker evaluation, including carcinoembryonic antigen (CEA), carbohydrate antigen (CA 19-9), and CA 50, may help determine the effectiveness of treatment.

COMPLICATIONS

- Pyloric obstruction
- Bleeding
- Severe pain
- Gastric perforation

For more information, see Chapter 23 in Pellico, L.H. (2013). *Focus on adult health. Medical-surgical nursing.* Philadelphia: Wolters Kluwer Health | Lippincott Williams & Wilkins.

Cancer of the Testis

Testicular cancer is the most common cancer in men aged 15 to 40 years, although it can occur in males of any age. It is a highly treatable and usually curable form of cancer, with a cure rate of greater than 90% for all stages of the disease.

PATHOPHYSIOLOGY

Classification of Testicular Tumors

Germinal Tumors

- More than 90% of all cancers of the testicle are germinal and may be further classified as seminomas or nonseminomas.
- Seminomas develop from the sperm-producing cells of the testes and account for 50% of tumors; they tend to remain localized, whereas nonseminomatous tumors grow quickly.
- Nonseminomas tend to develop earlier in life than seminomas, usually occurring in men in their 20s.
- Many tumors are mixtures of at least two different tumor types.

Nongerminal Tumors

- These develop in the supportive and hormone-producing tissues, or stroma, of the testicles.
- Two main types of stromal tumors are Leydig cell tumors and Sertoli cell tumors, which infrequently spread beyond the testicle.

RISK FACTORS

- Undescended testicles (cryptorchidism)
- Family history of testicular cancer
- Personal history of testicular cancer
- Caucasian Americans have a fivefold greater risk than do African Americans and double the risk of Asian American men.

CLINICAL MANIFESTATIONS AND ASSESSMENT

- Symptoms appear gradually, with a mass or lump on the testicle.
- Painless enlargement of the testis occurs; patient may complain of heaviness in the scrotum, inguinal area, or lower abdomen.
- Backache, pain in the abdomen, weight loss, and general weakness may result from metastasis.
- Testicular tumors tend to metastasize early, spreading from the testis to the lymph nodes in the retroperitoneum and to the lungs.

DIAGNOSTIC METHODS

- Testicular self-examination (TSE) can detect cancer; recent recommendations argue against this practice due to low incidence of discovering cancer and high anxiety associated with self-examination.
- Levels of human chorionic gonadotropin (HCG) and alpha fetoprotein (AFP) may be elevated.
- Levels of lactate dehydrogenase (LDH) may be elevated
- Chest X-ray is used to assess for metastasis in the lungs.
- Transscrotal testicular ultrasound may be used.
- CT of abdomen and pelvis determines extent of disease.
- Tissue biopsy is performed at time of surgery.

MEDICAL AND NURSING MANAGEMENT

The goals of management are to eradicate the disease and achieve a cure. Therapy is based on the cell type, the stage of the disease, and risk classification tables (determined as good, intermediate, and poor risks).

- Orchiectomy and retroperitoneal lymph node dissection (RPLND) if evidence of lymph node metastasis; libido and

climax are usually unimpaired after RPLND, but the patient may develop ejaculatory dysfunction.
- Sperm banking is offered before surgery.
- In radiation therapy for seminomatous tumors, the other testis is shielded from radiation to preserve fertility.
- Chemotherapy is reserved for the treatment of stage IIC testicular cancer, as well as for more advanced stages, using a cisplatin-based regimen.
- Follow-up studies may include chest X-rays; HCG, AFP, and LDH level testing, and serial CT scans to detect recurrent malignancy.

Nursing Management

See also "Nursing Management" under "Cancer" on pages 120–123 for additional information.

- Assess the patient's physical and psychological status, and monitor for response to and possible effects of surgery, chemotherapy, and radiation therapy.
- Address issues related to body image and sexuality. Inform the patient that radiation therapy will not necessarily prevent him from fathering children, and unilateral excision of a testis will not necessarily decrease virility.

Banking Sperm

- Cryopreserving semen in a sperm bank is an option for men who are about to undergo a procedure or treatment (eg, radiation therapy to the pelvis, chemotherapy, RPLND) that may affect their fertility.
- This requires visits to the facility where the sperm is obtained by masturbation and collected in a sterile container for storage.

For more information, see Chapter 34 in Pellico, L.H. (2013). *Focus on adult health. Medical-surgical nursing.* Philadelphia: Wolters Kluwer Health | Lippincott Williams & Wilkins.

Cancer of the Thyroid and Thyroid Tumor

Classification of thyroid gland tumors include benign or malignant, presence or absence of associated thyrotoxicosis, and diffuse or irregular quality of the glandular enlargement.

C

PATHOPHYSIOLOGY

A goiter is present if thyroid enlargement is sufficient to cause visible swelling in the neck. Toxic goiters are often accompanied by hyperthyroidism. Nontoxic goiters are associated with a euthyroid (normal) state and do not result from inflammatory or neoplastic causes. Simple or colloid goiter, the most common type, is often encountered in geographic regions where there is lack of iodine (eg, the great lakes areas of the United States). Insufficient iodine decreases the level of thyroxine (T_4), encouraging the production of thyroid-stimulating hormone (TSH) from the anterior pituitary; thyroid enlargement results. Simple goiter may also be caused by intake of large quantities of goitrogenic substances such as excess iodine or lithium in susceptible patients. Thyroid cancer is less prevalent than other forms of cancer; only about 1 in 20 thyroid nodules is cancerous. External radiation of the head, neck, or chest in infancy and childhood increases the risk for thyroid carcinoma.

Some thyroid glands are nodular due to hyperplasia (overgrowth). No symptoms may arise, unless these nodules increase in size and descend into the thorax, where local pressure symptoms may manifest. Some nodules become malignant, and some are associated with a hyperthyroid state. The patient with many thyroid nodules may eventually require surgery

RISK FACTORS

- Female
- As above

CLINICAL MANIFESTATIONS AND ASSESSMENT

- Simple goiters are asymptomatic, or the patient may complain of pressure in the neck.
- Patient may present with a soft, diffusely enlarged nodule over the neck.
- As the goiter progresses, the patient may experience symptoms such as difficulty breathing and swallowing.
- Lesions that are single, hard, and fixed on palpation or associated with cervical lymphadenopathy suggest malignancy.
- Thyroid function tests are rarely conclusive.

DIAGNOSTIC METHODS

- Needle biopsy or aspiration biopsy of thyroid with local anesthetic
- Thyroid function tests
- Ultrasound, MRI, CT scan, thyroid scans, radioactive iodine uptake studies, and thyroid suppression tests

MEDICAL AND NURSING MANAGEMENT

Goiter

- Most patients with small simple goiters and euthyroid states do not require treatment.
- Patients with large goiters generally receive exogenous thyroid hormones and iodine to reduce thyroid growth.
- Surgery is not required unless the goiter continues to grow despite pharmacological treatment, airway difficulties arise, or malignancy is suspected.

Thyroid Cancer

- Surgery is treatment of choice for thyroid cancer (total or near-total thyroidectomy).

- Modified or extensive radical neck dissection is done for lymph node involvement; efforts are made to spare parathyroid tissue, thus reducing risk for postoperative hypocalcemia.
- Oral radioactive iodine is used for radiosensitive tumors to eradicate residual thyroid tissue.
- Exogenous thyroid hormone is prescribed to prevent hypothyroidism.
- Life-long thyroxine is required if remaining thyroid tissue is inadequate to produce sufficient hormone.
- Post-hospitalization follow-up includes clinical assessment for recurrence of nodules or masses in the neck and signs of hoarseness, dysphagia, or dyspnea.
- Total body scans are performed 2 to 4 months after surgery to detect residual thyroid tissue or metastatic disease, with repeat scans at 1 year; if stable, a final scan is obtained in 3 to 5 years.

Nursing Management

See also "Nursing Management" under "Cancer" on pages 120–123 for additional information.

Providing Preoperative Teaching

- Provide preoperative teaching to reduce anxiety.
- When increased metabolic activity is present, instruct the patient about to eat a diet high in carbohydrates and proteins due to rapid depletion of glycogen reserves. Supplemental vitamins, particularly thiamine and ascorbic acid, may be prescribed. Advise the patient to avoid tea, coffee, cola, and other stimulants.
- Preoperatively, teach the patient how to support the neck after surgery; the patient should raise the elbows placing the hands behind the neck to provide support and reduce strain and tension on neck muscles and surgical incision.

Assessing the Postoperative Patient

- Postoperatively, assess surgical dressings and reinforce as necessary.

- Observe sides and back of the neck and the anterior dressing for bleeding. Observe for a sensation of pressure or fullness at incision site, and for frequent swallowing or choking, which may indicate subcutaneous hemorrhage and hematoma formation.
- Monitor the pulse and blood pressure for any indication of internal bleeding.
- Note vocal changes or hoarseness, as this may indicate injury to the laryngeal nerve or laryngeal edema, which may develop postoperatively.
- Record color, amount, and consistency of the drainage and maintain function of the device.

Maintaining the Airway

- Monitor for respiratory difficulties secondary to edema of the glottis, hematoma formation, or injury to the recurrent laryngeal nerve.
- Keep a tracheostomy set by the bedside; in the event of significant edema, endotracheal intubation may be unsuccessful due to narrowed airway.
- Plan for surgical evacuation if respiratory distress is caused by hematoma.

Managing Pain

- Assess intensity of pain and administer analgesics as prescribed.
- Anticipate apprehension and inform the patient that oxygen will assist breathing.
- Carefully support the patient's head and avoid tension on the sutures when moving and turning.
- Place patient in semi-Fowler's position, which is most comfortable, with the head elevated and supported by pillows.

Administering Hydration Therapy

- Administer IV fluids during the immediate postoperative period.
- When PO fluids are allowed, patients report little difficulty in swallowing. Serving cold fluids and ice is recommended.

Managing Safety

- Advise the patient to talk as little as possible to reduce edema to the vocal cords.
- Keep frequently needed items within easy reach, so the patient does not need to turn the head to reach for them.

Encouraging Nutrition and Physical Activity

- The patient is permitted to get out of bed as soon as possible, but must support his or her neck.
- Encourage soft foods. A well-balanced, high-calorie diet may be prescribed to promote weight gain if increased metabolism was present.

Providing Postoperative Patient Education

- Plan for discharge from the hospital on the day of surgery or soon afterward if the postoperative course is uncomplicated.
- Instruct patients undergoing radiation therapy how to assess and manage side effects of treatment.

Managing Post-Thyroidectomy Complications

- Hemorrhage, hematoma formation, edema of the glottis, and injury to the recurrent laryngeal nerve are complications discussed above.
- Observe for hypocalcemia secondary to inadvertent removal of the parathyroid glands, which causes hyperirritability of the nerves (spasms of the hands and feet and muscle twitching, called tetany). Plan to administer IV calcium gluconate and emergency airway management.
- Hypocalcemia is temporary after thyroidectomy unless all parathyroid tissue was removed.

For more information, see Chapter 31 in Pellico, L.H. (2013). *Focus on adult health. Medical-surgical nursing.* Philadelphia: Wolters Kluwer Health | Lippincott Williams & Wilkins.

Cancer of the Vulva

Vulvar cancer is a rare cancer occurring only 2.2 out of 100,000 cases annually; its incidence has been slowly increasing and is thought to be due to its link with HPV.

PATHOPHYSIOLOGY

There is increased evidence of young women with HPV being diagnosed with vulvar intraepithelial neoplasia but with a high cure rate after surgical resection and radiotherapy. Women with vulvar cancer are usually between the ages of 70 and 80, the majority (~80–90%) will be diagnosed in an early stage (I or II). The majority (90%) of vulvar cancer is squamous cell carcinoma (SCC), which can be superficial but invasive. Vulvar intraepithelial neoplasia (VIN) is more complex, deeply invasive, and is considered the precancerous condition of HPV types 16, 18, 31, and 33.

RISK FACTORS

- 70 to 80 years
- History of condyloma, HPV, abnormal cervical cytology
- Cigarette smoking
- Numerous sexual partners

CLINICAL MANIFESTATIONS AND ASSESSMENT

- External genitalia itching or burning are early signs, and are often self-treated by patients with over-the-counter (OTC) cortisone or anti-itch creams.
- Dyspareunia, vulvar edema, or pain is present in half of affected women.
- Later-stage manifestations include ulcerated lesions that are indicative of cancer; lesions may extend into the perianal and rectal areas and into non-hair-bearing areas.

DIAGNOSTIC METHODS

A Keyes punch biopsy or tissue biopsy is the gold standard for diagnosing vulvar cancer.

MEDICAL AND NURSING MANAGEMENT

- Vulvar colposcopy may be performed, but wide excision of the affected area or a vulvectomy (removal of the vulva) with lymph node sampling for clear margins is dependent upon the size, depth, and focality of lesions.
- Surgical alternative for early-stage lesions is imiquimod (Aldara), a topical immune-response modifier with antiviral and antitumor properties, typically used for external genital warts. Use for early vulvar cancer lesions is not FDA approved and is considered off label.
- Depending upon the extent of vulvectomy, chemotherapy and radiation treatments may also be indicated.
- There is a statistically significant correlation between extent of reconstructive surgery and disease outcomes; local reconstructive surgery demonstrates better prognosis with significant reduction in relapse rate.

Nursing Management

- Monitor patients postoperatively for wound infections, fever, discharge; avoid cross-contamination of body fluids (such as urine or feces) to reduce this occurrence.
- Foley care and assessment of skin is important to identify any potential site of entry for infection.
- Assess for DVT and PE due to prolonged bed rest postoperatively, required to avoid tension on the surgical site and promote healing.
- Encourage frequent position changes, use of compression stockings and intermittent pneumatic compression boots, and use of the incentive spirometry.
- Be sensitive to perceptions of distorted body image, decreased sensation affecting a woman's ability to enjoy sexual relations, and pelvic floor dysfunction, which occur when nerve supply in the vulvar area is disrupted.

- Involve the partner, social work, or mental health referral as needed to allow patients and their partners to understand what to expect after discharge from the hospital.

> For more information, see Chapter 33 in Pellico, L.H. (2013). *Focus on adult health. Medical-surgical nursing.* Philadelphia: Wolters Kluwer Health | Lippincott Williams & Wilkins.

Cardiomyopathies

Cardiomyopathy is a disorder of the myocardium (heart muscle) associated with mechanical and/or electrical dysfunction.

PATHOPHYSIOLOGY

All cardiomyopathies result in impaired cardiac output. Decreased stroke volume stimulates the sympathetic nervous system and the renin–angiotensin–aldosterone response, causing increased systemic vascular resistance, and sodium and fluid retention. This increases myocardial workload and leads to heart failure, myocardial destruction, and necrosis. The five most common cardiomyopathies are dilated cardiomyopathy (DCM), hypertrophic cardiomyopathy (HCM), restrictive cardiomyopathy, arrhythmogenic right ventricular cardiomyopathy (ARVC), and stress-induced cardiomyopathy.

RISK FACTORS

Genetic predisposition to cardiomyopathy is the greatest risk factor.

CLINICAL MANIFESTATIONS AND ASSESSMENT

Regardless of cause, cardiomyopathy can lead to severe heart failure, lethal arrhythmias, and death.

DIAGNOSTIC METHODS

- Echocardiogram
- Electrocardiogram (ECG)
- Myocardial biopsy

MEDICAL AND NURSING MANAGEMENT

Patients with cardiomyopathy may remain stable and asymptomatic for many years. As the disease progresses, so do symptoms. Treatment is specific to the type of cardiomyopathy, but often overlaps.

Pharmacologic Therapy

- Angiotensin-converting enzyme (ACE) inhibitors, aldosterone antagonists, and diuretics should be administered for all cardiomyopathies.
- Beta blockers are avoided in the early phases of decompensated heart failure but improve mortality benefit after the patient stabilizes. Beta blockers and calcium channel blockers are used to reduce catecholamine response to minimize the risk of left ventricular outflow tract obstruction in patients with HCM.
- Nitrates and dehydration should be avoided in HCM to maintain cardiac output.
- Antiarrhythmics are used to prevent and treat arrhythmias.
- Systemic anticoagulation is needed to prevent thromboembolic events.

Additional Interventions

- Monitor neurologic status as embolization can occur from mural thrombi (clot that is attached to the endocardium or wall of the blood vessel) and from venous thrombosis, especially in patients on bed rest.
- Screen all first-degree blood relatives using echocardiography and ECG (eg, parents, siblings, and children) for HCM, idiopathic DCM, and ARVC, as early diagnosis and treatment can prevent or delay significant symptoms and sudden cardiac death.

- Plan for pacemaker insertion if patient presents with heart block; atrial-ventricular and biventricular pacing have been used to improve symptoms of HCM and RCM. Implantable defibrillators are recommended for persistent cardiac dysfunction and/or ventricular arrhythmias, particularly with ARVC.
- Intra-aortic balloon pumps, left ventricular assist devices, and consideration of heart transplantation may be necessary in the most severe cases.
- For stress-induced cardiomyopathy, accurate diagnosis and differentiation from ST elevation myocardial infarction (STEMI) is critical to avoid unnecessary treatments, such as administration of fibrinolytics. Diuretics, ACE inhibitors, and beta blockers are frequently prescribed. Unstable patients may require positive inotropic medications, vasopressors, and intra-aortic balloon pumps. Overall prognosis is favorable. Recurrence can occur, although it is uncommon.

Nursing Management

- Perform careful cardiovascular assessment for signs of worsening heart failure; particularly dyspnea, congested lungs, peripheral edema, and the presence of abnormal heart sounds.
- Observe for arrhythmias, which occur frequently; continuous cardiac monitoring is recommended with personnel and equipment readily available to treat life-threatening arrhythmias.
- Maintain bed rest to decrease cardiac workload. Advise patient to increase physical activity slowly and to report symptoms that occur with increasing activity.
- Evaluate for anxiety, and guide patient in stress management practices for stress-induced cardiomyopathy.

Surgical Management

When medical treatment is no longer effective, the following surgical interventions are considered:

- Heart transplantation
- Mechanical circulatory assist devices
- Ventricular assist devices
- Total artificial hearts

For more information, see Chapter 16 in Pellico, L.H. (2013). *Focus on adult health. Medical-surgical nursing*. Philadelphia: Wolters Kluwer Health | Lippincott Williams & Wilkins.

Cataract

A cataract is a lens opacity or cloudiness.

PATHOPHYSIOLOGY

Cataracts can develop in either or both eyes at any age. By 80 years of age, over half of Americans have cataracts or have had cataract surgery. Visual impairment typically progresses at the same rate in both eyes. The extent of visual impairment depends on cataract size, density, and location in the lens. More than one type can be present in one eye.

Nuclear cataracts are caused by central opacity in the lens and are associated with myopia (nearsightedness), which worsens as the cataract progresses. Cortical cataracts involve the anterior, posterior, or equatorial cortex of the lens; equatorial or peripheral cataracts do not interfere with light passing through the center of the lens and have little effect on vision; however, vision is worse in very bright light.

Posterior subcapsular cataracts occur in front of the posterior capsule and typically develop in younger people. These may be associated with prolonged corticosteroid use, diabetes, or ocular trauma. Near vision is diminished, and increasing sensitivity to glare/bright lights occurs (sunlight, headlights).

RISK FACTORS

- Aging
- Myopia
- Retinal detachment and injury
- Infection

- Corticosteroids especially long term, high doses
- Cigarette smoking
- Sunlight and ionizing radiation
- Diabetes
- Obesity, poor nutrition
- Eye injuries

CLINICAL MANIFESTATIONS AND ASSESSMENT

- Painless, blurry vision
- Perception that surroundings are dimmer (as if glasses need cleaning)
- Light scattering; reduced contrast sensitivity, sensitivity to glare, and reduced visual acuity
- Other effects include myopic shift (return of ability to do close work [eg, reading fine print] without eyeglasses), astigmatism, monocular diplopia (double vision), color shift (the aging lens becomes progressively more absorbent at the blue end of the spectrum), brunescens (color values shift to yellow-brown), and reduced light transmission.
- Degree of lens opacity does not always correlate with the patient's functional status.

DIAGNOSTIC METHODS

- Snellen visual acuity test
- Ophthalmoscopy
- Slit-lamp biomicroscopic examination

MEDICAL AND NURSING MANAGEMENT

- Nonsurgical (medications, eyedrops, eyeglasses) treatment is not curative, nor does it prevent age-related cataract.
- In early stages of cataract development, glasses, contact lenses, strong bifocals, or magnifying lenses may improve vision.

Surgical Management

Surgical management of cataracts is considered when reduced vision interferes with normal activity. Surgery is performed on an outpatient basis and usually takes less than 1 hour.

- For bilateral cataracts, one eye is treated first, with several weeks to months separating the procedures; delay allows patient and surgeon to evaluate the results.
- Intracapsular cataract extraction: Entire lens (ie, nucleus, cortex, and capsule) is removed and fine sutures are used to close the incision. Performed infrequently, unless there is a need to remove entire lens, as in a dislocated lens.
- Extracapsular cataract extraction: Involves smaller incisional wounds (less trauma to the eye) and maintains the posterior capsule of the lens, reducing aphakic retinal detachment and cystoid macular edema. An intraocular lens (IOL) is implanted.
- Phacoemulsification: Ultrasonic device liquefies the nucleus and cortex, which are then suctioned out. The posterior capsule is left intact. Due to small incision, the wound heals rapidly; early stabilization of refractive error and less astigmatism occur.
- Aphakia (without a lens) develops after cataract surgery. Since the lens focuses light on the retina, it must be replaced for clear vision. Three lens replacement options exist: Aphakic eyeglasses, contact lenses, and intraocular lens (IOL) implants.
- Postoperatively, toxic anterior segment syndrome, characterized by corneal edema less than 24 hours after surgery and an accumulation of white cells in the anterior chamber of the eye, may occur. Symptoms include reduction in visual acuity and pain; if no microorganism growth exists, topical steroid treatment may be used.

Nursing Management

The patient with cataracts should receive the usual preoperative care for ambulatory surgical patients undergoing eye surgery.

Providing Preoperative Care

- Withhold anticoagulants and antiplatelets (eg, aspirin, warfarin [Coumadin]) to reduce the risk for retrobulbar hemorrhage for 5 to 7 days preoperatively.

- Administer dilating drops every 10 minutes for four doses at least 1 hour before surgery.
- Antibiotic, corticosteroid, and anti-inflammatory drops may be administered prophylactically to prevent postoperative infection and inflammation.

Providing Postoperative Care

- Provide verbal and written instructions about how to protect the eye, administer medications, recognize signs of complications, and obtain emergency care.
- Avoid lying on the side of the affected eye the night after surgery.
- Keep activity light (eg, walking, reading, watching television). Resume the following activities only as directed by the physician: Driving, sexual activity, unusually strenuous activity.
- Remember not to lift, push, or pull objects heavier than 15 lb.
- Avoid bending or stooping for an extended period.
- Explain that there should be minimal discomfort after surgery; instruct patient to take a mild analgesic agent, such as acetaminophen, as needed.
- Antibiotic, anti-inflammatory, and corticosteroid eye drops or ointments are prescribed postoperatively.

Teaching Patients Self-Care

- Teach patient to wear a protective eye patch to prevent accidental rubbing or poking of the eye for 24 hours after surgery, followed by eyeglasses worn during the day and a metal shield worn at night for 1 to 4 weeks.
- Sunglasses should be worn while outdoors during the day because the eye is sensitive to light.
- Explain that slight morning discharge, some redness, and a scratchy feeling may be expected for a few days. A clean, damp washcloth may be used to remove slight morning eye discharge.
- Ensure that the patient knows to notify the surgeon if new floaters (dots) in vision, flashing lights, decrease in vision, pain, or increase in redness occurs, due to risk for retinal detachment.

Continuing Care

- Eye patch is removed after the first follow-up appointment.
- Blurring of vision may be present for several days to weeks. Sutures, if used, are left in the eye but alter the curvature of the cornea, resulting in temporary blurring and some astigmatism.
- Vision gradually improves as the eye heals (typically within 6 to 12 weeks), when final corrective prescription is completed.
- Visual correction is needed for any remaining nearsightedness or farsightedness (even in patients with IOL implants).

For more information, see Chapter 49 in Pellico, L.H. (2013). *Focus on adult health. Medical-surgical nursing.* Philadelphia: Wolters Kluwer Health | Lippincott Williams & Wilkins.

Cerebral Vascular Accident (Stroke)

A cerebrovascular accident (CVA) results from the interruption of cerebral blood flow, leading to brain cell death and functional disability. Stroke is currently the fourth leading cause of death behind heart disease, cancer, and chronic respiratory diseases in the United States.

- Ongoing efforts aimed at reducing long-term complications of stroke are directed toward promoting secondary prevention through public education initiatives, researching innovative medical and surgical therapies in acute care, and implementing strategies for reducing modifiable risks in the primary care setting.
- Several studies have shown that a majority of people cannot name many of the typical stroke symptoms or do not consider calling 911 in the event they or a family member are experiencing stroke.
- Primary Stroke Centers, certified by the Joint Commission, provide care based on evidence-based clinical practice guidelines.
- Important support services included availability and interpretation of CT scans 24/7 and rapid laboratory testing.

PATHOPHYSIOLOGY

Ischemic Stroke

In an ischemic infarction, the disruption of the cerebral blood flow occurs due to obstruction of a blood vessel. As ischemia continues, neurons cannot maintain aerobic respiration. Anaerobic metabolism ensues, generating large amounts of lactic acid, and the neuron becomes incapable of producing sufficient adenosine triphosphate (ATP) to fuel the depolarization processes. Cellular death ensues.

- Ischemic strokes are subdivided into five subtypes, which direct therapeutic interventions and predict long-term prognosis.
- Large-artery thrombotic strokes (20%) are caused by atherosclerotic plaques in the large blood vessels of the brain.
- Small penetrating artery thrombotic strokes (25%) are most common and affect one or more vessels; typically caused by longstanding hypertension, hyperlipidemia, or diabetes. Small-artery thrombotic strokes are frequently referred to as *lacunar strokes* because of the small cavities that are created after the death of infarcted brain tissue.
- Cardiogenic embolic strokes (25%) are associated with cardiac arrhythmias, such as atrial fibrillation, valvular heart disease, or left ventricular thrombus. Emboli from the heart most commonly enter the left middle cerebral artery, causing ischemia and subsequent infarction.
- Cryptogenic strokes (30%) have no known cause, and include strokes from other causes, such as illicit drug use (cocaine), coagulopathies, migraine, and spontaneous dissection of the carotid or vertebral arteries (5%).

Transient Ischemic Attacks

A transient ischemic attack (TIA, "mini stroke," "warning" stroke) is currently defined as a brief episode of neurologic dysfunction caused by focal brain or retinal ischemia, with clinical symptoms typically lasting less than 1 hour and without evidence of acute infarction. For purposes of clarity in this handbook, ischemic stroke and TIA are considered one disease process due to the need in both instances to determine cause, plan care, and apply secondary stroke prevention measures.

Hemorrhagic Strokes

Hemorrhagic strokes include bleeding into the brain tissue (parenchyma), the ventricles, or the subarachnoid space. Blood outside the vasculature forms a mass that compresses brain tissue, causing increased intracranial pressure, secondary hemorrhage, ischemia, and possibly herniation. If blood extends into the ventricles, it can cause acute hydrocephalus. These events can impair level of consciousness and lead to coma and death.

Hemorrhagic stroke subtypes include intracerebral hemorrhage, subarachnoid hemorrhage, hemorrhage due to intracranial aneurysms, and hemorrhage due to arteriovenous malformations (AVMs). Uncontrolled hypertension, intracranial neoplasms, certain medications such as anticoagulants or amphetamines, and amyloid angiopathy are other causes of hemorrhagic stroke.

RISK FACTORS

The conditions or risk factors are diverse and often correlate to cardiac risk factors.

- Modifiable risk factors include hypertension, smoking and secondary exposure, diabetes, dyslipidemia, atrial fibrillation, diet (including excess sodium intake), obesity, sleep apnea, and sedentary lifestyle.
- Nonmodifiable risk factors include family history, older age and African American or Hispanic ethnicity.

CLINICAL MANIFESTATIONS AND ASSESSMENT

Stroke syndromes produce a wide variety of neurologic deficits, depending on the location of the lesion, which vessels are obstructed, the size and area of underperfused brain tissue, and the amount of collateral (secondary or accessory) blood flow to the affected area.

Common Symptoms

- Numbness or weakness of the face, arm, or leg, especially on one side of the body
- Confusion or change in mental status
- Trouble speaking or understanding speech
- Visual disturbances
- Difficulty walking, dizziness, or loss of balance or coordination
- Sudden, severe headache-most common
- Other symptoms that can be observed are vomiting, a slow or sudden change in level of consciousness, or focal seizures. When AVM ruptures, severe bleeding occurs; there can be extensive cerebral injury, coma, and death.

Motor Loss

- Hemiplegia, hemiparesis
- Because the upper motor neurons decussate (cross over), a disturbance of voluntary motor control on one side of the body may reflect damage to the upper motor neurons on the opposite side of the brain.

Communication Loss

- Dysarthria is difficulty speaking, caused by paralysis of the muscles responsible for producing speech (also referred to as *slurred speech*).
- Dysphasia (impaired speech) or aphasia (loss of speech) is partial or complete impairment of language resulting from brain injury; it affects spoken language, comprehension.
- Apraxia (inability to perform a previously learned action) is seen when a patient makes verbal substitutions for desired syllables or words.

Perceptual Disturbances

- Visual-perceptual dysfunctions include homonymous hemianopia (loss of half of the visual field).
- Disturbances in visual-spatial relations (perceiving the relation of two or more objects in spatial areas) are frequently seen in patients with right hemispheric damage.

Sensory Losses

- May present as slight impairment of touch or more severe with loss of proprioception; patient has difficulty in interrupting visual, tactile, and auditory stimuli.
- Agnosias are deficits in the ability to recognize previously familiar objects perceived by one or more of the senses.

Impaired Cognitive and Psychological Effects

- Frontal lobe damage: Learning capacity, memory, or other higher cortical intellectual functions may be impaired. Such dysfunction may be reflected in a limited attention span, difficulties in comprehension, forgetfulness, and lack of motivation.
- Emotional lability, hostility, frustration, resentment, lack of cooperation, and other psychological problems may occur at some point during the recovery period.

Acute Stroke Assessment

- The American Heart/Stroke Association's Stroke Chain of Survival is a rapid prehospital and acute care approach to the evaluation of patients with acute stroke symptoms. Also known as the "7 Ds," these components highlight key areas in the recognition and evaluation of a suspected stroke patient to reinforce an efficient method for a rapid approach to acute stroke care.
- The Emergency Nurses Association and the American College of Emergency Physicians recommend that stroke be labeled as level 2/5 meaning "needs immediate assessment," consistent with unstable trauma or critical-care cardiac patient.
- Acute stroke care can be divided into two phases: The hyperacute phase (the first 24 hours of care) and phase 2 (acute care during the hospitalization).
- Many of the same motor, sensory, cranial nerve, and cognitive functions are disrupted in both ischemic and hemorrhagic strokes; however, changes in level of consciousness, vomiting, sudden severe headache, and seizure are frequently associated with hemorrhagic strokes.

- During triage, elicit a detailed history and determine time of onset of symptoms. When the time of symptom onset is not definitive, the time the patient was last known to be at baseline becomes the default time of onset; drug treatment options and interventional procedures for ischemic stroke are time-dependent.
- Assess airway, breathing, and circulation (ABCs) with an initial set of vital signs.

DIAGNOSTIC METHODS

- CT scan to rule out hemorrhage
- MRI
- The National Institutes of Health Stroke Scale (NIHSS) has become an accepted assessment tool to quantify stroke severity and to assess patient outcome.

MEDICAL AND NURSING MANAGEMENT

- Thrombolysis is begun with recombinant tissue plasminogen activator (rtPA) for acute ischemic stroke within a 3-hour window of symptom onset, unless contraindicated; monitor for bleeding, angioedema (oral/lingual swelling), and anaphylaxis (allergic reaction).
- Hemorrhagic stroke treatment focuses on ABCs and level of consciousness. Immediate complications of a hemorrhage include extension of bleeding with increased intracranial pressure (ICP), acute hydrocephalus, potential for herniation, and secondary brain injury.
- Intubation is required for Glasgow Scores of 8 or lower. Maintain NPO until swallowing evaluation is completed, elevate head of bed, and maintain normothermia.
- Surgical evacuation of hematoma may be needed. Provide antihypertensive and anticonvulsants as indicated.

Nursing Management

- Perform neurological assessment and frequent vital signs
- Treat hyperthermia with acetaminophen as ordered.

- Notify provider for changes in vital signs, worsening of stroke symptoms, or other decline in neurological status.
- Administer O_2 by cannula at 2 to 3 L/min or maintain mechanical ventilation.
- Maintain continuous cardiac monitoring.
- Measure intake and output.
- Keep patient on bed rest.
- Administer IV fluids as ordered.
- Hemorrhagic stroke: Avoid heparin, warfarin, aspirin, clopidogrel, or aspirin/extended-release dipyridamole.

Prevention

- Help healthy individuals identify and address risk factors for stroke: Decrease the development of obesity, increase exercise, and provide a well-balanced diet.
- Encourage stroke patients and families to manage hypertension, dyslipidemia, stop smoking, decrease alcohol consumption, attain/maintain a healthy weight, manage obesity, and exercise.
- Teach patient about optimal pharmacologic management, including antiplatelet medications (such as aspirin, clopidogrel, or aspirin/extended-release dipyridamole), a statin (such as atorvastatin or simvastatin), and an antihypertensive (thiazide diuretic, ACE inhibitor, or beta blocker).
- Explain to patients with paroxysmal or permanent atrial fibrillation that anticoagulation (with warfarin or other anticoagulant) is recommended.
- For patients with hemorrhagic stroke, blood pressure control is critical. Inform patient about management of TIA or stroke caused by significant carotid artery stenosis; teach about carotid endarterectomy (CEA) when recommended.

NURSING PROCESS

The Patient With a Stroke

Assessment

- Maintain a nursing flow sheet documenting complete neurologic assessment, including mental status evaluation

(continues on page 216)

(orientation, affect, perception, memory, attention span, speech and language), motor control, swallowing ability, hydration status, fluid output, skin integrity, and activity level.
- Ongoing nursing assessment focuses on alterations in cognition and functional impairment and directs the appropriate nursing diagnoses.

Diagnosis

- Altered hemodynamics related to cardiac arrhythmias, hyper-/hypotension, fluid/electrolyte imbalances
- Impaired physical mobility related to hemiparesis, sensory loss, loss of balance or coordination, or visual field deficit
- Impaired verbal communication related to dysarthria, aphasia, altered cognition
- Impaired swallowing/risk for aspiration related to inability to protect airway or altered level of consciousness
- Risk for infection related to smoking history, invasive lines, Foley catheter, NG tube
- Risk for ineffective peripheral tissue perfusion related to risk for DVT/immobility
- High risk for injury related to visual field, motor, or perception deficits
- Knowledge deficit related to lack of awareness of stroke risk factors, secondary stroke prevention medications, potential lifestyle changes, physical and occupational therapies

Planning

Although rehabilitation begins on the day the patient has the stroke, the process is intensified during convalescence and requires a coordinated team effort.

- It is helpful for the team to know the patient's baseline function, past medical history, mental and emotional state, behavioral characteristics, and activities of daily living (ADLs).
- Consider predictors of stroke outcome (age, comorbidities such as diabetes, and presenting NIHSS score) in order to provide stroke survivors and their families with a realistic recovery trajectory. For example, a direct correlation exists between a NIHSS score of over 15 and poor 3-month outcomes.

Nursing Interventions

Nursing interventions include a comprehensive approach to physical care, preventing complications, and fostering recovery through listening to elicit the meaning of the stroke experience.

Improving Mobility and Preventing Joint Deformities

- Maintain correct positioning to prevent contractures; use measures to relieve pressure, assist in maintaining good body alignment, and prevent compressive neuropathies, especially of the ulnar and peroneal nerves.
- Apply a posterior splint at night to prevent flexion during sleep as flexor muscles are stronger than extensor muscles. Assess the skin for evidence of impaired circulation, sensation, and/or mobility, as well as for any evidence of altered skin integrity.

☼ NURSING ALERT

The supine position is used only for conscious patients because of the possibility of aspiration or occlusion of the airway with the tongue. Position the unconscious patient lying on the side, with the head of the bed elevated 10 to 30 degrees to facilitate the drainage of secretions from the mouth.

Preventing Shoulder Adduction

- Place a pillow in the axilla when there is limited external rotation to keep the arm away from the chest.
- Maintain arm in a neutral (slightly flexed) position, with distal joints positioned higher than proximal joints (ie, the elbow is positioned higher than the shoulder and the wrist higher than the elbow) to prevent edema and contracture.

Positioning the Hand and Fingers

- Position the fingers so that they are barely flexed, with the palm facing upward.
- Apply a splint if the upper extremity is flaccid.
- Prevent hand edema.
- Spasticity in the hand can be a disabling complication after stroke; intramuscular injections of botulinum toxin A into wrist and finger muscles may reduce spasticity.

(continues on page 218)

- Reinforce mirror therapy, in which the patient watches the mirror as movements with the unaffected hand are performed, leaving the impression that his or her affected hand is moving. This purportedly activates a bihemispheric cortical motor network that supports recovery.

Changing Positions
- Change the patient's position every 2 hours, limiting time spent on the affected side.
- For lateral position, place a pillow between the legs before the patient is turned.
- Avoid acutely flexing the upper thigh; this will promote venous return and prevent edema.

Establishing an Exercise Program
- Perform passive range-of-motion (ROM) exercises to affected extremities four or five times a day.
- Explain that repetition of an activity forms new pathways in the CNS and encourages new patterns of motion.
- Reminded the patient to exercise the unaffected side at intervals throughout the day; a written schedule is helpful.
- Quadriceps muscle and gluteal setting exercises are started early to improve the muscle strength needed for walking; these are performed at least five times daily for 10 minutes at a time.

Preparing for Ambulation
- Assist the patient out of bed as soon as possible.
- Begin an active rehabilitation program as soon as the patient regains consciousness: First teach patient to maintain balance while sitting, then standing.
- For difficulty in achieving standing balance, a tilt table can be used. Monitor for orthostatic hypotension while gradually elevating the head and assessing blood pressure, pulse, skin color, and any complaints of dizziness or lightheadedness. If hypotension, tachycardia, pallor, diaphoresis, dizziness, or lightheadedness are noted, lower the head of the bed until the symptoms resolve.
- Plan for the patient to ambulate using parallel bars; have a chair or wheelchair readily available in case the patient suddenly becomes fatigued or dizzy.

- A three- or four-pronged cane provides a stable support in the early phases of rehabilitation.

Preventing Shoulder Pain

- Observe for painful shoulder, subluxation (partial dislocation) of the shoulder, and shoulder–hand syndrome or reflex sympathetic dystrophy syndrome (RSDS):
  - RSDS features burning pain, tenderness, swelling, vasoconstrictive-related coldness of the affected extremity, and trophic changes to the hair, nails, skin.
- Avoid lifting the patient by the flaccid shoulder or pulling on the affected arm or shoulder.
- Position the flaccid arm on a table or pillows while the patient is seated; provide a sling, when mobile, to prevent the extremity from dangling without support.
- Monitor for post stroke pain; patient may require addition of analgesia to his treatment program. Opioids are generally prescribed for acute pain and are considered for chronic pain. Assess for side effects, tolerance, dependency, and abuse.
- Adjuvant drugs such as antidepressants, anticonvulsants, and anxiolytics may also be considered. Tricyclic antidepressants are often prescribed for neuropathic pain, whereas anticonvulsants are used for their ability to stabilize neuronal membranes.
- Topical analgesics, such as lidocaine cream or patch, may be prescribed.

Enhancing Self-Care

- As soon as the patient can sit up, personal hygiene activities are encouraged.
- Assist the patient in setting realistic goals, adding a new task daily. The first goal is to complete self-care activities on the unaffected side.
- Ensure that the patient does not neglect the affected side.
- Teach the patient about assistive devices; a small towel is easier to control while drying after bathing, and boxed paper tissues are easier to use than a roll of toilet tissue.
- Conduct an early baseline assessment of functional ability with an instrument like the Functional Independence Measure (FIM).

(continues on page 220)

C

- Instruct family to bring in clothing to improve morale (preferably a size larger than usual). Front or side fasteners or Velcro closures are the most suitable. Teach the patient that dressing is easiest while seated.
- Assist the patient with perceptual problems to match clothing to the body and keep the environment organized and uncluttered, due to easy distractibility. Provide support and encouragement to prevent the patient from becoming overly fatigued and discouraged; even with intensive training, not all patients can achieve independence in dressing.

Managing Sensory-Perceptual Difficulties

- Approach patients with decreased fields of vision on their unaffected side; place all visual stimuli (eg, clock, calendar, television) on this side.
- Teach the patient to turn the head in the direction of the defective visual field to compensate for this loss. Make eye contact with the patient and draw his or her attention to the affected side by encouraging the patient to move the head; the nurse stands such that the patient must move or turn to visualize who is in the room.
- Increasing the natural or artificial lighting in the room and providing eyeglasses are important aids to increasing vision.
- For homonymous hemianopsia (loss of half of the visual field) be aware the patient may neglect that side and the space on that side; this referred to as *amorphosynthesis.* Remind patient of the other side of the body, maintain alignment of the extremities, and, if possible, place the extremities where the patient can see them.

Assisting With Nutrition

- Observe for paroxysms of coughing, food dribbling out of or pooling in one side of the mouth, food retained for long periods in the mouth, or nasal regurgitation when swallowing liquids, indicative of dysphagia.
- Monitor for aspiration, pneumonia, dehydration, and malnutrition.
- Consult with speech therapist to evaluate the patient's gag reflexes and ability to swallow; if partially impaired, it may

return over time. The patient may be taught alternative swallowing techniques, advised to take smaller boluses of food, place food on the unaffected side of the mouth, and taught about types of foods that are easier to swallow.

- The patient may be started on a thick liquid or puréed diet because these foods are easier to swallow than thin liquids. Position the patient upright (chair preferred), and instruct him or her to tuck the chin toward the chest while swallowing, to prevent aspiration. The diet may be advanced as the patient becomes more proficient at swallowing.
- If the patient cannot resume oral intake, a GI feeding tube will be placed. Elevate the head of the bed at least 30 degrees to prevent aspiration, check the position of the tube before feeding, assess residuals, and ensure that the cuff of the tracheostomy tube (if present) is inflated.

Attaining Bowel and Bladder Control

- Observe for urinary incontinence due to confusion, inability to communicate needs, and inability to use the urinal or bedpan because of impaired motor and postural control.
- For atonic bladder or loss of control of external urinary sphincter, intermittent catheterization with sterile technique may be required. Persistent urinary incontinence or urinary retention may be symptomatic of bilateral brain damage. Analyze voiding pattern and offer urinal or bedpan on this pattern or schedule. Upright posture and standing position are helpful for male patients.
- Constipation and loss of bowel control may occur. Unless contraindicated, a high-fiber diet and adequate fluid intake (2 to 3 L/day) should be provided, and a regular time (usually after breakfast) should be established for toileting.

Improving Thought Processes

- Monitor for cognitive, behavioral, and emotional deficits related to brain damage.
- In many instances, a considerable degree of function can be recovered because not all areas of the brain are equally damaged; some remain more intact and functional than others.

(continues on page 222)

C

- After assessment of the patient's deficits, the neuropsychologist, in collaboration with the primary care physician, psychiatrist, nurse, and other professionals, structures a training program using cognitive-perceptual retraining, visual imagery, reality orientation, and cueing procedures to compensate for losses.
- Review the results of neuropsychological testing, observe the patient's performance and progress, provide positive feedback, and convey an attitude of confidence and hope.
- Interventions capitalize on the patient's strengths and remaining abilities while attempting to improve performance of affected functions.

Improving Communication

- Assess for aphasia, which impairs expression and understanding of what is being said. Damage to Broca's area, located in a convolution adjoining the middle cerebral artery, is responsible for control of muscular movements needed to speak each word.
- Patients with right hemiplegia (due to damage or injury to the left side of the brain) may not speak, whereas those with left hemiplegia are less likely to have speech disturbances.
- The speech therapist assesses the communication needs of the stroke patient, describes the precise deficit, and suggests the best overall method of communication. Most language intervention strategies can be tailored to the individual patient. The patient is expected to take an active part in establishing goals.
- Nursing interventions include strategies to make the atmosphere conducive to communication. This includes being sensitive to the patient's reactions and needs and responding to them in an appropriate manner.
- Provide a consistent schedule, routines, and repetition to help the patient to function despite deficits. A written copy of the daily schedule, a folder of personal information (birth date, address, names of relatives), checklists, and an audiotaped list help improve the patient's memory and concentration.
- A communication board, with pictures of common needs and phrases, may be used. When talking with the patient, gain the patient's attention, speak slowly, and keep the language

of instruction consistent. Give one instruction at a time, and allow for the patient to process what has been said. The use of gestures may enhance comprehension.

- In working with the patient with aphasia, the nurse must remember to talk to the patient during care activities. This provides social contact for the patient.

Maintaining Skin Integrity

- Prevent skin and tissue breakdown related to altered sensation and inability to respond to pressure and discomfort by turning and moving the patient frequently.
- Frequently assess the skin, with emphasis on bony areas and dependent parts of the body.
- During the acute phase, a specialty bed (eg, low-air-loss bed) may be used until the patient can move independently or assist in moving.
- Maintain a regular turning schedule (at least every 2 hours), even if pressure-relieving devices are used to prevent tissue and skin breakdown.
- Minimize shear and friction forces when turning and moving.
- Keep the skin clean and dry; gentle massage of healthy (non-reddened) skin and adequate nutrition are other factors that help to maintain normal skin and tissue integrity.

Improving Family Coping

- Encourage family members to participate in counseling and to use support systems that will help with emotional and physical stress of caring for the patient. Involving others in the patient's care and teaching stress management techniques and methods for maintaining personal health also facilitate family coping.
- Give the family realistic information to promote acceptance of the patient's disability and prevent unrealistic expectations. Information about expected outcomes and counseling to avoid doing activities for the patient that he or she can do are included. Assure that their love and interest are part of the patient's therapy.
- Teach the family that rehabilitation for hemiplegia requires many months and that progress may be slow. The rehabilitation

(continues on page 224)

team, the medical and nursing team, the patient, and the family must all be involved in developing attainable goals for the patient at home.

- Prepare the family to expect occasional episodes of emotional lability. The patient may laugh or cry easily, or be irritable, demanding, depressed, or confused. The nurse can explain to the family that the patient's laughter does not necessarily connote happiness, nor does crying reflect sadness, and that emotional lability usually improves with time.

Helping the Patient Cope With Sexual Dysfunction

- Explain that sexual dysfunction after stroke is multifactorial. Medical reasons, such a neurologic and cognitive deficits, previous diseases, and medications, as well as various psychosocial factors may exist. Loss of self-esteem and value as a sexual being play an important role in determining sexual drive, activity, and satisfaction after a stroke.
- Begin dialogue between the patient and his or her partner about sexuality. In-depth assessments to determine sexual history before and after the stroke should be followed by appropriate interventions.
- Interventions for the patient and partner focus on providing relevant information, education, reassurance, adjustment of medications, counseling regarding coping skills, suggestions for alternative sexual positions, and a means of sexual expression and satisfaction.

Providing Patient Education and Preparing the Patient for the Home

- The nurse teaches the patient and family about stroke, its causes and prevention, and the rehabilitation process.
- During rehabilitation, the focus is on teaching the patient to resume as much self-care as possible. Assistive devices or modification to the home may be necessary for the disability.
- An occupational therapist may be helpful in assessing the home environment and recommending modifications for independence. A shower is more convenient than a tub for the patient with hemiplegia due to loss of strength. Using a stool of medium height with rubber suction tips allows the patient

to wash with greater ease. A long-handled bath brush with a soap container is helpful to the patient who has only one functional hand. If a shower is not available, a stool may be placed in the tub and a portable shower hose attached to the faucet. Handrails may be attached alongside the bathtub and the toilet. Other assistive devices include special utensils for eating, grooming, dressing, and writing.

- Physical therapy can be beneficial in the home environment.
- Counseling and antidepressant therapy may help if depression develops. As progress is made in the rehabilitation program, some problems will diminish; positive reinforcement for the progress that is being made is helpful.
- Community-based stroke support in the form of in-person meetings, as well as Web-based support programs, is helpful. Encourage the patient to continue hobbies, recreational and leisure interests, and to maintain contact with friends to prevent social isolation.
- Recognize the potential effects of caregiving on the family. Not all families have the adaptive coping skills and adequate psychological functioning necessary for the long-term care of another person. The patient's spouse may be elderly, with his or her own health concerns; in some instances, the patient may have been the provider of care to the spouse.
- Assess for depression in caregivers; they are more likely to resort to physical or emotional abuse and are more likely to place the patient in a nursing home. Suggest respite care, which may be available from an adult day care center.
- The home care nurse reminds the patient and family to continue health promotion and screening practices.

Evaluation

Expected patient outcomes may include the following:
- Demonstrates intact neurologic status and normal vital signs and respiratory patterns
- Demonstrates understanding of diagnostic procedures and treatment plan
- Keeps follow-up appointments with stroke neurologist or primary care provider

> For more information, see Chapter 47 in Pellico, L.H. (2013). *Focus on adult health. Medical-surgical nursing.* Philadelphia: Wolters Kluwer Health | Lippincott Williams & Wilkins.

C Cholelithiasis (and Cholecystitis)

Calculi, or gallstones, usually form in the gallbladder from the solid constituents of bile; they vary greatly in size, shape, and composition.

PATHOPHYSIOLOGY

Two major types of gallstones exist, those composed predominantly of pigment and those composed primarily of cholesterol. Pigment stones form when unconjugated pigments in the bile precipitate to form stones. The risk is increased in patients with cirrhosis, hemolysis, and infections of the biliary tract. Pigment stones cannot be dissolved and must be removed surgically.

In gallstone-prone patients, decreased bile acid synthesis and increased cholesterol synthesis in the liver supersaturates bile, causing precipitation and stone formation. Gallstones act as an irritant that produces inflammatory changes.

RISK FACTORS

- Age over 40 years
- Female
- Native American or Hispanic women
- Multiple pregnancies
- Obesity; frequent changes in weight or rapid weight loss
- Treatment with high-dose estrogen (eg, in prostate cancer) or low-dose estrogen therapy
- Ileal resection or disease, gastric bypass surgery
- Total parental nutrition
- Cystic fibrosis

- Diabetes mellitus
- Family history

CLINICAL MANIFESTATIONS AND ASSESSMENT

- May be silent, producing no pain and only mild GI symptoms; stones may be detected incidentally during surgery or evaluation for unrelated problems.
- Epigastric distress, such as fullness, abdominal distention, and vague pain in the right upper quadrant of the abdomen, may occur, particularly following rich, fried, or fatty foods.
- Pain and biliary colic with repeated episodes of obstruction may occur. Increased frequency of biliary colic typically will result in cholecystitis. Continued obstruction may result in abscess, necrosis, and perforation with generalized peritonitis.

☀ N U R S I N G   A L E R T

Be alert for signs and symptoms of peritonitis including vague, generalized abdominal pain that becomes increasingly severe and constant; abdominal distention and tenderness with rebound tenderness; anxiety, pallor; diaphoresis; anorexia; nausea; vomiting; inability to pass feces and flatus; rigidity of the abdomen; an absence of bowel sounds; cautious movement; knee-chest position for comfort.

- With cystic duct obstruction, gallbladder becomes distended, inflamed, and eventually infected (acute cholecystitis):
  - Fever and palpable abdominal mass may be present along with biliary colic and excruciating upper right abdominal pain, radiating to the back or right shoulder.
  - Nausea and vomiting may be present, often several hours after a heavy meal.
  - Other symptoms include nausea, chills, and gastric distress including belching and bloating.
- Murphy's sign: Tenderness in the right upper quadrant on deep inspiration, preventing full inspiratory excursion when the examiner's fingers are under the liver border.
- See management under cholecystitis.

CHOLECYSTITIS

Cholecystitis is acute inflammation of the gallbladder. An empyema of the gallbladder develops if the gallbladder becomes filled with purulent fluid (pus). Repeated episodes of cystic duct obstruction by gallstones will cause cholecystitis.

PATHOPHYSIOLOGY

Gallstones are the cause of more than 90% of cases of acute cholecystitis. When a stone obstructs bile outflow, bile remaining in the gallbladder initiates a chemical reaction that causes autolysis and edema. The gallbladder becomes inflamed and distended; the pressure causes vascular compromise, ischemia, and necrosis. Secondary infection with bacteria complicate the course of this disorder in up to 75% of patients.

Acalculous cholecystitis describes acute gallbladder inflammation in the absence of obstruction by gallstones. It occurs after major surgical procedures, severe trauma, or burns. Cystic duct obstruction, primary bacterial infections of the gallbladder, multiorgan failure, and acute renal failure may also cause this. Bile stasis (lack of gallbladder contraction) and increased viscosity of the bile are also thought to play a role.

CLINICAL MANIFESTATIONS AND ASSESSMENT

- Pain, tenderness, and rigidity of the right upper abdomen; pain usually radiates to the back, right shoulder, or scapula.
- Nausea and vomiting are common.
- Leukocytosis (elevated WBCs) is present.
- Positive Murphy's sign or right subcostal tenderness is present.

MEDICAL MANAGEMENT

The major objectives of medical therapy are to reduce the incidence of acute episodes of gallbladder pain and cholecystitis with supportive and dietary management.

Pharmacologic Therapy

- Ursodeoxycholic acid (UDCA [Urso, Actigall]) and chenode-oxycholic acid (chenodiol or CDCA [Chenix]) are effective in dissolving primarily cholesterol stones.
- Patients with significant, frequent symptoms; cystic duct occlusion, or pigment stones are not candidates for therapy with UDCA.

Surgical Management

- Laparoscopic cholecystectomy: Performed through a small incision or puncture made through the abdominal wall in the umbilicus.
- Cholecystectomy: Gallbladder is removed through an abdominal incision (usually right subcostal) after ligation of the cystic duct and artery. May be used if problems are encountered during laparoscopic procedure.

For more information, see Chapter 25 in Pellico, L.H. (2013). *Focus on adult health. Medical-surgical nursing.* Philadelphia: Wolters Kluwer Health | Lippincott Williams & Wilkins.

Chronic Obstructive Pulmonary Disease

Chronic obstructive pulmonary disease is a disease characterized by airflow limitation that is not fully reversible. The airflow limitation is usually progressive and associated with an abnormal inflammatory response of the lung.

PATHOPHYSIOLOGY

Chronic obstructive pulmonary disease is characterized by an increase in mucus-producing cells, and chronic lung and structural changes resulting from a continuing cycle of destruction and repair. Affected are the proximal and peripheral airways, lung parenchyma, and pulmonary vasculature. Inflammation in COPD is thought to be an amplification of the normal inflammatory response; oxidative stress and an excess of destructive cytokines in the lungs may amplify this. Individuals may have predominantly emphysema, chronic bronchitis, or heightened airway responsiveness. Many people have a combination of these processes.

Emphysema

Emphysema describes an abnormal enlargement of the air spaces beyond the terminal bronchioles, with destruction of the walls of the alveoli. The alveolar and interstitial attachments are reduced, predisposing them to collapse during exhalation. External airway compression and obstruction is caused by hyperinflation and air trapping. The panacinar or panlobular form causes uniform destruction of acinus, where alveoli are located (hereditary form is related to deficiency of alpha$_1$-antitrypsin). A centrilobular form is related to smoking; alveolar ducts and bronchioles in the center of lobules of the upper lobes are primarily affected.

Chronic Bronchitis

Chronic obstructive bronchitis is defined as the presence of cough and sputum production for at least 3 months in each of 2 consecutive years. In simple chronic bronchitis, pulmonary function remains normal. Chronic mucus hypersecretion causes lung function decline; exacerbations and infections occur. Thickening of the epithelium, smooth muscle hypertrophy, and airway inflammation are implicated in remodeling of the airways, causing the airway lumen to be smaller.

Most patients have elements of both emphysema and chronic bronchitis. In the later stages of COPD, gas exchange is often impaired. As the alveolar walls continue to break down, the pulmonary capillary bed is reduced in size. Resistance to pulmonary blood flow is increased, increasing pressure in the pulmonary artery; chronic hypoxemia increases pulmonary artery pressures as well. Right-sided heart hypertrophy and failure (*cor pulmonale*) may result. Additionally, decreased carbon dioxide elimination results in increased arterial carbon dioxide tension (hypercapnia), causing respiratory acidosis and chronic respiratory failure. In acute illness, worsening hypercapnia can lead to acute respiratory failure.

Damage to bronchioles result in altered function of the alveolar macrophages, making the individual more susceptible to respiratory infection, including acute bronchitis. Chronic obstructive pulmonary disease is now considered a systemic disease and may affect skeletal muscle, cardiovascular, neurologic, psychiatric, and endocrine system functions.

RISK FACTORS

- Cigarette smoking
- Environmental tobacco smoke (second-hand smoke, fetal exposure due to smoking during pregnancy)
- Occupational dust and chemicals (organic dusts, inorganic dusts, chemical agents, fumes)
- Indoor and outdoor air pollution (cooking or heating in poorly ventilated areas)
- History of severe respiratory infections, history of tuberculosis in those over 40 years old

CLINICAL MANIFESTATIONS AND ASSESSMENT

- Chronic obstructive pulmonary disease is characterized by dyspnea, chronic cough and sputum production; begins with dyspnea on exertion and worsens over time. In severe COPD, dyspnea may occur at rest.
- Chronic cough and sputum production often precede the development of airflow limitation by many years. In early-stage disease, an early morning productive cough of white to clear sputum may be present. During exacerbations, increased sputum quantity and viscosity may occur, with changes in sputum color.
- A positive history of progressive dyspnea and/or a productive cough in a cigarette smoker leads to a suspicion of COPD.
- Hyperinflation causes increased anterior to posterior diameter of the chest, called "barrel chest."
- Bilateral intercostal retractions at the posterior axillary line, horizontal fixation of the ribs in the inspiratory position, and

hyperresonance to percussion (particularly in thin individuals) develops.

- Diminished breath sounds with prolonged exhalation (bronchovesicular breath sounds) and adventitious sounds (coarse crackles, rhonchi, and wheezes) are often heard when the patient has increased secretions, bronchial hyperreactivity, or an exacerbation.
- Symptoms are specific to the disease. See "Clinical Manifestations" under "Bronchitis" on page 100 and "Emphysema" on pages 286–287.

DIAGNOSTIC METHODS

- Pulmonary function tests include spirometry and forced expired volume in 1 second (FEV_1), total lung capacity (TLC), and diffusion capacity.
- Bronchodilator reversibility testing may be performed to rule out asthma and to guide initial treatment. Spirometry is first obtained; the patient is given an inhaled bronchodilator and spirometry is repeated. The patient demonstrates a degree of reversibility if the pulmonary function values improve significantly (>12%) after administration of the bronchodilator.
- Arterial blood gas measurements may be obtained to assess baseline oxygenation and gas exchange and are especially important in advanced COPD.
- Chest X-ray may be obtained to establish the patient's baseline and to exclude alternative diagnoses. A chest X-ray is seldom diagnostic in COPD unless obvious bullous (large, air-filled "blisters") disease or severe hyperinflation is present. Chest X-rays are used in exacerbations to determine if the patient has an infiltrate or a concomitant lung mass.
- A CT scan is not routinely obtained in the diagnosis of COPD, but a high-resolution CT scan may help in the differential diagnosis or to evaluate patients for surgical procedures, such as bullectomy or lung volume reduction surgery (LVRS).
- Screening for alpha$_1$-antitrypsin deficiency is usually recommended for symptomatic patients younger than 45 years and for those with a strong family history of COPD.

MEDICAL AND NURSING MANAGEMENT

The goals of medical therapy are to stabilize, manage, and monitor the disease; reduce symptoms; reduce exacerbation risk and rate; promote maximal functional ability; prevent premature disability; and assist the individual to adapt to handicap and limited prognosis as the disease progresses.

The management of the patient depends on the severity of the COPD. In early-stage disease, clinical strategies are aimed at maximizing pulmonary function, keeping the patient active, preventing exacerbations, and engaging the patient in self-management. In progressive stages, more intensive therapies are added.

- Smoking cessation slows disease progression; assist patients to set a "quit date" and follow-up within a few days to address problems.
- Pharmacotherapy increases long-term smoking abstinence rates when used in conjunction with smoking cessation counseling. Nicotine replacement (gum, inhaler, nasal spray, transdermal patch, sublingual tablet, or lozenges) may be used as a single agent or in combination with other pharmacologic agents.
- Antidepressants such as bupropion SR (Zyban, Wellbutrin) and nortriptyline (Aventyl) also have been shown to increase long-term quit rates. Bupropion is useful in those concerned with weight gain during smoking abstinence as it may result in weight loss.
- Varenicline (Chantix) reduces nicotine withdrawal symptoms and has been associated with increased quit rates.

⚡ NURSING ALERT
Bupropion is contraindicated in patients with a history of seizures as it may lower the seizure threshold.

Pharmacologic Therapy

- Bronchodilators, corticosteroids, or anticholinergics via metered dose inhaler or nebulizer may be prescribed.

- Influenza and pneumococcal vaccinations reduce incidence of pneumonia, hospitalizations for cardiac conditions, and deaths. A vaccine to protect against *Haemophilus influenzae,* a common cause of COPD exacerbations, is currently in development.
- Other pharmacologic treatments that may be used in COPD include alpha$_1$-antitrypsin augmentation therapy for those with a diagnosed deficiency.
- Antibiotics are given for acute infection, and mucolytic agents are given for help with secretion clearance.
- Cough suppressants are usually reserved for nighttime use, when cough interferes with sleep.
- Oxygen therapy is prescribed for SaO$_2$ levels of less than 90%; it is used in acute exacerbations, continuously for chronic hypoxemia, and during exercise and sleep for select patients; oxygen decreases the workload of the cardiopulmonary system, prevents polycythemia and pulmonary hypertension.

NURSING ALERT

A small subset of patients with COPD and chronic hypercapnia (elevated PaCO$_2$ levels) may be at some risk for respiratory failure if they receive too high an oxygen concentration. Concern persists that such patients would lose their "drive to breathe" also called "hypoxic drive." Overconcern may lead to giving patients too little oxygen, worsening hypoxemia. Although hypercapnic patients are at increased risk for respiratory failure, the risk is related to the severity of their COPD. Adequate oxygenation is important in their management and should never be withheld.

Surgical Interventions

- Bullectomy to reduce dyspnea
- Lung volume reduction surgery is an option for a subset of patients with severe upper lobe emphysema. A portion of the diseased lung parenchyma is removed, reducing hyperinflation and improving the elastic recoil and diaphragmatic mechanics. Not curative, but may decrease dyspnea and improve quality of life.

- Lung transplantation is an alternative surgical treatment for patients with end-stage emphysema with an FEV_1 of less than 25% of the predicted and who have complications such as pulmonary hypertension, marked hypoxemia, and hypercapnia.

Pulmonary Rehabilitation

- The primary goals of rehabilitation are to reduce symptoms, improve quality of life, and increase participation in everyday activities using a multidisciplinary approach.
- Breathing exercises, learning to pace activities, physical reconditioning and endurance, energy conservation, skills training, and psychological support are included.
- Nutritional counseling and medication education are other important components of rehabilitation.

Preventing and Managing Exacerbations and Complications

- Exacerbations are characterized by a change in the patient's baseline dyspnea, cough, and/or sputum production, which warrants a change in management.
- Exacerbations are associated with worsening prognosis and an accelerated decline in pulmonary function.
- Signs and symptoms may include increased dyspnea, increased sputum production and purulence, respiratory failure, changes in mental status, or worsening blood gas abnormalities.
- The primary causes of acute exacerbations include infection (bacterial and viral), heart failure, and response to pollutants and allergens.
- Prevention of exacerbations is associated with preservation of pulmonary function and a decrease in hospitalizations. Some pharmacological agents, such as inhaled long-acting beta adrenergics (LABAs) combined with steroids (Advair, Symbicort) and the anticholinergic agent Spiriva, have been associated with a prolonged time between exacerbations.
- Bronchodilators, inhaled or systemic corticosteroids, antibiotics, oxygen therapy, and intensive respiratory interventions may be used.

- Early treatment with antibiotics in patients needing hospitalization for an acute exacerbation may result in improved outcomes.
- Indications for hospitalization for acute exacerbation include severe dyspnea that does not respond adequately to initial therapy, confusion or lethargy, respiratory muscle fatigue, paradoxical chest wall movement, peripheral edema, worsening or new onset of central cyanosis, persistent or worsening hypoxemia, and the need for noninvasive or invasive assisted mechanical ventilation.
- Ventilatory support may be required until the underlying cause, such as infection, can be treated.
- Other complications of COPD include pneumonia, atelectasis, pneumothorax, and pulmonary arterial hypertension.
- Suspect pulmonary hypertension in patients complaining of dyspnea and fatigue disproportionate to pulmonary function abnormalities; enlargement of the central pulmonary arteries on chest X-ray, echocardiography suggestive of right ventricular enlargement, and elevated plasma B-type natriuretic peptide (BNP) may be present. Anticipate stabilization of the underlying lung disease, with administration of long-term supplemental oxygen and diuretics.

☀ *N U R S I N G   A L E R T*

The hormone BNP is produced by the ventricles of the heart. Elevation of BNP occurs when ventricular volume expands and/or ventricular pressure increases. Thus, it is a marker of ventricular dysfunction. A normal BNP is less than 100 pg/mL or less than 100 ng/L.

Nursing Management

In all settings, nurses play a key role in the care of the patient with COPD.

Assessing the Patient

- Obtain information about shortness of breath (dyspnea), cough, and sputum production; change in sputum color, quantity, or thickness, or increased fatigue and a decreased ability to perform one's usual activities is noted.

- To assess progress of the disease, use a numerical scale based on 0 to 10 (with 0 being no shortness of breath and 10 being the worst) when quantifying dyspnea.
- Assess for the presence of other medical problems (cardiovascular, diabetes, stroke, history of pneumonia, cancer), allergies, history of smoking in pack years, current smoking, a history of past exacerbations and pulmonary hospitalizations including a history of intubations, a description of how the patient spends a usual day, sleep quality and amount, problems with mood (anxiety and/or depression), and what self-care measures the patient is currently using.
- Observe breathing pattern and body position; accessory muscle use, shoulder elevation, use of the tripod position (leaning forward with the arms braced on the knees), and increased respiratory rate are indicative of respiratory distress
- Assess for quality (good aeration or diminished) of breath sounds, the presence of adventitious sounds (crackles or wheezes), and whether the adventitious sounds clear with cough.
- Review laboratory data: Pulmonary function tests, tests of oxygenation, and radiological studies.

Promoting Smoking Cessation

- Teach the patient that smoking cessation is not futile; continued smoking promotes lung function decline and disabling symptoms.
- Relate the cause of the hospitalization to smoking behavior to personalize the message to the patient.
- Discuss pharmacological agents that increase successful cessation.

Managing Chronic Dyspnea

- Recognize that chronic dyspnea is different from acute dyspnea in that the patient may exhibit no visible signs of distress. Analogous to pain, dyspnea occurs when the patient says it does and feels like the patient says it does.
- Assess underlying causes and manage dyspnea with bronchodilators, assisting with activities of daily living, providing oxygen therapy for hypoxemia, and teaching strategies for relieving increased shortness of breath and for limiting future episodes.

- Assist patient with breathing retraining; pursed-lip breathing helps slow exhalation and is thought to prevent the collapse of the small airways, decreasing hyperinflation. It may promote relaxation and allow patients to gain control of their breathing and reduce feelings of panic. A simple explanation to patients is that pursed-lip breathing makes "more room to breathe."
- Suggest the use of a small hand-held fan directing flow onto the cheek to reduce the sensation of dyspnea.
- Teach relaxation techniques, such as progressive muscle relaxation.
- Teach patients how to pace activities with their breathing and plan for dyspnea-producing activities. For climbing stairs, climb more slowly and only during exhalation; use a pause-breathe in, exhale and climb one to two steps.
- When dyspnea is not adequately responsive to medications and breathing techniques, opioids may be needed; concerns over physical dependence, addiction, and respiratory depression should be addressed. Opioids should not be withheld in very severe patients for whom palliative care is the goal.

Managing Impaired Gas Exchange

- Monitor for hypoxemia with pulse oximetry and arterial blood gas measurements; administer supplemental oxygen as indicated. Maintain oxygen saturation at 90% or higher to protect vital organ function.
- Teach importance of adhering to the oxygen prescription; the presence or absence of dyspnea is an unreliable symptom of hypoxemia.
- Monitor for cognitive impairment, which is increased in hypoxemic patients; administer long-term oxygen to improved cardiac and cognitive function and prognosis.
- Teach patient the number of hours per day to wear oxygen, the dose of oxygen (usually given as number of liters per minute), and special instructions for using oxygen for sleep and exercise.

Managing Cough and Ineffective Airway Clearance

- Monitor patients with chronic bronchitis and those experiencing an acute exacerbation for increased sputum, quantity, viscosity, and weakness or fatigue, which impairs effective airway clearance.

- Assist patient in eliminating or reducing pulmonary irritants including cigarette smoking, second-hand smoke, aerosol cleaning and household products, and cooking fumes.
- Teach directed or controlled coughing and to drink enough fluid to prevent dehydration.
- Provide chest physiotherapy with postural drainage and/or mechanical percussion and vibration and suctioning.

Improving Exercise Tolerance

- Observe for exercise intolerance secondary to exacerbations, hospitalizations, and systemic corticosteroids (associated with myopathy, especially of legs), which add to decreased activity, muscle weakness, and fatigue.
- Assist patient with early mobilization during acute exacerbation, including those in intensive care.
- Teach patient to alternate high-energy with low-energy activities throughout the day; consider use of walking aids and consultation with occupational and physical therapists.

Promoting Nutrition

- Nutrition therapy is aimed at assessing the nutritional status of the patient, treating the underlying cause, and stabilizing weight and body composition. Patients may be underweight, of normal weight but have decreased muscle mass, or be overweight because of increased fat mass or increased fluid retention.
- Provide oral nutritional supplements to increase body weight and respiratory function. Caution patients to avoid negating the effectiveness of supplements by using them as meal substitutes.
- Time bronchodilators before meals; assist severely dyspneic patients during meal times to minimize energy spent eating; teach patients to eat small, frequent meals to help them avoid becoming too full; and encourage the choice of calorie-rich foods when indicated.
- Consider referring patients to dieticians and encouraging progressive periods of exercise aimed at increased muscle mass. Overweight patients may need the help of nutrition education by a dietician to help them lose weight safely. Exercise should be encouraged to help patients increase muscle mass.

C

☀ *N U R S I N G   A L E R T*

Carbohydrates generate CO_2 production, thus may be limited in COPD patients; however, experts suggest that low-carbohydrate, high-lipid feeds (to reduce CO_2 generation) are rarely necessary. Rather, body mass index (BMI) should be used to evaluate nutritional status and should be maintained in the range over 20 but less than 25. If the BMI is less than 20, improved nutritional status is associated with respiratory muscle strength and prognosis. Weight reduction (if the BMI is >25) is associated with decreased dyspnea and improved functional status.

Managing Exacerbations and Complications

- Prevention and early recognition of exacerbations of COPD are important self-care measures for patients to learn.
- Instruct patients to prevent infection through hand-washing, avoiding or minimizing contact with sick individuals, and receiving immunizations against influenza and pneumococcal pneumonia.
- Patients should be able to report signs of infection: Increased dyspnea, fever, or change in sputum color, character, consistency, or amount.
- Teach patient that any marked worsening of symptoms (chest tightness, dyspnea, fatigue) suggests infection and should be reported to the health care provider. Viral infections may make patients more susceptible to more serious bacterial infections.

☀ *N U R S I N G   A L E R T*

High fevers of 102°F or greater accompanied by shaking chills are signs of a more serious infection, such as pneumonia. Patients should be instructed to go to the nearest emergency room immediately.

- Acknowledge the patient's past response to "bad breathing" days to guide patient teaching; changes in normal routines, increased activity, family events, increased stress, and fatigue are some of the causes of "bad breathing days."

For more information, see Chapter 11 in Pellico, L.H. (2013). *Focus on adult health. Medical-surgical nursing.* Philadelphia: Wolters Kluwer Health | Lippincott Williams & Wilkins.

Cirrhosis, Hepatic

Cirrhosis of the liver occurs when the normal liver tissue is replaced by fibrotic or scar tissue in response to damage. Cirrhosis represents the final stage of all chronic liver diseases and is one of the leading causes of death in the United States.

PATHOPHYSIOLOGY

Cirrhosis of the liver occurs when the normal liver tissue is replaced by fibrotic or scar tissue in response to damage to the liver, resulting in the loss of normal structure. The progression and severity of chronic liver disease can be classified as either compensated or decompensated cirrhosis.

RISK FACTORS

- Alcohol and other hepatotoxins
- Hepatitis and other infections
- Autoimmune disorders
- Toxins
- Metabolic disorder

CLINICAL MANIFESTATIONS AND ASSESSMENT

- Compensated cirrhosis is typically asymptomatic but may include intermittent mild fever, vascular spiders, palmar erythema (reddened palms), unexplained epistaxis, ankle edema,

vague morning indigestion, flatulent dyspepsia, abdominal pain, hepatomegaly, and splenomegaly.
- Decompensated cirrhosis results in the development of jaundice, ascites, GI bleeding from esophageal varices, and hepatic encephalopathy:
  - Spontaneous bacterial peritonitis, hepatorenal syndrome, and hepatopulmonary syndrome cause symptoms such as shortness of breath and hypoxemia.
- Weakness, muscle wasting, weight loss, continuous mild fever, clubbing of fingers, purpura (due to decreased platelet count)

MEDICAL AND NURSING MANAGEMENT

Medical management is based on presenting symptoms.

- Treatment includes antacids, vitamins and nutritional supplements, balanced diet, potassium-sparing diuretics (for ascites), and avoidance of alcohol.
- Colchicine may increase the length of survival in patients with mild to moderate cirrhosis.

NURSING PROCESS

The Patient With Cirrhosis

Assessment

- Assess onset of symptoms and history of precipitating factors such as long-term alcohol abuse, dietary intake, and changes in the patient's physical and mental status.
- Explore past and current patterns of alcohol use (duration and amount).
- Document exposure to hepatotoxic including medications, illicit IV/injection drugs, inhalants, and general anesthetic agents.
- Assess mental status, orientation to person place and time
- Note abdominal distention and bloating, GI bleeding, bruising, and weight changes.

- Assess nutritional status and daily weights, and monitor plasma proteins, transferrin, and creatinine levels.

Diagnosis

Nursing diagnoses may include the following:

- Activity intolerance related to fatigue, general debility, muscle wasting, and discomfort
- Imbalanced nutrition, less than body requirements, related to chronic gastritis, decreased GI motility, and anorexia
- Impaired skin integrity related to compromised immunologic status, edema, and poor nutrition
- Risk for injury and bleeding related to altered clotting mechanisms
- Potential complications may include the following:
  - Bleeding and hemorrhage
  - Hepatic encephalopathy
  - Fluid volume excess

Planning

The goals for the patient may include increased participation in activities, improvement of nutritional status, improvement of skin integrity, decreased potential for injury, improvement of mental status, and absence of complications.

Nursing Interventions

Promoting Rest

- Position the patient in bed for maximal respiratory efficiency and adequate thoracic expansion (especially important if ascites is marked). Patient should use incentive spirometer every hour while awake.
- Administer oxygen as needed.
- Prevent respiratory, circulatory, and vascular disturbances through range of motion exercises, turning every 2 hours, and encouraging the patient to increase activity gradually.
- Activity and mild exercise, as well as rest, are planned.

(continues on page 244)

Improving Nutritional Status

- Provide a nutritious, high-protein diet supplemented by B-complex vitamins and others, including A, C, and K; provide protein supplements, if indicated.
- Provide small, frequent meals, considering patient preferences; protein supplements may be indicated.
- Provide enteral or parenteral nutrition if patient is vomiting or eating poorly.
- Provide patients having fatty stools (steatorrhea) with water-soluble forms of fat-soluble vitamins A, D, and E,
- Administer folic acid and iron to prevent anemia.
- Provide a low-protein diet if encephalopathy develops; incorporating vegetable protein may reduce the risk of encephalopathy.
- Restrict sodium to prevent ascites.

Providing Skin Care

- Change patient's position frequently due to edema immobility, jaundice, and increased susceptibility to skin breakdown and infection.
- Avoid using irritating soaps and adhesive tape.
- Provide lotion to soothe irritated skin; take measures to prevent patient from scratching the skin.

Reducing Risk of Injury

- Protect the patient from falls and other injuries.
- Use padded side rails if patient becomes agitated or restless.
- Orient to time, place, and procedures to minimize agitation.
- Instruct patient to ask for assistance to get out of bed.
- Carefully evaluate any injury because of risk for internal bleeding.
- Provide safety measures to prevent injury or cuts (electric razor, soft toothbrush) due to abnormal clotting.
- Apply pressure to venipuncture sites to minimize bleeding.

Monitoring and Managing Potential Complications

- Observe for and protect from bleeding and hemorrhage due to decreased production of prothrombin and clotting factors:
  - Avoid intramuscular injections.
  - Observe stool for melena and blood.

- Monitor vital signs.
- Prevent rupture of esophageal varices by avoiding increases in portal pressure; administer stool softeners to prevent straining.
- Keep readily available equipment (eg, balloon tamponade tube), IV fluids, and medications needed to treat hemorrhage from esophageal and gastric varices.
- Administer fluids and blood for bleeding; may require transfer to ICU or emergency surgery.
- Hepatic encephalopathy:
  - Observe for deteriorating mental status and dementia or physical signs, such as abnormal voluntary and involuntary movements. Hepatic encephalopathy is mainly caused by the accumulation of ammonia in the blood.
  - Administer lactulose and nonabsorbable intestinal tract antibiotics to decrease ammonia levels, modify medications to eliminate those that may precipitate or worsen hepatic encephalopathy, and promote bed rest to minimize energy expenditure.
- Monitor mental status.
- Evaluate for electrolyte disturbances that can contribute to encephalopathy.
- Monitor for fluid volume excess and pulmonary compromise.
- Administer diuretics, implement fluid restrictions, and enhance patient positioning to optimize pulmonary function.
- Monitor intake and output, changes in daily weight, abdominal girth, and edema formation.
- Patients are also monitored for any changes in renal function.

Promoting Home- and Community-Based Care

- Provide diet teaching: *No alcohol,* restrict sodium to 2 g/day, provide a well-balanced diet.
- Refer to Alcoholics Anonymous, psychiatric care, counseling, or spiritual advisor if indicated.
- Encourage rest.
- Avoid consumption of raw shellfish.
- Instruct family about symptoms of impending encephalopathy and possibility of bleeding and susceptibility to infection.

(continues on page 246)

C

Evaluation

Expected patient outcomes may include the following:

- Participates in activities
- Increases nutritional intake
- Exhibits improved skin integrity
- Avoids injury
- Is free of complications

COMPLICATIONS

- Bleeding and hemorrhage
- Hepatic encephalopathy

For more information, see Chapter 25 in Pellico, L.H. (2013). *Focus on adult health. Medical-surgical nursing.* Philadelphia: Wolters Kluwer Health | Lippincott Williams & Wilkins.

Constipation

Constipation refers to an abnormal infrequency or irregularity of defecation, abnormal hardening of stools that makes their passage difficult and sometimes painful, decrease in stool volume, or prolonged retention of stool in the rectum.

PATHOPHYSIOLOGY

The pathophysiology of constipation is poorly understood, but it is thought to include interference with one of three major functions of the colon: Mucosal transport (ie, mucosal secretions facilitate the movement of colon contents), myoelectric activity (ie, mixing of the rectal mass and propulsive actions), or the processes of defecation.

If all organic causes are eliminated, idiopathic constipation is diagnosed. When the urge to defecate is ignored, the rectal mucous membrane and musculature become insensitive to the presence of fecal masses, and consequently a stronger stimulus is required to produce the necessary peristaltic rush for defecation. The initial effect of fecal retention is irritability of the colon, which at this stage frequently goes into spasm, especially after meals, giving rise to colicky midabdominal or low abdominal pains. After several years of this process, the colon loses muscular tone and becomes essentially unresponsive to normal stimuli. Atony or decreased muscle tone occurs with aging. This also leads to constipation because the stool is retained for longer periods.

RISK FACTORS

- Medications: Tranquilizers, anticholinergics, antidepressants, antihypertensives, bile acid sequestrants, opioids, aluminum-based antacids, iron preparations
- Rectal or anal disorders (eg, hemorrhoids, fissures); obstruction (eg, bowel tumors); metabolic, neurologic, and neuromuscular conditions (eg, Hirschsprung's disease, Parkinson's disease, multiple sclerosis); endocrine disorders (eg, diabetes mellitus, hypothyroidism, pheochromocytoma)
- Lead poisoning
- Connective tissue disorders (eg, scleroderma, systemic lupus erythematosus)
- Diseases of the colon, such as IBS and diverticular disease, are commonly associated with constipation.
- Acute disease process in the abdomen (eg, appendicitis or cholecystitis) or with any abdominal surgery
- Older adults tend to have decreased food intake, reduced mobility, weak abdominal and pelvic muscles, and multiple chronic illnesses requiring medications that can cause constipation.
- Ill-fitting dentures or poor dentition increases difficulty in chewing, and patients frequently will choose softer, processed foods that are lower in fiber.
- Low-fiber, convenience foods

- Reduced fluid intake
- Depression, weakness, or prolonged bed rest
- Overuse and dependency on laxatives
- Inability to increase intra-abdominal pressure, or not taking time or ignoring the urge to defecate

CLINICAL MANIFESTATIONS AND ASSESSMENT

- Fewer than three bowel movements per week, abdominal distention, and pain and pressure
- Decreased appetite, headache, fatigue, indigestion, sensation of incomplete emptying
- Straining at stool; elimination of small volume of lumpy, hard, dry stool
- Complications such as hypertension, hemorrhoids and fissures, fecal impaction, and megacolon

DIAGNOSTIC METHODS

The nurse elicits information about the onset and duration of constipation, current and past elimination patterns, the patient's expectation of normal bowel elimination, and lifestyle information (eg, exercise and activity level, occupation, food and fluid intake, and stress level). Past medical and surgical history, current medications, and laxative and enema use, information about the sensation of rectal pressure or fullness, abdominal pain, excessive straining at defecation, and flatulence are included.

MEDICAL AND NURSING MANAGEMENT

- Treatment should target the underlying cause of constipation and prevention of recurrence; education, bowel habit training, increased fiber and fluid intake, and judicious use of laxatives is included.

- Encourage routine exercise to strengthen abdominal muscles.
- Recommend daily intake of 6 to 12 teaspoons of unprocessed bran, especially for the treatment of the elderly.
- If a laxative is necessary, use bulk-forming agents, saline and osmotic agents, lubricants, stimulants, or fecal softeners. Enemas and rectal suppositories are not recommended for treating constipation.
- Specific medication therapy to increase intrinsic motor function include cholinergic agents (eg, bethanechol [Urecholine]), cholinesterase inhibitors (eg, neostigmine [Prostigmin]), or prokinetic agents (eg, metoclopramide [Reglan]).
- The nurse focuses on restoring or maintaining a regular pattern of elimination by responding to the urge to defecate, ensuring adequate intake of fluids and high-fiber foods, learning methods to avoid constipation, relieving anxiety about bowel elimination patterns, and avoiding complications.

COMPLICATIONS

- Hypertension
- Fecal impaction
- Hemorrhoids (dilated portions of anal veins)
- Fissures (tissue folds)
- Megacolon (abnormal enlargement of the colon)

For more information, see Chapter 24 in Pellico, L.H. (2013). *Focus on adult health. Medical-surgical nursing.* Philadelphia: Wolters Kluwer Health | Lippincott Williams & Wilkins.

Contact Dermatitis

Contact dermatitis is an inflammatory reaction of the skin to physical, chemical, or biologic agents.

PATHOPHYSIOLOGY

The epidermis is damaged by repeated physical and chemical irritations. Contact dermatitis may be of the primary irritant type, in which a nonallergic reaction results from exposure to an irritating substance, or it may be an allergic reaction resulting from exposure of sensitized people to contact allergens.

RISK FACTORS

- Allergic reaction
- Soaps, detergents, scouring compounds, and industrial chemicals
- Extremes of heat and cold
- Frequent use of soap and water
- Preexisting skin disease

CLINICAL MANIFESTATIONS AND ASSESSMENT

- Itching, burning, and erythema is present, followed by edema, papules, vesicles, and oozing or weeping as first reactions.
- In the subacute phase, the vesicular changes are less marked and alternate with crusting, drying, fissuring, and peeling.
- If repeated reactions occur or the patient continually scratches the skin, lichenification and pigmentation occur; secondary bacterial invasion may follow.

MEDICAL AND NURSING MANAGEMENT

The objectives of management are to rest the involved skin and protect it from further damage.

- Soothe and heal the involved skin and protect it from further damage.
- Determine the distribution pattern of the reaction to differentiate between allergic type and irritant type.

- Identify and remove the offending irritant; soap is generally not used on the site until healed.
- Use bland, unmedicated lotions for small patches of erythema; apply cool wet dressings over small areas of vesicular dermatitis; a corticosteroid ointment may be used.
- Medicated baths at room temperature are prescribed for larger areas of dermatitis.
- In severe, widespread conditions, a short course of systemic steroids may be prescribed.

For more information, see Chapter 52 in Pellico, L.H. (2013). *Focus on adult health. Medical-surgical nursing.* Philadelphia: Wolters Kluwer Health | Lippincott Williams & Wilkins.

Coronary Atherosclerosis and Coronary Artery Disease

The most common cause of cardiovascular disease in the United States is atherosclerosis, an abnormal accumulation of lipid, or fatty substances, and fibrous tissue in the lining of arterial blood vessel walls.

PATHOPHYSIOLOGY

Coronary artery disease (CAD) begins early in life as fatty streaks of lipids deposited in the intima of the arterial wall. The continued development of atherosclerosis involves an inflammatory response beginning with injury to the vascular endothelium. The presence of inflammation has multiple effects on the arterial wall, including the attraction of inflammatory cells (macrophages or monocytes, WBCs). Macrophages infiltrate the injured vascular endothelium and ingest lipids, creating "foam cells," which are present in all stages of atherosclerotic plaque formation. Activated macrophages also release biochemical substances that can further damage the endothelium, attracting platelets and initiating clotting.

The abnormal accumulation of lipid or fatty substances and fibrous tissue in the vessel wall, or atheroma, protrude into the lumen of the blood vessel, reducing blood flow to the myocardium. Rupture of this plaque forms a focus for thrombus formation leading to sudden cardiac death or acute myocardial infarction (MI).

RISK FACTORS

- Age (men >45 years old, women >55 years old)
- Gender (men <55 years old are at greater risk; after 55 years of age, men and women are at the same risk)
- Race (African Americans, Mexican Americans, Native Americans, and some Asian Americans demonstrate increased risk)
- Family history of first-degree relative with premature diagnosis of heart disease
- Presence of metabolic syndrome, which includes three of the following conditions: Insulin resistance, abdominal obesity, dyslipidemia, hypertension, proinflammatory state (high levels of C-reactive protein), prothrombotic state (high fibrinogen)

✴ N U R S I N G   A L E R T
C-reactive protein (CRP) is released into the blood during inflammatory states. The normal value is less than 0.1 mg/dL or less than 1 mg/L.

CLINICAL MANIFESTATIONS AND ASSESSMENT

Symptoms and complications develop according to the location and degree of narrowing of the arterial lumen, thrombus formation, and obstruction of blood flow to the myocardium. Symptoms include the following:

- Ischemia manifested as angina or MI
- Dysrhythmias, sudden death

✦ᴺᵁᴿˢᴵᴺᴳ ᴬᴸᴱᴿᵀ

Classic signs and symptoms of myocardial ischemia include an acute onset of substernal chest pain, described as crushing and/or pain and radiation to the chest, jaw, back, or arms; dyspnea; extreme fatigue; diaphoresis; nausea; and vomiting. Myocardial infarction pain differs from anginal pain in that pain of MI persists despite rest and nitroglycerine. Women often complain of atypical chest pain and nonspecific signs and symptoms.

Gerontologic Considerations

- Teach elderly patients to recognize that their chest pain–like symptoms (such as weakness) are indications that they should rest or take prescribed medications.
- Pharmacologic stress testing may be used to diagnose CAD in elderly patients because other conditions (eg, peripheral vascular disease, arthritis, degenerative disk disease, physical disability, foot problems) may limit the patient's ability to exercise.
- Sometimes "silent CAD" exists, in which there are no symptoms.

MEDICAL AND NURSING MANAGEMENT

See "Medical and Nursing Management" under "Acute Coronary Syndrome and Myocardial Infarction" on pages 20–23 for additional information including percutaneous coronary intervention (PCI) and coronary artery revascularization through coronary artery bypass grafting (CABG).

Controlling cholesterol and treating hyperlipidemia, and managing hypertension and diabetes mellitus are discussed here; additional medical and nursing management is discussed under angina.

Controlling Cholesterol Abnormalities

- Encourage all adults 20 years of age or older to undergo fasting lipid profile (total cholesterol, LDL, HDL, and triglyceride) at least once every 5 years and more often if the profile is abnormal. Patients younger than 20 years of age with a known family history of hyperlipidemia and/or vascular disease should probably be tested earlier.

- Patients who have had MI, a PCI, or a CABG require assessment of the LDL cholesterol level within a few months of the event, then every 6 weeks until the desired level is achieved; after that every 4 to 6 months.
- Set a goal with the patient to achieve an HDL level over 40 to 60 mg/dL. A high HDL level is a strong negative risk factor for heart disease (protects against disease). The goal is to have low LDL values and high HDL values.
- Assist the patient in planning to control serum cholesterol and LDL levels with diet and physical activity; antilipemics may be prescribed

Treating Hyperlipidemia

- Lipid-lowering medications can reduce CAD mortality in patients with elevated lipid levels and in at-risk patients with normal lipid levels. Monitor for adherence to the therapeutic plan, the effect of cholesterol-lowering medications, and the development of side effects.
- Encourage lifestyle changes that include a heart-healthy diet, increased physical activity for 30 minutes per day, smoking cessation, stress management, hypertension management, and diabetes management.

Managing Hypertension

- Encourage early detection, monitoring, and treatment for hypertension.
- Teach that adherence to a therapeutic regimen can prevent the serious consequences associated with untreated elevated blood pressure.

Controlling Diabetes Mellitus

- Teach the patient that hyperglycemia fosters dyslipidemia, increased platelet aggregation, and altered red blood cell function, which can lead to thrombus formation.
- Effective treatment with appropriate antihyperglycemic agents and diet improves endothelial function and endothelial-dependent dilation.

See "Nursing Management" under "Angina Pectoris" on pages 59–60 and "Acute Coronary Syndrome and Myocardial Infarction" on pages 20–23 or additional information.

> For more information, see Chapter 14 in Pellico, L.H. (2013). *Focus on adult health. Medical-surgical nursing.* Philadelphia: Wolters Kluwer Health | Lippincott Williams & Wilkins.

C

Cushing's Syndrome and Cushing's Disease

Cushing's syndrome, or hypercortisolism, is a disorder characterized by high levels of serum cortisol.

PATHOPHYSIOLOGY

Cushing's syndrome is commonly caused by use of synthetic corticosteroid medications and, infrequently, due to excessive corticosteroid production secondary to hyperplasia or tumor of the adrenal cortex. Overproduction of endogenous corticosteroids may be caused by several mechanisms, including a tumor of the pituitary gland that produces adrenocorticotropic hormone (ACTH). Primary hyperplasia of the adrenal glands in the absence of a pituitary tumor is less common. Another less common cause of Cushing's syndrome is the ectopic production of ACTH by malignancies; bronchogenic carcinoma is the most common.

RISK FACTORS

- Chronic use of corticosteroids
- Women between 20 and 40 years
- Primary hyperplasia of the adrenal gland in absence of a pituitary tumor
- Ectopic production of ACTH by malignancies

CLINICAL MANIFESTATIONS AND ASSESSMENT

- Arrested growth, weight gain and obesity, musculoskeletal changes, and glucose intolerance
- Classic features: Central-type obesity, a protruding abdomen with a fatty "buffalo hump" in the neck and supraclavicular areas, a round "moon-faced" appearance; skin is thin, fragile, easily traumatized, with ecchymoses and striae. Muscle wasting and thin extremities develop.
- Weakness and lassitude; sleep is disturbed because of altered diurnal secretion of cortisol.
- Excessive protein catabolism with muscle wasting and osteoporosis; kyphosis, backache, and compression fractures of the vertebrae are possible.
- Retention of sodium and water, producing hypertension, hypokalemia, and heart failure.
- Increased susceptibility to infection; slow healing of minor cuts, oiliness of skin, and acne
- Hyperglycemia or overt diabetes
- Virilization in females (due to excess androgens) with appearance of masculine traits and recession of feminine traits (eg, excessive hair on face, breasts atrophy, menses cease, clitoris enlarges, and voice deepens); libido is lost in males and females.
- Changes occur in mood and mental activity; psychosis may develop, and distress and depression are common.
- If pituitary tumor is present, visual disturbances may occur due to pressure on the optic chiasm.

DIAGNOSTIC METHODS

- Overnight dexamethasone suppression test to measure plasma cortisol level (stress, obesity, depression, and medications may falsely elevate results)
- Laboratory studies including serum sodium, blood glucose, serum potassium; 24-hour urine to assess free cortisol level
- CT, ultrasound, or MRI scan or ultrasound may localize adrenal tissue and detect adrenal tumors.

MEDICAL AND NURSING MANAGEMENT

Treatment is usually directed at the pituitary gland because most cases are due to pituitary tumors rather than to tumors of the adrenal cortex.

- Surgical removal of the tumor by transsphenoidal hypophysectomy is the treatment of choice (78% success removal rate).
- Radiation of the pituitary gland is successful but takes several months for symptom control.
- Adrenalectomy is performed in patients with primary adrenal hypertrophy.
- Postoperatively, temporary replacement therapy with hydrocortisone for several months may be necessary until the adrenal glands begin to respond.
- If bilateral adrenalectomy was performed, lifetime replacement of adrenal cortex hormones is necessary.
- Adrenal enzyme inhibitors (eg, metyrapone, aminoglutethimide, mitotane, ketoconazole) may be used for ectopic ACTH-secreting tumors that cannot be totally removed; monitor closely for inadequate adrenal function and side effects.
- If Cushing syndrome results from exogenous corticosteroids, attempts are made to taper the drug to the minimum required dose.

Nursing Management

Decreasing Risk of Injury

- Provide a protective environment to prevent falls, fractures, and other injuries to bones and soft tissues.
- Assist the patient who is weak in ambulating to prevent falls or colliding into furniture.
- Recommend foods high in protein, calcium, and vitamin D to minimize muscle wasting and osteoporosis; refer to dietitian for assistance.

Decreasing Risk of Infection

- Avoid unnecessary exposure to people with infections.
- Assess frequently for subtle signs of infections; corticosteroids mask signs of inflammation and infection.

Encouraging Rest and Activity

- Encourage moderate activity to prevent complications of immobility and promote self-esteem.
- Plan rest periods throughout the day and promote a relaxing, quiet environment for rest and sleep.

Promoting Skin Integrity

- Use meticulous skin care to avoid traumatizing fragile skin.
- Avoid adhesive tape, which can tear and irritate the skin when removed.
- Assess skin and bony prominences frequently.
- Encourage and assist patient to change positions frequently.

Improving Body Image

- Discuss the impact that changes have had on patient's self-concept and relationships with others. Major physical changes will disappear in time if the cause of Cushing's syndrome is treated.
- Weight gain and edema may be modified by a low-carbohydrate, low-sodium, and high-protein diet.

Improving Thought Processes

- Explain to patient and family the cause of emotional instability, and help them cope with mood swings, irritability, and depression.
- Report any psychotic behavior.
- Encourage patient and family members to verbalize feelings and concerns.

Monitoring and Managing Addisonian Crisis

Withdrawal of corticosteroids, by adrenalectomy, or by removal of a pituitary tumor places patient at risk for adrenal hypofunction and Addisonian crisis.

- Monitor the patient closely for hypotension, rapid weak pulse, rapid respiratory rate, pallor, and extreme weakness.
- Administer fluid and electrolytes, especially potassium and corticosteroids before, during, and after treatment or surgery.
- Anticipate and treat circulatory collapse and shock.
- Monitor blood glucose levels.

Teaching Patients Self-Care

- If indicated, stress to patient and family that stopping corticosteroid use abruptly and without medical supervision can result in adrenal insufficiency and reappearance of symptoms.
- Emphasize the need to keep an adequate supply of the corticosteroid available to prevent running out or skipping a dose because this could result in Addisonian crisis.
- Stress the need for dietary modifications to ensure adequate calcium intake without increasing risk for hypertension, hyperglycemia, and weight gain.
- Teach patient and family to monitor blood pressure, blood glucose levels, and weight.
- Stress the importance of wearing a medical alert bracelet and notifying other health professionals (eg, dentist) that he or she has Cushing's syndrome.

For more information, see Chapter 31 in Pellico, L.H. (2013). *Focus on adult health. Medical-surgical nursing.* Philadelphia: Wolters Kluwer Health | Lippincott Williams & Wilkins.

D

Diabetes Insipidus

Diabetes insipidus (DI) is a disorder of the posterior lobe of the pituitary gland characterized by a deficiency of antidiuretic hormone (ADH, vasopressin).

PATHOPHYSIOLOGY

Lack of ADH from the posterior pituitary results in loss of large volumes of dilute urine resulting in dehydration. Nephrogenic DI results from damage to the renal tubules, and psychogenic DI is caused by excessive water intake.

RISK FACTORS

- Head trauma, brain tumor, or surgical ablation or irradiation of the pituitary gland
- Infections of the central nervous system (CNS; meningitis, encephalitis, tuberculosis)
- Metastatic disease or cancers of the breast or lung. Nephrogenic diabetes insipidus may be related to hypokalemia, hypercalcemia, and medications such as lithium or demeclocycline (Declomycin) that impair the kidney's ability to reabsorb water.

CLINICAL MANIFESTATIONS AND ASSESSMENT

- Polyuria: Enormous daily output of very dilute urine, from 3 to 20 L/day
- Polydipsia: Patient experiences intense thirst, drinking 2 to 20 L of fluid daily, with a craving for cold water
- Hypotension, tachycardia
- Dry mucous membranes, poor skin turgor
- Weight loss

DIAGNOSTIC METHODS

There is no one diagnostic test for diabetes insipidus.

- A 24-hour urine collection is obtained to measure for volume and creatinine. A urine volume of less than 2 L/24 hours (without hypernatremia) rules out diabetes insipidus.
- Desmopressin (DDAVP; desamino-arginine vasopressin) challenge test; DDAVP is administered intranasally, subcutaneously, or intravenously with subsequent measurement of urine volumes, specific gravity, and/or urine osmolality. Elevation of urine osmolarity by more than 50% indicates neurogenic DI.
- Other diagnostic procedures include concurrent measurements of plasma levels of ADH and plasma and urine osmolality, as well as a trial of desmopressin (synthetic vasopressin) therapy, fluid deprivation test, and IV infusion of hypertonic saline solution.

MEDICAL AND NURSING MANAGEMENT

The objectives of therapy are (1) long-term replacement of ADH, (2) to ensure adequate fluid replacement, and (3) to identify and correct the underlying intracranial pathology.

Pharmacologic Therapy

- Desmopressin (DDAVP), intranasally, once or twice daily to control symptoms

- Vasopressin tannate in oil (ADH) intramuscularly, when intranasal route is not possible. Shake the vial vigorously or warm; administer in the evening; rotate injection sites to prevent lipodystrophy.
- Chlorpropamide (Diabinese), thiazide diuretics, and prostaglandin inhibitors such as ibuprofen, indomethacin, and aspirin may be used to potentiate the action of vasopressin.

Nursing Management

- Monitor vital signs, fluid volume status, intake and output (I & O) and weight.
- Demonstrate correct medication administration and observe return demonstration.
- Instruct patient and family about follow-up care and emergency measures, giving specific verbal and written instructions.
- Provide support for patients undergoing studies for possible cranial lesions.
- Advise patient to wear a medical identification bracelet and to carry medication and information about the disorder at all times.

For more information, see Chapter 31 in Pellico, L.H. (2013). *Focus on adult health. Medical-surgical nursing.* Philadelphia: Wolters Kluwer Health | Lippincott Williams & Wilkins.

Diabetes Mellitus

Diabetes mellitus is a group of metabolic disorders characterized by elevated levels of blood glucose (hyperglycemia). Diabetes affects nearly 24 million people in the United States, or approximately 8% of the population.

PATHOPHYSIOLOGY

Diabetes results from defects in insulin secretion, lack of response to insulin, or both. Insulin, produced by the pancreas, regulates the production, use, and storage of glucose. Insulin moves glucose from the bloodstream into cells and assists with storage of glucose in the liver as glycogen. Type 1 diabetes, an autoimmune process, is characterized by destruction of the pancreatic beta cells; type 2 results from insulin resistance and impaired insulin secretion. Long-term hyperglycemia may contribute to microvascular complications including kidney failure, neuropathy, and retinopathy. An increased incidence of macrovascular diseases lead to atherosclerosis of the coronary arteries and myocardial infarction (MI), cerebrovascular disease and stroke, or peripheral arterial disease.

Type 1 Diabetes

- About 5% to 10% of patients with diabetes have type 1 diabetes, which is an autoimmune process in which autoantibodies against islet cells cause immune destruction of the beta cells. It is believed to be initiated by genetic or environmental factors such as viruses or toxins.
- Type 1 diabetes has an acute onset and most commonly affects children and young adults, but it can occur at any age.
- Individuals with type 1 diabetes are dependent upon insulin injections for blood glucose control and prevention of ketoacidosis.

Type 2 Diabetes

- About 90% to 95% of patients with diabetes have type 2 diabetes. While commonly associated with older age and obesity, the incidence is increasing in children and young adults as the epidemic of obesity grows.
- Key problems are insulin resistance, in which tissues are less sensitive to insulin, or decreased insulin production.
- Associated with a slow, progressive glucose intolerance; its onset may go undetected for many years.
- Sufficient insulin usually is present to prevent the breakdown of fat ketone acids; diabetic ketoacidosis (DKA) does not typically occur; however, uncontrolled type 2 diabetes may lead to hyperglycemic hyperosmolar nonketotic syndrome (HHNS).
- Type 2 diabetes is first treated with diet and exercise, then with oral hypoglycemic agents, later with insulin if needed.

Gestational Diabetes Mellitus

- Gestational diabetes is characterized by any glucose intolerance with onset during pregnancy; occurs in up to 14% of women, increasing the risk for hypertensive and other complications.
- Risks for gestational diabetes include marked obesity, a personal history of gestational diabetes, glycosuria, or a strong family history of diabetes
- Many women with gestational diabetes develop type 2 diabetes later in life; they should be encouraged to maintain ideal body weight and reduce risks for type 2 diabetes.

RISK FACTORS

Because diabetes is frequently not diagnosed until complications develop, screening is recommended for overweight adults and children with risk factors for type 2 diabetes.

- High incidence in Native Americans, Alaska Natives, blacks, Hispanics, Asian Americans, and Pacific Islanders
- Patient previously identified with impaired glucose tolerance, prediabetes (fasting glucose of 100 to 125 mg/dL), gestational diabetes, or birth to a baby weighing more than 9 lbs
- Family history, obesity, hypertension, or elevated HDL cholesterol or triglycerides

Gerontologic Considerations

The incidence of hyperglycemia in the elderly is increasing; elderly adults are more likely to have coexisting illness such as hypertension, heart disease, stroke, and age-related problems that may complicate diabetes management.

CLINICAL MANIFESTATIONS AND ASSESSMENT

- Diagnosis of diabetes is based on fasting plasma glucose (FPG), with levels of 126 mg/dL or random plasma glucose levels exceeding 200 mg/dL on more than one occasion being diagnostic.

- Polyuria, polydipsia, polyphagia, and unexpected weight loss
- Dehydration, fatigue and weakness, vision changes, tingling or numbness in hands or feet, dry skin, skin lesions or wounds that are slow to heal, and recurrent infections

DIAGNOSTIC METHODS

- Fasting plasma glucose levels of 126 mg/dL or greater, or random plasma glucose or 2-hour postload glucose levels greater than 200 mg/dL
- Evaluation for complications, which may appear prior to diagnosis

MEDICAL AND NURSING MANAGEMENT

The main goal of treatment is to achieve normal blood glucose levels (euglycemia) without hypoglycemia while maintaining a high quality of life.

- Diabetes management has five components: Nutrition, exercise, monitoring, medication, education

Pharmacologic Therapy

- Patients with type 1 diabetes require daily insulin injections to control blood glucose levels. Type 2 diabetes is associated with insulin obesity and resistance; the primary treatment of type 2 diabetes is exercise and weight loss.
- Rapid- and short-acting insulins are expected to cover increases in glucose levels after meals soon after injection; the patient should eat no more than 15 minutes after injecting a rapid-acting insulin. Intermediate-acting insulins are expected to cover subsequent meals, and the long-acting insulins provide a relatively constant (or basal) level of insulin.
- Conventional insulin therapy requires a mixture of short- and intermediate-acting insulins once or more daily; the patient must maintain constant meal patterns and activity levels. Intensive insulin regimen involves three to four injections of

insulin a day and is beneficial in reducing the risk of complications; not all people with diabetes are candidates for this approach.
- Oral antidiabetic agents or insulin may be added if diet and exercise are not successful in controlling blood glucose levels in patients with type 2 diabetes.
- Oral antidiabetic agents include sulfonylureas, biguanides, alpha-glucosidase inhibitors, non-sulfonylurea insulin secretagogues (meglitinides and phenylalanine derivatives), and thiazolidinediones (glitazones).
- Insulin vials in use should be kept at room temperature, all others should be refrigerated. A 3-week supply of insulin syringes may be prepared and kept in the refrigerator.
- Insulin may be administered by traditional subcutaneous injection, jet injection, or continuous insulin pump.

Surgical Intervention

Transplantation of the pancreas or a portion of the pancreas, including islet cell transplantation, has been used on a limited basis.

NURSING PROCESS

The Patient With Diabetes

Assessment

- Assess blood glucose values and hemoglobin A1C.
- Determine if patient has and is able to use glucometer for pre-meal and bedtime glucose monitoring.
- Assess for signs and symptoms, and for patients knowledge of hyperglycemia, hypoglycemia, diabetes self-care, skin assessments, and long-term complications.
- Observe patient preparing and injecting insulin, and assess knowledge of signs, symptoms, and treatment of hyper- and hypoglycemia.
- Assess knowledge of vascular complications, smoking, the use of preventive health measures such as an annual influenza vaccination, pneumonia vaccination, and a daily dose of aspirin, unless contraindicated, as well as current medication regimen.

Nursing Diagnoses

- Imbalanced nutrition related to increase in stress hormones, secondary to the primary medical problem and imbalances in insulin, food, and physical activity
- Risk for impaired skin integrity related to immobility and decreased sensation
- Deficient knowledge about diabetes self-care skills related to new diagnosis, lack of basic diabetes education, or lack of continuing in-depth diabetes education

Potential complications from inadequate control of blood glucose may include:

- Hyperglycemia, hypoglycemia
- DKA or HHNS

Planning

The major goals for the patient include improved nutritional status, maintenance of skin integrity, and ability to perform basic diabetes self-care skills, as well as preventive care for the avoidance of chronic complications of diabetes and absence of complications.

Nursing Interventions

Nutrition

- Nutrition is the foundation of diabetes management. Total caloric intake is designed to attain or maintain reasonable body weight, control blood glucose levels, and normalize lipid levels and blood pressure to prevent heart disease.
- Meal planning should consider the patient's food preferences, lifestyle, usual eating times, and ethnic and cultural background. Recent advances in diabetes management and insulin therapy allow greater flexibility in the timing and content of meals.
- Calorie prescription is based on energy needs, age, and size; 50% to 60% of calories should be derived from carbohydrates, 20% to 30% from fat, and the remaining 10% to 20% from protein.
- Fats should be reduced to less than 30% of total calories, saturated fats to less than 7% of total calories, and dietary cholesterol to less than 200 mg/day.

(continues on page 268)

- The majority of carbohydrates should come from whole grain, fruits, and vegetables. Sucrose should be limited.
- To reduce saturated fat and cholesterol intake, some nonanimal sources of protein (eg, legumes and whole grains) should be included.
- Increasing dietary fiber, such as that found in legumes, oats, and fruits, increases satiety, helps with weight loss, and assists with lowering glucose and lipid levels.
- To assist with meal planning, counting carbohydrates, exchange lists, or the Diabetes Food Guide Pyramid may be used.
- Alcohol should be limited to one beverage daily for women and two for men. Alcohol may cause dangerous hypoglycemia, weight gain, hyperglycemia, and hyperlipidemia.
- Sweeteners may assist with dietary adherence and should be used in moderation.
- Patients should read food labels evaluating total calories in "sugarless," "sugar-free," "dietetic," or "healthy" foods that may contain honey, brown sugar, corn syrups, and/or saturated or hydrogenated vegetable fats or animal fats.

Exercise

- Moderate to vigorous regular exercise is necessary in lowering blood glucose, reducing cardiovascular risks, stress management, and providing a feeling of well-being.
- Patients should not exercise if blood glucose is over 250 mg/dL and ketones are in the urine.
- Prevent hypoglycemia during exercise by eating a 15 g carbohydrate or complex carbohydrate/protein snack prior to exercising, at the end of exercise, and at bedtime.
- Individuals with diabetes should discuss exercise with their health care providers and undergo medical evaluation before starting an exercise program.

Blood Glucose Monitoring

- Self-monitoring of blood glucose and interpretation of results is a cornerstone of diabetes management and prevention of long-term complications.
- Factors affecting self-monitoring of blood glucose performance include visual acuity, fine motor coordination, cognitive ability, comfort with technology and willingness to use it, and cost.

- Self-monitoring of blood glucose is recommended two to four times daily, usually before meals and at bedtime. All patients, should test their glucose when hypoglycemia or hyperglycemia is suspected; with changes in medications, activity, or diet; and with stress or illness.

Developing a Diabetic Teaching Plan

The focus of diabetes education is on patient empowerment, highlighting the knowledge, skills, and attitudes needed to maintain and improve one's health.

- The American Diabetes Association recommends that teaching include three levels of care: Survival skills, home management, and advanced skills to improve lifestyle and individualization of diabetes self-care.
- Survival skills should be taught as early as possible, including simple pathophysiology, treatment modalities, recognition of hypoglycemia/hyperglycemia, where to purchase and store insulin, and practical information such as when to contact the health care provider.
- Assess the patient's (and family's) readiness to learn; recognize patients will progress through stages of the grieving process.
- In-depth and continuing education involves more detailed information about preventive measures for avoiding long-term diabetic complications, such as foot care, eye care, and risk factor management.
- Directly observe patient skills; do not depend on self-report of abilities and skills.

Promoting Self-Care

- If problems exist with glucose control or the patient develops preventable complications, assess for physical or emotional factors interfering with self-care or need for more complete information.
- Assess for physical factors including decreased visual acuity, or emotional factors such as denial or depression, which may impair the patient's ability to perform self-care skills.

(continues on page 270)

- Assist the patient to identify if family, personal, or work have been given priority over diabetes management.
- Assess the patient for infection or emotional stress, which may lead to elevated blood glucose levels despite adherence to the treatment regimen.

NURSING ALERT

When stressed, the "flight-or-flight" response increases catecholamine release, which stimulates glucose production and inhibits insulin release, which elevates serum glucose levels.

Continuing Care

- Continuing care of patients with diabetes is critical in managing and preventing complications. Home health nurses can provide diabetes education, wound care, insulin preparation, or assistance with glucose monitoring.
- The patient should participate in recommended health promotion activities such as immunizations and age-appropriate health screenings.
- Participation in support groups is encouraged for patients who have had diabetes for many years, as well as for those who are newly diagnosed and their families.

Evaluation

- Achieves optimal control of blood glucose; reports absence of acute complications
- Maintains skin integrity, demonstrates proper foot care
- Demonstrates/verbalizes diabetes survival skills and preventive care
- Exhibits understanding of treatment modalities
- Takes steps to prevent eye disease
- States measures to control risk factors

COMPLICATIONS

- Hypoglycemia
- DKA
- HHNS

- Cardiovascular diseases such as peripheral artery disease (PAD), angina/MI, cerebrovascular accident (CVA)
- Retinopathy
- Neuropathy

> For more information, see Chapter 30 in Pellico, L.H. (2013). *Focus on adult health. Medical-surgical nursing.* Philadelphia: Wolters Kluwer Health | Lippincott Williams & Wilkins.

Diabetic Ketoacidosis

Diabetic ketoacidosis is caused by an absence or markedly inadequate amount of insulin resulting in hyperglycemia, ketosis, dehydration, electrolyte loss, and metabolic acidosis.

PATHOPHYSIOLOGY

Without insulin, the amount of glucose entering the cells is reduced, and output of glucose by the liver is increased, causing hyperglycemia. The kidneys excrete excess glucose, causing an osmotic diuresis; dehydration and electrolyte loss ensue. Lipolysis or breakdown of fats to ketoacids leads to the development of metabolic acidosis. Kussmaul respirations develop in response to acidemia, leading to rapid deep respirations. The breath may have a fruity odor as ketones are exhaled. Causes of DKA include insufficient or missed doses of insulin, physical or emotional stress, and illness or infection

CLINICAL MANIFESTATIONS AND ASSESSMENT

- Polyuria, polydipsia, polyphagia, weakness, and malaise
- Orthostatic or frank hypotension with rapid weak pulse in patients with volume depletion

- Gastrointestinal symptoms of acidosis, include anorexia, nausea/vomiting, and abdominal pain
- Blurred vision, weakness, and headache
- Acetone breath (fruity odor); Kussmaul respirations: Hyperventilation with very deep, but not labored, respirations as compensation for metabolic acidosis
- Mental status varies widely from alert to lethargic or comatose based on plasma osmolality.

DIAGNOSTIC METHODS

- Blood glucose level of more than 250 mg/dL
- Low pH: 6.8 to 7.3
- Low $PaCO_2$: 10 to 30 mm Hg
- Low serum bicarbonate level: 0 to 15 mEq/L
- Abnormal serum electrolyte levels (sodium, potassium, and chloride)

MEDICAL AND NURSING MANAGEMENT

In addition to treating hyperglycemia, management of DKA is aimed at correcting dehydration, electrolyte loss, and acidosis. For prevention of DKA related to illness, patients must be taught "sick day" rules for managing diabetes when ill.

Rehydration

- Initially, isotonic fluid replacement with 0.9% normal saline is administered at a rate of 0.5 to 1 L/hr for 2 to 3 hours, to replace fluid loss caused by polyuria, hyperventilation, and vomiting. Moderate to high rates of infusion (200 to 500 mL/hr) may continue for several more hours depending on patient's vital signs, physical assessment findings, and urinary output.
- When the blood glucose level reaches 250 mg/dL (16.6 mmol/L) or less, the IV solution may be changed to one containing dextrose 5% to prevent a precipitous decline in the blood glucose level.

Restoring Electrolytes

Potassium may be low related to diureses or high if related to acidemia. Serum levels of potassium will decrease as insulin facilitates the movement of potassium into the cells. Timely replacement of potassium is needed to prevent cardiac dysrhythmias.

☀ NURSING ALERT

Signs and symptoms of hypokalemia are not seen until the serum level is less than 3.0 mEq/L. The most profound effects are on cardiac function and may lead to dysrhythmia or weakness and fatigue.

Reversing Acidosis

Acidosis of DKA is reversed with insulin, which puts glucose back in the cell and inhibits the breakdown of fat that cause ketone production. Regular insulin is used by slow, continuous infusion (0.1 units/kg/hr) to reduce glucose by 50 to 100 mg/dL/hr. Subcutaneous insulin is resumed when acidosis is corrected and the patient can tolerate oral feeding.

☀ NURSING ALERT

To minimize the effect of adsorption of insulin to the IV container or tubing, it is recommended that the nurse "coat the IV line" by flushing the tubing with a priming volume of 20 mL before connecting it to the patient.

NURSING PROCESS

The Patient With Diabetic Ketoacidosis

Assessment

- Monitor hourly blood glucose for patients receiving insulin infusion.
- Monitor the electrocardiogram (ECG) for dysrhythmias indicating abnormal potassium levels.
- Assess vital signs, arterial blood gases, breath sounds, and mental/neurological status every hour and record.

(continues on page 274)

Diagnosis

- Fluid volume deficit related to polyuria and dehydration
- Fluid and electrolyte imbalance related to fluid loss or shifts
- Deficient knowledge about diabetes self-care skills/information

Planning

The major goals for the patient may include maintenance of fluid and electrolyte balance, optimal control of blood glucose levels, ability to perform diabetes self-care activities, and absence of complications.

Nursing Interventions

Maintaining Fluid and Electrolyte Balance

- Administer IV fluids, insulin, and electrolytes as prescribed.
- Encourage oral fluid intake when permitted.
- Measure intake and output.
- Monitor laboratory values of serum electrolytes (especially sodium and potassium).
- Explore factors that may have led to the development of DKA with the patient and family; review management strategies to prevent future complications.

Monitoring and Managing Potential Complications

- Fluid overload: Monitor cardiac rate and rhythm, breath sounds, venous distention, skin turgor, and urine output; monitor fluid intake and keep careful records of IV and other fluid intake, along with urine output measurements.
- Hypokalemia: Monitor cardiac rate, cardiac rhythm, ECG due to effects of hypokalemia on cardiac function.
- Cerebral edema: When serum osmolality is decreased too rapidly, fluid shifts into the CNS causing cerebral edema. Patients may complain of headache and exhibit changes in the level of consciousness (LOC) and cranial nerve dysfunction.

Evaluation

Expected Outcomes

- Achieves fluid, electrolyte, and acid–base balance
- Has absence of complications

For more information, see Chapter 30 in Pellico, L.H. (2013).
Focus on adult health. Medical-surgical nursing. Philadelphia:
Wolters Kluwer Health | Lippincott Williams & Wilkins.

D

Diarrhea

Diarrhea is a condition defined by an increased frequency of
bowel movements (more than three per day), increased amount of
stool (>200 g/day), and altered consistency (liquid stool).

PATHOPHYSIOLOGY

Diarrhea can result from any condition that causes increased intestinal secretions, decreased mucosal absorption, or altered (increased)
motility. Types of diarrhea include secretory, osmotic, malabsorptive, infectious, and exudative. It can be acute (self-limiting and
often associated with infection) or chronic (persists for a long period
and may return sporadically). It can be caused by certain medications, tube feeding formulas, metabolic and endocrine disorders,
and viral and bacterial infections. Other causes are nutritional and
malabsorptive disorders, anal sphincter deficit, Zollinger-Ellison
syndrome, paralytic ileus, AIDS, and intestinal obstruction.

CLINICAL MANIFESTATIONS AND ASSESSMENT

- Increased frequency and fluid content of stool
- Abdominal cramps, distention, intestinal rumbling (borboryg-
mus), anorexia, and thirst

- Often associated with urgency, perianal discomfort, incontinence, or a combination of these factors
- Painful spasmodic contractions of the anus and ineffectual straining (tenesmus) with each defecation
- Other symptoms, depending on the cause and severity and related to dehydration and fluid and electrolyte imbalances, include the following:
- Watery stools, which may indicate small bowel disease
- Loose, semisolid stools, which are associated with disorders of the large bowel
- Voluminous greasy stools, which suggest intestinal malabsorption
- Blood, mucus, and pus in the stools, which denote inflammatory enteritis or colitis
- Oil droplets on the toilet water, which are diagnostic of pancreatic insufficiency
- Nocturnal diarrhea, which may be a manifestation of diabetic neuropathy

DIAGNOSTIC METHODS

- When the cause is not obvious: Complete blood cell count, serum chemistries, urinalysis, routine stool examination, and stool examinations for infectious or parasitic organisms, bacterial toxins, blood, fat, electrolytes, and white blood cells
- Endoscopy or barium enema may assist in identifying the cause.

MEDICAL AND NURSING MANAGEMENT

- Primary medical management is directed at controlling symptoms, preventing complications, and eliminating or treating the underlying disease.
- Certain medications (eg, antibiotics, anti-inflammatory agents) and antidiarrheals (eg, loperamide [Imodium], diphenoxylate [Lomotil]) may reduce the severity of diarrhea and the disease.

- Increase oral fluids; oral glucose and electrolyte solution may be prescribed if tolerated; IV therapy is used for intolerance to oral replacement or rapid hydration in very young or elderly patients.
- Antimicrobials are prescribed when the infectious agent has been identified or diarrhea is severe.

NURSING PROCESS

Care of the Patient with Diarrhea

Assessment

- Elicit a complete health history to identify character and pattern of diarrhea, any related signs and symptoms, current medication therapy, daily dietary patterns and intake, past related medical and surgical history, and recent exposure to an acute illness or travel to another geographic area.
- Perform a complete physical assessment, paying special attention to auscultation of bowel sounds, palpation for abdominal tenderness, inspection of stool (obtain a sample for testing).
- Inspect mucous membranes and skin to determine hydration status, and assess perianal area.

Diagnosis

- Fluid volume deficit
- Impaired skin integrity

Planning

The nurse collaborates to restore fluid and electrolyte balance, identify cause(s) of diarrhea, and monitor frequency and consistency of stool.

Nursing Interventions

- Encourage bed rest, liquids, and foods low in bulk until acute period subsides.

(continues on page 278)

- Recommend bland diet (semisolids to solids) when food intake is tolerated.
- Encourage patient to limit intake of caffeine and carbonated beverages, and avoid very hot and cold foods, which increase intestinal motility.
- Advise patient to restrict intake of milk products, fat, whole-grain products, fresh fruits, and vegetables for several days.
- Administer antidiarrheal drugs as prescribed.
- Monitor serum electrolyte levels closely.
- Report evidence of dysrhythmias or change in level of consciousness immediately.
- Encourage patient to follow a perianal skin care routine to decrease irritation and excoriation.

Evaluation

- Brisk skin turgor, moist mucus membranes
- Electrolytes within normal range
- Patient reports decreasing liquidity, frequency of stool

⚡ N U R S I N G   A L E R T

Skin in elderly patients is sensitive to rapid perianal excoriation because of decreased turgor and reduced subcutaneous fat layers.

COMPLICATIONS

- Cardiac dysrhythmias due to fluid and electrolyte imbalance, especially hypokalemia
- Urinary output less than 30 mL/hr, muscle weakness, paresthesia, hypotension, anorexia, drowsiness
- Skin care issues related to irritant dermatitis, and death if fluid or electrolyte imbalances become severe.

For more information, see Chapter 24 in Pellico, L.H. (2013). *Focus on adult health. Medical-surgical nursing.* Philadelphia: Wolters Kluwer Health | Lippincott Williams & Wilkins.

Disseminated Intravascular Coagulation

Disseminated intravascular coagulation (DIC) is a potentially life-threatening disorder of bleeding and clotting. It is a sign of an underlying disorder, not a disease itself.

PATHOPHYSIOLOGY

In DIC, the normal hemostatic mechanisms are altered so that tiny clots form within the microcirculation of the body. These clots consume platelets and clotting factors, eventually causing coagulation to fail and bleeding to result The primary prognostic factor is the ability to treat the underlying condition that precipitated DIC.

RISK FACTORS

- Cancer
- Shock
- Abruption placenta
- Toxins or allergic reactions

CLINICAL MANIFESTATIONS AND ASSESSMENT

- Clinical manifestations of DIC are bleeding, ischemia, and organ failure, secondary to clot formation.
- Patient may bleed from mucous membranes, venipuncture sites, and gastrointestinal and urinary tracts.
- Bleeding can range from minimal occult internal bleeding to profuse hemorrhage from all orifices.
- Patients typically develop multiple organ dysfunction syndrome (MODS), including renal failure, respiratory failure, and multifocal CNS infarctions as a result of microthromboses, macrothromboses, or hemorrhages.

DIAGNOSTIC METHODS

- Characterized by low platelet and fibrinogen levels; prolonged prothrombin time (PT), partial thromboplastin time (PTT), and thrombin time; and elevated fibrin degradation products (D-dimers and clotting inhibitors; eg, antithrombin [AT]).
- The International Society on Thrombosis and Hemostasis has developed a highly sensitive and specific scoring system using the platelet count, fibrin degradation products, PT, and fibrinogen level to diagnose DIC. This system is also useful in predicting the severity of the disease and subsequent mortality.

MEDICAL AND NURSING MANAGEMENT

The most important focus of management is treating the underlying cause of DIC. A second goal is to correct the effects of tissue ischemia by improving oxygenation, replacing fluids, correcting electrolyte imbalances, and administering vasopressor medications. If serious hemorrhage occurs, the depleted coagulation factors and platelets may be replaced (cryoprecipitate to replace fibrinogen and factors V and VII; fresh-frozen plasma to replace other coagulation factors).

Heparin infusion, a controversial management method, may be used to interrupt the thrombosis process. Other therapies include recombinant activated protein C and AT infusions.

Nursing Management

- Assess coagulation studies, platelets, D-dimer
- Observe for occult or gross bleeding, including petechiae

Nursing Diagnoses

- Fluid volume deficit
- Impaired gas exchange

Nursing Interventions

Maintaining Hemodynamic Status

- Closely monitor vital signs, including neurologic checks, and assess for the amount of external bleeding.
- Avoid procedures and activities that can increase intracranial pressure, such as coughing and straining.
- Avoid medications that interfere with platelet function, if possible (eg, beta-lactam antibiotics, acetylsalicylic acid, nonsteroidal anti-inflammatory drugs [NSAIDs]).
- Avoid rectal probes or rectal medications and intramuscular injection medications.
- Use low pressure with any suctioning.
- Administer oral hygiene carefully: Use sponge-tipped swabs, salt or soda mouth rinses; avoid lemon-glycerine swabs, hydrogen peroxide, commercial mouthwashes.
- Avoid dislodging any clots, including those around IV sites, injection sites, and so forth.

Maintaining Skin Integrity

- Assess skin, with particular attention to bony prominences and skin folds.
- Reposition carefully; use pressure-reducing mattress and lamb's wool between digits and around ears, and soft absorbent material in skin folds, as needed.
- Perform skin care every 2 hours; administer oral hygiene carefully.
- Use prolonged pressure (5 minutes minimum) after essential injections.

Monitoring for Imbalanced Fluid Volume

- Auscultate breath sounds every 2 to 4 hours.
- Monitor extent of edema.
- Monitor volume of IV medications and blood products; decrease volume of IV medications if possible.
- Administer diuretics as prescribed.

Assessing for Ineffective Tissue Perfusion Related to Microthrombi

- Assess neurologic, pulmonary, and skin systems.
- Monitor response to heparin therapy; monitor fibrinogen levels.

- Assess extent of bleeding.
- Stop epsilon-aminocaproic acid (an anti-fibrinolytic), if symptoms of thrombosis occur.

Reducing Fear and Anxiety

- Identify previous coping mechanisms, if possible; encourage patient to use them as appropriate.
- Explain all procedures and rationale in terms that the patient and family can understand.
- Assist family in supporting patient.
- Use services from behavioral medicine and clergy, if desired.

For more information, see Chapter 24 in Pellico, L.H. (2013). *Focus on adult health. Medical-surgical nursing.* Philadelphia: Wolters Kluwer Health | Lippincott Williams & Wilkins.

Diverticular Disease

A diverticulum is a saclike herniation of the lining of the bowel that extends through a defect in the muscle layer. Diverticula may occur anywhere in the small intestine or colon but most commonly occur in the distal sigmoid colon. Diverticulosis exists when multiple diverticula are present without inflammation or symptoms.

PATHOPHYSIOLOGY

Diverticula form when the mucosa and submucosal layers of the colon herniate through the muscular wall because of high intraluminal pressure, low volume in the colon (ie, fiber-deficient contents), and decreased muscle strength in the colon wall. Inflammation and subsequent infection of the diverticulum (ie, diverticulitis), can cause the development of abscesses, which may eventually perforate, leading to peritonitis and erosion of the arterial blood vessels, causing bleeding. Diverticulitis may occur as an acute attack or may persist as a continuing, smoldering infection. The symptoms manifested generally result from complications: abscess, fistula formation, obstruction, perforation, peritonitis, and hemorrhage.

Diverticulosis exists when multiple diverticula are present without inflammation or symptoms. A low intake of dietary fiber is considered a predisposing factor, but the exact cause has not been identified. Most patients with diverticular disease are asymptomatic, so its exact prevalence is unknown.

RISK FACTORS

- Congenital predisposition is likely when the disorder is present in those younger than 40 years.
- Low intake of dietary fiber

CLINICAL MANIFESTATIONS AND ASSESSMENT

Diverticulosis

- Chronic constipation often precedes development; however, it may be asymptomatic.
- Bowel irregularity is characterized by intervals of diarrhea, nausea, and anorexia, and bloating or abdominal distention.
- Cramps, narrow stools, and increased constipation or at times intestinal obstruction with repeated inflammation is noted.
- Weakness, fatigue, and anorexia are present.

Diverticulitis

- Acute onset of mild to severe pain in the left lower quadrant
- Nausea, vomiting, fever, chills, and leukocytosis
- If untreated, septicemia

DIAGNOSTIC METHODS

- Colonoscopy with biopsy to rule out other diseases, when indicated
- Computed tomography (CT) scan to detect abscesses
- Abdominal X-ray may show free air under diaphragm if perforation developed
- Barium enema (BE) may be done, but has largely been replaced by colonoscopy; when symptoms of diverticulitis present, BE is contraindicated due to risk of perforation.
- Laboratory tests: Complete blood cell count, revealing an elevated white blood cell count, and elevated erythrocyte sedimentation rate (ESR)

Gerontologic Considerations

The incidence of diverticular disease increases with age because of degeneration and structural changes in the circular muscle layers of the colon and cellular hypertrophy. Symptoms are less pronounced among elderly patients, who may not experience abdominal pain until infection occurs. They may delay reporting symptoms because they fear surgery or cancer. Blood in stool may frequently be overlooked because of failure to examine the stool or inability to see changes because of impaired vision.

MEDICAL AND NURSING MANAGEMENT

Dietary and Pharmacologic Management

- Diverticulitis can usually be treated on an outpatient basis with diet and medication; symptoms are treated with rest, analgesics, and antispasmodics.
- The patient is instructed to ingest clear liquids until inflammation subsides, then a high-fiber, low-fat diet. A bulk-forming laxative is also prescribed.
- Antibiotics are prescribed for 7 to 10 days.
- Hospitalization is indicated for patients with significant symptoms, those who are elderly, immunocompromised, or taking

corticosteroids. The bowel is rested by withholding oral intake, administering IV fluids, and instituting nasogastric suctioning if vomiting or abdominal distention is present.

- An opioid is prescribed for pain relief. NSAIDs, however, are associated with increased risk of perforation and should be avoided.
- Oral intake is increased as symptoms subside. A low-fiber diet may be necessary until signs of infection decrease.
- Antispasmodics such as propantheline bromide and oxyphen-cyclimine (Daricon) may be prescribed.
- Normal stools can be achieved by administering bulk preparations (psyllium), stool softeners, warm oil enemas, or suppository (bisacodyl [Dulcolax]).

Surgical Management

- Immediate surgical intervention is necessary if complications (eg, perforation, peritonitis, hemorrhage, obstruction) occur.
- CT-guided percutaneous drainage of an abscess and IV antibiotics are administered for abscess formation without peritonitis, hemorrhage, or obstruction.
- Surgery may take place in one-stage resection, in which the inflamed area is removed and a primary end-to-end anastomosis is completed.
- Multiple-stage procedures may be performed for complications such as obstruction or perforation; a temporary or "double-barrel" colostomy may be created.
- See Chapter 24 for further discussion on fecal diversion procedures.

COMPLICATIONS

- Peritonitis
- Abscess formation
- Bleeding

For more information, see Chapter 24 in Pellico, L.H. (2013). *Focus on adult health. Medical-surgical nursing.* Philadelphia: Wolters Kluwer Health | Lippincott Williams & Wilkins.

E

Emphysema, Pulmonary

Emphysema describes an abnormal enlargement of the air spaces beyond the terminal bronchioles, with destruction of the walls of the alveoli.

PATHOPHYSIOLOGY

In emphysema, the alveolar and interstitial attachments are reduced and predisposed to collapse during exhalation. External airway compression and obstruction is caused by hyperinflation and air trapping. This results in "less room to breathe."

Emphysema is divided into two main types: panacinar or panlobular (hereditary form related to deficiency of alpha$_1$-antitrypsin, which causes uniform destruction of acinus [where alveoli are located]) and centrilobular (related to smoking, in which the alveolar ducts and bronchioles in the center of lobules of the upper lobes are primarily affected).

RISK FACTORS

- Smoking
- Inhalation of irritants
- Inherited disorders

MEDICAL AND NURSING MANAGEMENT

See "Nursing Management" under "Chronic Obstructive Pulmonary Disease" on pages 233–240 for additional information.

For more information, see Chapter 11 in Pellico, L.H. (2013). *Focus on adult health. Medical-surgical nursing*. Philadelphia: Wolters Kluwer Health | Lippincott Williams & Wilkins.

E

Empyema

Empyema is a collection of thick, purulent fluid accumulating in the pleural space and is often loculated (walled-off) where the infection is located.

RISK FACTORS

Pneumonia and other pulmonary infections

CLINICAL MANIFESTATIONS AND ASSESSMENT

- Patient is acutely ill with signs and symptoms similar to those of an acute respiratory infection or pneumonia (fever, night sweats, pleural pain, cough, dyspnea, anorexia, weight loss).
- Symptoms may be vague if the patient is immunocompromised or less obvious if patient has received antimicrobial therapy.

DIAGNOSTIC METHODS

- Chest auscultation, which demonstrates decreased or absent breath sounds over the affected area; dullness on chest percussion; decreased fremitus
- Chest computed tomography (CT) and thoracentesis (under ultrasound guidance)

MEDICAL AND NURSING MANAGEMENT

- The objectives of treatment are to discover the underlying cause of the empyema, prevent reaccumulation of fluid, and relieve dyspnea and respiratory compromise.
- Thoracentesis to remove fluid, to obtain a specimen for analysis, and to relieve dyspnea and respiratory compromise is performed; ultrasound may be used for guidance.
- A chest tube may be inserted to evacuate the pleural space and reexpand the lung.
- For malignancy, chemical pleurodesis to obliterate the pleural space may be performed. Talc, bleomycin, or doxycycline is instilled into the pleural space via chest tube or thorascopic route. Alternatively, surgical pleurectomy, decortication, or pleuroperitoneal shunt may be performed.
- A small catheter attached to a drainage bottle for outpatient management ((Pleurx catheter [Denver Biomedical]) may be used.

Nursing Management

- Prepare and position the patient for thoracentesis, offering support during the procedure.
- Ensure quantity of pleural fluid is recorded and sent for testing.
- Monitor chest tube and water-seal drainage system.
- Provide nursing care specific to the underlying cause of the effusion.
- Provide analgesia and/or antianxiety medications pre- and post-pleurodesis; reposition patient to facilitate distribution of the sclerosing agent throughout the pleural surface. Encourage the patient to splint the chest wall with hand or pillow.

For more information, see Chapter 10 in Pellico, L.H. (2013). *Focus on adult health. Medical-surgical nursing.* Philadelphia: Wolters Kluwer Health | Lippincott Williams & Wilkins.

Endocarditis, Infective

Infective endocarditis (IE) is an infection of the endocardium.

PATHOPHYSIOLOGY

E

Staphylococci and streptococci account for most IE. These pathogens colonize at the site of an abnormality or injury of the endocardium, such as a prosthetic valve site. Inflammation and infection result in endothelial damage and platelets, fibrin, blood cells, and microorganisms forming clusters or vegetations on the endocardium. The vegetations can embolize to other tissues throughout the body. The infection may erode through the endocardium into the underlying structures (eg, valve leaflets), causing tears or deformities of valve leaflets, dehiscence of prosthetic valves, deformity of the chordae tendineae, or paravalvular abscesses.

Acute IE is often caused by *Staphylococcus* infection and its onset is rapid, occurring within days to weeks. Subacute IE, usually caused by *Streptococcus,* occurs more slowly, and its course is prolonged. Systemic emboli occur with left-sided heart infective endocarditis; pulmonary emboli can occur when the right heart is infected, typically from IV drug use.

RISK FACTORS

- Nosocomial infection in patients with bacteremia and indwelling catheter, prolonged IV therapy with central venous catheters or hemodialysis patients
- Patients taking immunosuppressive medications or corticosteroids are more susceptible to fungal endocarditis.

- Intravenous drug use
- Body piercings
- Prosthetic heart valves or structural cardiac defects (eg, valve disorders, septal defects, hypertrophic cardiomyopathy [HCM])

CLINICAL MANIFESTATIONS AND ASSESSMENT

- Symptoms are often vague, such as anorexia, myalgias, fever, chills, weight loss, back and joint pain, and night sweats; fever may be intermittent or absent, especially in patients receiving antibiotic, corticosteroids, the elderly, or those with CHF or renal failure.
- Heart murmur may be absent initially but develops in almost all patients; murmurs that worsen over time indicate progressive damage from vegetations or perforation of the valve or chordae tendineae.
- Osler nodes, painful, erythematous nodules, may be present in the pads of fingers or toes.
- Janeway lesions, painless red or purple macules, may be present on the palms and soles.
- Roth spots, seen on funduscopic exam, are oval retinal hemorrhages with pale centers.
- Splinter hemorrhages may be seen under the fingernails and toenails.
- Petechiae appear on the neck, chest, abdomen, conjunctiva, and mucous membranes.
- Central nervous system manifestations include headache, transient cerebral ischemia, and strokes secondary to embolization; embolization may affect other organ systems.
- Cardiomegaly, heart failure, tachycardia, or splenomegaly may occur.

DIAGNOSTIC METHODS

A diagnosis of acute infective endocarditis is made when the onset of infection and resulting valvular destruction are rapid, occurring within days to weeks.

- Positive blood cultures; however, negative blood cultures do not rule out infective endocarditis, especially if a patient has received antibiotics or if slow-growing bacteria are present.
- Echocardiography to detect vegetations or abscesses, prosthetic valve dehiscence, new regurgitation or heart failure
- Anemia, elevated white blood cell (WBC) counts, elevated sedimentation rate (ESR), and elevated C-reactive protein
- Electrocardiographic (ECG) may demonstrate atrioventricular blocks, bundle branch blocks, and fascicular blocks.

MEDICAL AND NURSING MANAGEMENT

Prevention

- Modifications for antibiotic prophylaxis: Prophylaxis is no longer recommended with routine dental procedures, unless highest risk of adverse outcomes. For respiratory procedures involving incision (ie, tonsillectomy), prophylaxis is given. Gastrointestinal/genitourinary procedures no longer require antibiotic prophylaxis.
- Objectives of treatment are to eradicate the infection and prevent complications.
- Long-term, parenteral antibiotic therapy is given in doses that produce a high serum concentration to ensure eradication of the dormant bacteria within the dense vegetations. Initiate antibiotics as soon as blood cultures have been obtained.
- PICC or other long-term venous access devices may be needed: assess daily for redness, tenderness, warmth, swelling, drainage, or other signs of infection.
- Surgery is indicated in face of a persistent or recurrent infection, if heart failure occurs, or if patients have more than one serious systemic embolic episode, valve obstruction, valvular or myocardial abscess, or fungal endocarditis.
- Most patients who have prosthetic valve endocarditis require valve replacement, and this greatly improves the prognosis for patients with severe symptoms.

Nursing Interventions

- Monitor patient's temperature; a fever may persist for weeks.
- Assess heart sounds for new or worsening murmur.
- Monitor for signs and symptoms of systemic embolization and end-organ damage that may result, such as cerebrovascular accident, meningitis, heart failure, myocardial infarction, pulmonary embolism, glomerulonephritis, and splenomegaly.
- Instruct the patient and family about medications and signs and symptoms of infection.
- Educate patients who have previously received antibiotic prophylaxis regarding the updated recommendations.
- Blood cultures are taken periodically to monitor the effect of therapy, and serum levels of the selected antibiotic are monitored to ensure that the serum demonstrates bactericidal activity.
- Refer to home care nurse to supervise and monitor IV antibiotic therapy in the home.

For additional nursing interventions, see "Preoperative and Postoperative Nursing Management" in Chapter P on pages 531–554.

COMPLICATIONS

- Heart failure
- Cerebral vascular complications
- Valvular stenosis or regurgitation
- Myocardial damage
- Mycotic aneurysms

For more information, see Chapter 16 in Pellico, L.H. (2013). *Focus on adult health. Medical-surgical nursing.* Philadelphia: Wolters Kluwer Health | Lippincott Williams & Wilkins.

Endometriosis

Endometriosis is a progressive, benign gynecological disorder causing chronic inflammation and formation of adhesions.

PATHOPHYSIOLOGY

Endometriosis is the presence of endometrial-like tissue that proliferates outside of the uterine cavity, causing persistent pelvic pain, scarring, and infertility. The pathophysiology of this disease is largely unknown. It is thought to be caused by the retrograde flow of endometrial tissue through the fallopian tubes during menses and into the peritoneal cavity where this tissue seeds, forming adhesions in the pelvic, bladder, and bowel areas. The peritoneal endometrial tissues are influenced by the hormonal changes of the menstrual cycle and therefore swell, break down, and bleed; typically, the patients' symptoms worsen during the premenstrual phase.

E

RISK FACTORS

Affects women of childbearing years.

CLINICAL MANIFESTATIONS AND ASSESSMENT

- Chronic pelvic pain is the most common symptom.
- Low back pain, dyspareunia, dysmenorrhea, menorrhagia, dysuria, and dyschezia (pain with defecation); level of pain does not always correlate with stage of endometriosis.
- Cyclical bowel and bladder symptoms are difficult to differentiate between endometriosis, irritable bowel syndrome (IBS), or interstitial cystitis (IC) due to their similarity in presentation of symptoms.
- Tenderness of the fallopian tubes, ovaries, or uterus on bimanual exam would be an indication for further evaluation. The most common finding is tenderness with palpation of the posterior vaginal fornix, but a definitive diagnosis cannot be established without further diagnostic testing.
- Depression and pain that may lead to inability to work and difficulties in personal relationship is common.
- Infertility may occur.

DIAGNOSTIC METHODS

- A detailed health history regarding the patient's symptoms in relation to her menstrual cycle will help the health care provider establish a pattern.
- Transvaginal ultrasound visualizes the uterine cavity and endometrium for any adhesions.

MEDICAL AND NURSING MANAGEMENT

Treatment depends on symptoms, desire for pregnancy, and extent of disease. In asymptomatic cases, routine examination may be all that is required. Pregnancy often alleviates symptoms because neither ovulation nor menstruation occurs. Surgery may be indicated to relieve symptoms.

Pharmacologic Therapy

- NSAIDS for pain
- Continuous oral contraceptives suppress ovulation and growth of endometrial implants thereby decreasing inflammation and pain.
- Gonadotropin-releasing hormone (GnRH) agonists such as Lupron, androgenic agents (Danazol), and antiprogestogens (gestrinone) are considered second-line therapy. Side effects include hot flashes, vaginal dryness, and vasomotor symptoms associated with menopause.
- There are no differences in the outcomes of the use of combined oral contraceptives (COCs) over GnRH, although GnRH agonists have higher incidence of menopausal symptoms.

Surgical Management

- Surgical intervention is considered the last line of therapy.
- Exploratory laparoscopy with lysis of adhesions is considered the gold standard and temporarily decreases the pain and bleeding associated with endometriosis.
- Total abdominal hysterectomy remains the definitive therapy for those women who have completed their childbearing years.

- Complementary and alternative therapies include yoga, physical therapy, and massage.
- Due to the issues surrounding loss of fertility with this disease, stress management should be included.

For more information, see Chapter 33 in Pellico, L.H. (2013). *Focus on adult health. Medical-surgical nursing.* Philadelphia: Wolters Kluwer Health | Lippincott Williams & Wilkins.

Epididymitis

Epididymitis is an infection of the epididymis, which usually spreads from an infected prostate or urinary tract.

PATHOPHYSIOLOGY

In men younger than 35 years of age, the major cause of epididymitis is *C. trachomatis.* The infection passes upward through the urethra and the ejaculatory duct and then along the vas deferens to the epididymis, and can migrate to the testis as well.

RISK FACTORS

Sexually transmitted infection (STI)

CLINICAL MANIFESTATIONS AND ASSESSMENT

- Unilateral pain and soreness in the inguinal canal along the course of the vas deferens
- Pain and swelling in the scrotum and groin
- Bacteria (bacteruria) in the urine

- Chills and fever, along with nausea, urinary frequency, urgency, or dysuria
- Urinary frequency, urgency, or dysuria, and testicular pain aggravated by bowel movements
- Laboratory assessment includes urinalysis and Gram stain of urethral drainage if there is suspicion of STI.

MEDICAL AND NURSING MANAGEMENT

- Scrotal support, ice
- Antibiotics
- If associated with chlamydial infection, the patient's sexual partner must be treated with antibiotic.
- If no improvement occurs within 2 weeks, an underlying testicular tumor should be considered.
- Epididymectomy (excision of the epididymis from the testes) may be performed as a last resort for patients who have recurrent, refractory, incapacitating episodes of this infection.

Nursing Management

- Elevate scrotum with a scrotal bridge or folded towel to prevent traction on spermatic cord, to improve venous drainage, and to relieve pain.
- Administer antimicrobial medications until acute inflammation subsides.
- Provide intermittent cold compresses to scrotum to help ease pain; later, local heat or sitz baths may help resolve inflammation.
- Give analgesics as prescribed for pain relief.
- Instruct patient to avoid straining, lifting, and sexual stimulation until infection is under control.
- Instruct patient to continue with analgesic and antibiotic medications as prescribed and to use ice packs as necessary for discomfort.
- Explain that it may take 2 to 3 months for the epididymis to return to normal.

For more information, see Chapter 34 in Pellico, L.H. (2013). *Focus on adult health. Medical-surgical nursing.* Philadelphia: Wolters Kluwer Health | Lippincott Williams & Wilkins.

Epilepsy

Epilepsy is a group of syndromes characterized by unprovoked, recurring seizures.

PATHOPHYSIOLOGY

Seizures are temporary episodes of abnormal motor, sensory, autonomic, or psychic activity (or a combination of these) that result from sudden excessive electrical discharge from cortical neurons. A part or all of the brain may be involved. The most common syndromes are those with generalized seizures, which involve the brain diffusely, and those with partial-onset seizures, which are limited to one side of the cerebral hemisphere. Epilepsy can be idiopathic (formerly termed primary), in which no cause is identified, or symptomatic (formerly termed secondary), when the cause is known and the epilepsy is a symptom of another underlying condition, such as a brain tumor.

RISK FACTORS

- In most cases, the cause is unknown (idiopathic), some cases are inherited.
- Epilepsy may follow:
  - Traumas, head injuries, cerebrovascular diseases
  - Birth trauma, asphyxia neonatorum
  - Drug or alcohol intoxication
  - Fever, metabolic or nutritional disorders
  - Brain tumors, abscesses or infectious diseases, and congenital malformations

Not all seizures imply epilepsy. Although seizures are the cardinal symptom of epilepsy, seizures occur as a manifestation of an identifiable problem, such as hyponatremia or high fever. Once treated, the seizures cease. Epilepsy is a chronic disease and refers to recurrent, unpredictable, and unprovoked seizures.

CLINICAL MANIFESTATIONS AND ASSESSMENT

Seizures range from simple staring episodes to prolonged convulsive movements with loss of consciousness. Seizures are classified as partial, generalized, and unclassified according to the area of brain involved. Aura, a premonitory or warning sensation, may occur before a seizure (eg, seeing a flashing light, hearing a sound).

Simple Partial Seizures

In simple partial seizures, consciousness remains intact, whereas in a complex partial seizure, consciousness is impaired. Only a finger or hand may shake; the mouth may jerk uncontrollably; the patient may talk unintelligibly, may be dizzy, or may experience unusual or unpleasant sights, sounds, odors, or taste—all without loss of consciousness. However, it is understood that not all seizures or syndromes fit neatly into this classification, and patients may have more than one type of seizure.

Complex Partial Seizures

In complex partial seizures, the person either remains motionless or moves automatically but inappropriately for time and place, or he or she may experience excessive emotions of fear, anger, elation, or irritability. Whatever the manifestations, the person does not remember the episode when it is over.

Generalized Seizures (Formerly Grand Mal Seizures)

- Involve both hemispheres of the brain; intense rigidity of the entire body may occur, followed by alternating muscle relaxation and contraction (generalized tonic–clonic contraction)

- Simultaneous contractions of diaphragm and chest muscles produce characteristic epileptic cry.
- May bite tongue; patient is incontinent of urine and stool.
- Convulsive movements last 1 or 2 minutes.

Postictal State

The term *postictal* refers to the period after a seizure, when patients are often confused and hard to arouse and may sleep for hours. Many complain of headache, sore muscles, fatigue, and depression.

DIAGNOSTIC METHODS

- Medical history including previous seizure history, alcohol and drug use, medications, allergies, and family history.
- Question patient about illnesses that may have affected the brain, including head injury.
- Question women about last menstrual period (there is increased seizure frequency during menses) and pregnancy status.
- Ask the patient about common triggers associated with seizures; these can be olfactory, visual (flashing lights), or auditory (certain types of music), or related to fatigue, sleep deprivation, hypoglycemia, emotional stress, electrical shock, febrile illness, alcohol consumption, certain drugs, drinking too much water, constipation, and hyperventilation.
- Biochemical, hematologic, and serologic studies are performed.
- Magnetic resonance imaging (MRI), magnetic resonance spectroscopy (MRS), and positron emission tomography (PET) is performed to detect structural lesions such as focal abnormalities, cerebrovascular abnormalities, and cerebral degenerative changes.
- Single photon emission CT (SPECT) may be used to identify the epileptogenic zone.
- Electroencephalograms (EEGs) aid in classifying the type of seizure.
- Video recording of seizures taken simultaneously with EEG telemetry is useful in determining the type of seizure, duration and magnitude.

MEDICAL AND NURSING MANAGEMENT

The goals of treatment are to maintain the airway, stop the seizures as quickly as possible, ensure adequate cerebral oxygenation, and maintain a seizure-free state. Intravenous access is needed to administer medications and obtain blood samples.

Pharmacologic Therapy

Medications are used to achieve seizure control. The usual treatment is single-drug therapy.

- Intravenous diazepam, lorazepam, phenytoin, or fosphenytoin is administered slowly in an attempt to halt the seizures. General anesthesia with a short-acting barbiturate or neuromuscular blockade may be used if initial treatment is unsuccessful.
- To maintain a seizure-free state, other medications (phenytoin, phenobarbital) are prescribed after the initial seizure is treated.

Surgical Management

- Surgery is indicated when epilepsy results from intracranial tumors, abscesses, cysts, or vascular anomalies.
- Surgical removal of the epileptogenic focus is done for seizures that originate in a well-circumscribed area of the brain that can be excised without producing significant neurologic defects.

NURSING PROCESS

The Patient With Epilepsy

Assessment

- Obtain a complete seizure history. Ask about factors or events that precipitate the seizures; document alcohol intake.

Status Epilepticus

Status epilepticus (acute prolonged seizure activity) is a series of generalized seizures that occur without full recovery of consciousness between attacks. The condition is a medical emergency that is characterized by continuous clinical or electrical seizures lasting at least 30 minutes. Repeated episodes of cerebral anoxia and edema, along with loss of airway, may lead to irreversible brain damage. Common factors that precipitate status epilepticus include withdrawal of antiseizure medication, fever, and concurrent infection.

E

- Determine whether the patient has an aura before an epileptic seizure, which may indicate the origin of the seizure (eg, seeing a flashing light may indicate that the seizure originated in the occipital lobe).
- Observe and assess neurologic condition during and after a seizure. Assess vital and neurologic signs continuously.
- Assess effects of epilepsy on lifestyle.

Diagnosis

Nursing Diagnoses

- Risk for injury related to seizure activity
- Fear related to possibility of having seizures
- Ineffective coping related to stresses imposed by epilepsy
- Deficient knowledge about epilepsy and its control

Collaborative Problems/Potential Complications

Status epilepticus (see Box E-1 above) and toxicity related to medications

Planning

Major goals include prevention of injury, control of seizures, achievement of a satisfactory psychosocial adjustment, acquisition of knowledge and understanding about the condition, and absence of complications.

(continues on page 302)

Nursing Interventions

General Care and Injury Prevention

- Perform periodic physical examinations and laboratory tests for patients taking medications known to have toxic hematopoietic, genitourinary, or hepatic effects.
- Provide ongoing assessment and monitoring of respiratory and cardiac function.
- Monitor the seizure type and general condition of patient.
- Turn patient to side-lying position to assist in draining pharyngeal secretions.
- Have suction equipment available to maintain airway patency and prevent aspiration.
- Monitor IV line closely for dislodgment during seizures.
- Protect patient from injury during seizures with padded side rails, and keep under constant observation.
- Do not restrain patient's movements during seizure activity. Do not insert anything in patient's mouth.

Reducing Fear of Seizures

- Reduce fear that a seizure may occur unexpectedly by encouraging compliance with prescribed treatment.
- Emphasize that prescribed antiepileptic medication must be taken on a continuing basis and is not habit forming.
- Assess lifestyle and environment to determine factors that precipitate seizures, such as emotional disturbances, environmental stressors, onset of menstruation, or fever. Encourage patient to avoid such stimuli.
- Encourage patient to follow a regular and moderate routine in lifestyle, diet (avoiding excessive stimulants), exercise, and rest (regular sleep patterns).
- Advise patient to avoid photic stimulation (eg, bright flickering lights, television viewing); dark glasses or covering one eye may help.
- Encourage patient to attend classes on stress management.

Improving Coping Mechanisms

- Understand that epilepsy imposes feelings of stigmatization, alienation, depression, and uncertainty.
- Provide counseling to patient and family to help them understand the condition and limitations imposed.

- Encourage patient to participate in social and recreational activities.
- Teach patient and family about symptoms and their management.

Promoting Home- and Community-Based Care

Teaching Patients Self-Care

- For patients taking phenytoin (Dilantin), prevent or control gingival hyperplasia by teaching patient to perform thorough oral hygiene and gum massage and to seek regular dental care.
- Instruct patient to notify physician if unable to take medications due to illness.
- Instruct patient and family about medication side effects and toxicity.
- Provide specific guidelines to assess and report signs and symptoms of medication overdose.
- Teach patient to keep a drug and seizure chart, noting when medications are taken and any seizure activity.
- Instruct patient to take showers rather than tub baths to avoid drowning and to never swim alone.
- Encourage realistic attitude toward the disease; provide facts concerning epilepsy.
- Instruct patient to carry an emergency medical identification card or wear an identification bracelet.
- Advise patient to seek preconception and genetic counseling if desired (inherited transmission of epilepsy has not been proved).
- Encourage routine assessment of serum drug levels.

Continuing Care

- Financial considerations: Epilepsy Foundation of America offers a mail-order program for medications at minimum cost and access to life insurance, as well as information on vocational rehabilitation and coping with epilepsy.
- Vocational rehabilitation: The state Vocational Rehabilitation Agency, Epilepsy Foundation of America, and federal and state agencies may be of assistance in cases of job discrimination.

(continues on page 304)

Evaluation

Expected Patient Outcomes

- Sustains no injuries from seizure activity
- Indicates a decrease in fear
- Displays effective individual coping
- Exhibits knowledge and understanding of epilepsy
- Experiences no complications of seizures (injury) or complications of status epilepticus

For more information, see Chapter 46 in Pellico, L.H. (2013). *Focus on adult health. Medical-surgical nursing.* Philadelphia: Wolters Kluwer Health | Lippincott Williams & Wilkins.

Epistaxis (Nosebleed)

Epistaxis, a hemorrhage from the nose, is caused by the rupture of tiny, distended vessels in the mucous membrane of any area of nose. The anterior septum is the most common site.

RISK FACTORS

- Infections
- Drying of nasal mucous membranes
- Nasal inhalation of illicit drugs
- Trauma (including vigorous nose blowing and nose picking)
- Arteriosclerosis
- Hypertension
- Nasal or sinus tumors
- Thrombocytopenia
- Aspirin use
- Liver disease
- Hereditary hemorrhagic syndromes

MEDICAL AND NURSING MANAGEMENT

Management of epistaxis depends on its cause and the location of the bleeding site.

- Initial treatment includes applying direct pressure; sit patient upright with the head tilted forward to prevent swallowing and aspiration of blood, and pinch the soft outer portion of the nose against the midline septum for 5 or 10 minutes continuously.
- If pressure is unsuccessful, the nose is examined using good illumination; cotton applicators soaked in a vasoconstricting solution (ie, epinephrine, ephedrine, cocaine) may be inserted into the nose to reduce the blood flow.
- Visible bleeding sites may be cauterized with silver nitrate or electrocautery (high-frequency electrical current).
- Surgicel or Gelfoam may be used.
- If the origin of the bleeding cannot be identified, the nose may be packed with gauze impregnated with petrolatum jelly or antibiotic ointment. The packing may remain in place for 48 hours or up to 5 or 6 days if necessary to control bleeding.
- Antibiotics may be prescribed to prevent sinusitis and toxic shock syndrome.

Nursing Management

- Monitor vital signs, airway, and breathing, and assist in control of bleeding.
- Provide tissues and an emesis basin for expectoration of blood.
- Administer IV infusions of crystalloid solutions (normal saline), and maintain cardiac and pulse oximetry monitoring for significant hemorrhage.
- Once bleeding is controlled, instruct the patient to avoid vigorous exercise for several days and to avoid hot or spicy foods and tobacco; vasodilation may increase risk of rebleeding.
- Teach patient to provide self-care by reviewing ways to prevent epistaxis: Avoid forceful nose blowing, straining, high altitudes, and nasal trauma.
- Provide adequate humidification to prevent drying of nasal passages.

- Instruct patient how to apply direct pressure to nose with thumb and index finger for 15 minutes if nosebleed recurs.
- Instruct patient to seek medical attention if recurrent bleeding cannot be stopped.

> For more information, see Chapter 9 in Pellico, L.H. (2013). *Focus on adult health. Medical-surgical nursing.* Philadelphia: Wolters Kluwer Health | Lippincott Williams & Wilkins.

E

Esophageal Varices

Esophageal varices are dilated tortuous veins usually found in the submucosa of the lower esophagus; they may develop higher in the esophagus or extend into the stomach.

PATHOPHYSIOLOGY

- Caused by portal hypertension, secondary to cirrhosis or polycythemia. Scarring or thrombosis causes high pressures in the portal system, which may cause the varices to rupture. Bleeding can lead to hemorrhagic shock and increased nitrogen load from bleeding into the GI tract, which elevates ammonia levels and increases the risk for hepatic encephalopathy. Gastroesophageal varices are present in 50% of patients with cirrhosis, and hemorrhage is one of the major causes of death in patients with cirrhosis.

RISK FACTORS

- Alcohol intake
- Physical exercise
- Activities that increase intra-abdominal pressure: Lifting, straining at stool, coughing, or vomiting

CLINICAL MANIFESTATIONS AND ASSESSMENT

- Hematemesis, melena, or general deterioration in mental or physical status; often a history of alcohol abuse is present.
- Signs and symptoms of shock (cool clammy skin, hypotension, tachycardia) may be present.

☀ NURSING ALERT
Bleeding esophageal varices can quickly lead to hemorrhagic shock and should be considered an emergency.

DIAGNOSTIC METHODS

Endoscopic evaluation (or esophagogastroduodenoscopy [EGD]) is used in the diagnosis and treatment; should take place within 12 hours after stabilizing the patient.

MEDICAL AND NURSING MANAGEMENT

- Patient is critically ill, requiring intensive care for close monitoring and management.
- Airway protection with endotracheal intubation may be needed to prevent aspiration of blood.
- Obtain venous access administer isotonic fluids, volume expanders.
- Transfuse blood, blood components, and volume expander as indicated; avoid fluid overload as portal pressure rises and increased bleeding may develop.
- Evaluate vital signs frequently when hematemesis and melena are present.
- Monitor for hypovolemia using central venous catheter or pulmonary artery catheter as indicated.
- Administer oxygen to prevent hypoxemia; evaluate oxygenation via pulse oximetry or arterial blood gas (ABG).

- Indwelling urinary catheter is needed for frequent output monitoring.

Nonsurgical Treatment

Nonsurgical treatment is preferred due to high mortality associated with emergency surgery and the poor physical condition of most of these patients. Nonsurgical measures include pharmacologic therapy, endoscopic therapy, balloon tamponade, and transjugular intrahepatic portosystemic shunting (TIPS).

Pharmacologic Therapy

- Vasopressin (Pitressin), vasopressin with nitroglycerin, somatostatin and octreotide (Sandostatin), beta-blocking agents, and nitrates
- Antibiotic therapy (IV ciprofloxacin, or ceftriaxone in patients with advanced cirrhosis) to prevent infection and improve survival

Endoscopic Therapies

- Esophageal banding therapy and variceal band ligation
- Endoscopic injection sclerotherapy (EIS): A sclerosing agent is injected into the bleeding esophageal varices to promote thrombosis and eventual sclerosis.

Balloon Tamponade

- Used as a temporary measure to control bleeding in an active hemorrhage. In this procedure, pressure is exerted on the cardia (upper orifice of the stomach) and against the bleeding varices by a double-balloon tamponade (Sengstaken-Blakemore tube).
- Effective in controlling bleeding in 80% of patients; however is associated with lethal complications including esophageal rupture, aspiration, and rebleeding, and carries a high mortality risk; used as a temporary bridge to other treatments.

Transjugular Intrahepatic Portosystemic Shunting

- Transjugular intrahepatic portosystemic shunting (TIPS) procedure is indicated for the treatment of an acute episode of variceal bleeding refractory to pharmacologic or endoscopic therapy.

- TIPS rapidly lowers portal pressure in those who rebleed after pharmacologic or endoscopic prophylaxis has failed; may be a bridge to liver transplantation.
- Complications include bleeding, sepsis, increased hepatic encephalopathy, heart failure, organ perforation, shunt thrombosis, and progressive liver failure.

Nursing Management

- Closely monitor vital signs, with focus on pulse and blood pressure; after endoscopy observe for bleeding, perforation of the esophagus, aspiration pneumonia, and esophageal stricture.
- Administer antacids, histamine-2 antagonists, or proton pump inhibitors.
- After procedures, fluids are withheld until gag reflex returns; lozenges and gargles may be used to relieve throat discomfort if physical and mental status permit.
- Do not feed patient when bleeding: Assess nutritional status; initiate TPN as ordered.
- Perform a neurologic assessment, monitoring for signs of hepatic encephalopathy (findings may range from drowsiness to encephalopathy and coma).
- Thirst may be relieved by frequent oral hygiene and moist sponges to the lips.
- Administer vitamin K therapy for blood loss and coagulation abnormalities.
- Provide a quiet environment and calm reassurance.
- Observe for delirium secondary to alcohol withdrawal, which can complicate the situation.

COMPLICATIONS

- Hypovolemic or hemorrhagic shock
- Hepatic encephalopathy
- Electrolyte imbalances

For more information, see Chapter 25 in Pellico, L.H. (2013). *Focus on adult health. Medical-surgical nursing.* Philadelphia: Wolters Kluwer Health | Lippincott Williams & Wilkins.

Exfoliative Dermatitis

Exfoliative dermatitis is a serious condition characterized by progressive inflammation in which erythema and scaling occur.

PATHOPHYSIOLOGY

A profound loss of stratum corneum (ie, outermost layer of the skin) occurs, which causes capillary leakage, hypoproteinemia, and negative nitrogen balance. Because of widespread dilation of cutaneous vessels, large amounts of body heat are lost.

Exfoliative dermatitis has a variety of causes. It is considered to be a secondary or reactive process to an underlying skin or systemic disease.

RISK FACTORS

- It may appear as a part of the lymphoma group of diseases and may precede the appearance of lymphoma.
- Secondary or reactive process to an underlying skin or systemic disease.

CLINICAL MANIFESTATIONS AND ASSESSMENT

- Begins acutely as a patchy or a generalized erythematous eruption accompanied by fever, malaise, and occasionally gastrointestinal symptoms. The skin color changes from pink to dark red.
- After a week, the characteristic exfoliation (ie, scaling) begins, usually in the form of thin flakes that leave the underlying skin smooth and red, with new scales forming as the older ones come off.
- Hair loss may accompany this disorder. Relapses are common.

- Systemic effects include high-output heart failure, intestinal disturbances, breast enlargement, elevated levels of uric acid in the blood (ie, hyperuricemia), and temperature disturbances.

MEDICAL AND NURSING MANAGEMENT

Goals of management are to maintain fluid and electrolyte balance and to prevent infection. Treatment is individualized and supportive and is started as soon as condition is diagnosed.

- Patient may be hospitalized and placed on bed rest.
- Discontinue all medications that may be implicated.
- Maintain comfortable room temperature because of patient's abnormal thermoregulatory control.
- Maintain fluid and electrolyte balance because of considerable water and protein loss from skin surface.
- Give plasma expanders as indicated.

For more information, see Chapter 52 in Pellico, L.H. (2013). *Focus on adult health. Medical-surgical nursing.* Philadelphia: Wolters Kluwer Health | Lippincott Williams & Wilkins.

F

Fractures

A fracture is a break in the continuity of bone caused by direct blows, crushing forces, sudden twisting motions, and extreme muscle contractions.

PATHOPHYSIOLOGY

When a fracture occurs, adjacent structures may develop soft tissue edema or hemorrhage into the muscles and joints may occur. Joint dislocations, ruptured tendons, severed nerves, and damaged blood vessels may also result. When adjacent blood vessels and nerves are damaged, neurovascular complication may develop and the organs lying beneath the fracture may sustain secondary damage.

TYPES OF FRACTURES

- Complete fracture: A break across the entire cross section of the bone
- Incomplete fracture: Occurs when the break develops through only part of the cross-section of the bone (eg, a greenstick fracture)
- Oblique fracture: Runs across the bone at a diagonal angle of 45 to 60 degrees
- Comminuted fracture: Produces several bone fragments
- Impacted fracture: One whose ends are driven into each other
- Closed or simple fracture: Does not produce a break in the skin

- Open fracture, compound, or complex fracture: A break in which the skin or mucous membrane wound extends to the fractured bone
- Compression fractures: Caused by compression of vertebrae and are associated frequently with osteoporosis

CLINICAL MANIFESTATIONS AND ASSESSMENT

The diagnosis of a fracture is based on the patient's report of injury (if present) and symptoms, the physical signs, and the X-ray findings. Observe for:

- Acute pain and muscle spasm
- Loss of function due to pain and loss of bone integrity to which muscles attach
- Visible or palpable deformity; movement at fracture site where a joint is not present
- Shortening of extremity in fractures of long ones
- Crepitus or a grating sensation as bone fragments rub against one another
- Localized edema and ecchymosis secondary to trauma and bleeding into the tissues
- Five "P's" of neurovascular impairment: pain; poikilothermia or cold limb; pallor; paresthesia including numbness, "pins and needles," burning, itching, and/or tingling; and pulselessness or weak pulse
- Manifestations of blood loss, especially in fractures of the femur and pelvis

MEDICAL AND NURSING MANAGEMENT

Whenever a fracture is suspected, the affected body part should be immobilized before the patient is moved.

Emergency Management

- Splint the affected extremity/area or support the limb distal and proximal to the fracture.
- Cover open fracture sites with a sterile dressing.
- Do not attempt to reduce the fracture.

- Administer tetanus prophylaxis if last know booster is over 5 years ago.
- Maintain hemodynamic stability; a femur fracture may have an estimated blood loss (EBL) of 1,000 to 1,500 mL. An open fracture may increase the EBL by 50%.

Medical and Surgical Management

Goals include improving function by restoring motion and stability and relieving pain and disability.

- Reduction or "setting" the bone restores the fracture fragments to anatomic alignment and rotation.
- Closed reduction is achieved through manipulation and manual traction with application of cast, splint, or other device. Closed reduction with internal fixation (the fracture is reduced prior to surgery for internal fixation).
- Open reduction with internal fixation (ORIF). Internal fixation devices, metallic pins, wires, screws, plates, nails, or rods, are used to hold the bone fragments in position until bone healing occurs.
- Reduction under anesthesia with percutaneous pinning may be used.
- Traction (skin or skeletal) may be used to effect fracture reduction and immobilization.
- Wound irrigation and débridement is performed, often in the operating room, for open fractures.
- Administer analgesics.
- Amputation is reserved for severe extremity conditions (eg, massive trauma).
- Bone graft provide joint stabilization, defect filling, or stimulation of bone healing.
- Tendon transfer is used to improve motion.
- Note that open fractures are considered contaminated and carry risks for osteomyelitis, tetanus, and gas gangrene.

Nursing Management

The major goals for the patient with a fracture include knowledge of the treatment regimen, relief of pain, improved physical mobility, achievement of maximum level of self-care, healing of any trauma-associated lacerations and abrasions, maintenance of adequate neurovascular function, and absence of complications.

- Assess neurovascular status of immobilized extremity every hour initially, then every 4 hours, comparing to the nonaffected extremity.
- Assess for edema that can compromise circulation and nerve and motor function.
- Teaching and anticipatory guidance is given regarding treatment sensations and healing with restoration of full strength and mobility, which may take months.
- Manage pain with immobilization, elevation, cold packs, and analgesic medications.
- Monitor pain from patients in casts by evaluating for impaired tissue perfusion or pressure ulcer formation.
- Provide trapeze to facilitate repositioning.
- Provide range of motion (ROM) to joints and digits not immobilized.
- Prevent deep vein thrombosis (DVT) by encouraging the patient to perform active flexion–extension ankle exercises, calf-pumping exercises 10 to 20 times an hour, and to move digits and joints distal to injury to decrease venous stasis in the unaffected limb.
- Teach exercises to maintain health of unaffected muscles (see Box F-1 on page 316 for muscle setting exercises).
- Elastic stockings, intermittent compression devices such as Venodyne boots, and anticoagulant therapy may be prescribed to help prevent thrombus formation.
- Collaborate with physical therapist to teach patient to use crutches, walker, and assistive devices safely.

Monitoring and Managing Potential Complications

Fat Embolism Syndrome

- In fat embolism syndrome (FES), fat globules are released when a bone is fractured; these particles travel and may occlude

Muscle-Setting Exercises

Isometric contractions of the muscle maintain muscle mass and strength and prevent atrophy.

Quadriceps-Setting Exercise
- Position patient supine with leg extended.
- Instruct patient to push knee back onto the mattress by contracting the anterior thigh muscles.
- Encourage patient to hold the position for 5 to 10 seconds.
- Let patient relax.
- Have the patient repeat the exercise 10 times each hour when awake.

Gluteal-Setting Exercise
- Position the patient supine with legs extended, if possible.
- Instruct the patient to contract the muscles of the buttocks.
- Encourage the patient to hold the contraction for 5 to 10 seconds.
- Let the patient relax.
- Have the patient repeat the exercise 10 times each hour when awake.

the small blood vessels that supply the lungs, brain, kidneys, and other organs.
- Onset is rapid, within 24 to 72 hours after injury.
- Risk factors include trauma, fracture of long bones or pelvic bones, multiple fractures, or crush injuries; more typically seen in adults 20 to 30 years of age and in adults with fractures of proximal femur (hip).
- Presenting features include change in behavior and disorientation combined with respiratory compromise. Additional symptoms include hypoxia, axillary, subconjunctival or petechiae of the chest, tachypnea, tachycardia, and pyrexia. Respiratory manifestations include tachypnea, dyspnea, crackles, wheezes, and substernal chest pain.

- Arterial blood gas (ABG) findings reveal a PaO_2 below 60 mm Hg, with an early respiratory alkalosis (hyperventilation) and later respiratory acidosis (hypoventilation).
- The chest radiograph exhibits a typical "snowstorm" infiltrate.
- Acute pulmonary edema, acute respiratory distress syndrome (ARDS), and heart failure may develop.
- Cerebral disturbances due to hypoxia and fat embolization to the brain include mental status changes varying from headache and mild agitation to confusion, delirium, and coma.
- Free fat may be found in the urine if emboli are filtered by the renal tubules. Acute tubular necrosis and renal failure may develop.
- Measures to reduce incidence of FES include immediate immobilization with minimal manipulation, and maintenance of fluid and electrolyte balance.

N U R S I N G A L E R T

Subtle personality changes, restlessness, irritability, or confusion in a patient who has sustained a fracture are indications for immediate reassessment of the patient's vitals, O_2 sat, physical examination, and laboratory data.

Additional Complications

- Delayed union refers to prolonged healing, malunion refers to flawed union of fractured bone, nonunion results from failure of the ends of a fractured bone to unite in normal alignment.
- Venous thromboembolism, including DVT and pulmonary embolism (PE) may occur several days to weeks after the injury.
- Disseminated intravascular coagulation (DIC) results in widespread hemorrhage and microthrombosis with ischemia. The nurse watches for unexpected bleeding after surgery, bleeding from mucous membranes, venipuncture sites, the gastrointestinal (GI) and urinary tracts.
- Avascular necrosis of bone (AVN) refers to bone that has lost its blood supply and dies, causing pain and limited movement. Treatment generally consists of attempts to revitalize the bone with bone grafts, prosthetic replacement, or arthrodesis (joint fusion).

F

- Reaction to internal fixation devices may necessitate removal; these include faulty or damaged device, corrosion of the device, allergy to the metal, and osteoporotic remodeling adjacent to the fixation device.
- Infection in the area of external fixation device will demonstrate erythema, purulent drainage, warmth, leukocytosis, and fever. Perform pin care according to hospital and provider protocol.
- Complex regional pain syndrome (CRPS) formerly called RSD, is a painful sympathetic nervous system problem, manifested by severe burning pain, swelling, hyperesthesia, limited ROM, discoloration, vasomotor skin changes (ie, fluctuating warm, red, dry and cold, sweaty, cyanotic), and trophic changes (ie, glossy, shiny skin, increased hair and nail growth). Early effective pain relief is achieved with nerve blocks, tricyclic antidepressants, anticonvulsants, nonsteroidal anti-inflammatory drugs (NSAIDs), corticosteroids, muscle relaxants, and opioids for severe pain.
- Heterotopic ossification (myositis ossificans) is the abnormal formation of bone, near bones or in muscle, in response to soft-tissue injury. Muscle pain occurs and normal muscular movement are limited. Early mobilization and NSAIDs for deep muscle contusion may prevent its occurrence. The bone lesion usually resolves over time, but may need to be excised for persistent symptoms.

FRACTURES OF SPECIFIC SITES

The type and location of the fracture and the extent of damage to surrounding structures determine the therapeutic management. Maximum functional recovery is the goal of management.

CLAVICLE

- Fracture of the clavicle (collar bone) commonly results from a fall or a direct blow to the shoulder, such as during equestrian sports or cycling. Head or cervical spine injuries may accompany these fractures. They are also seen in the geriatric population after a low-impact fall.

- When the clavicle is fractured, the patient assumes a protective position, slumping the shoulders and immobilizing the arm to prevent shoulder movements.
- The treatment goal is to align the shoulder in its normal position by means of closed reduction and immobilization with a clavicular strap or arm sling; if displaced, an ORIF may be performed.
- Caution the patient not to elevate the arm above shoulder level until the fracture has healed (about 6 weeks) and to avoid vigorous activity for 3 months. Encourage the patient to exercise the elbow, wrist, and fingers as soon as possible and, when prescribed, to perform shoulder exercises. Tell the patient that vigorous activity is limited for 3 months.

HUMERAL SHAFT

- Fractures of the shaft of the humerus may injure the nerves and brachial blood vessels in the affected arm, therefore neurovascular assessment is essential to identify when immediate attention is required. A wrist drop is indicative of radial nerve injury. An ORIF of a fracture of the humerus is necessary if the patient has nerve palsy, blood vessel damage, comminuted fracture, or pathologic fracture.
- For uncomplicated fractures, a sling or collar and cuff support the forearm.
- Pendulum shoulder exercises are performed as prescribed to provide active movement of the shoulder, thereby preventing adhesions of the shoulder joint capsule.
- Complications that are seen with humeral shaft fractures include delayed union and nonunion (failure of the ends of a fractured bone to unite).

ELBOW

- Elbow fractures (distal humerus) may result in injury to the radial head, distal humerus, or proximal ulna with resulting damage to the median, radial, or ulnar nerves. Evaluate the patient for paresthesia and signs of compromised circulation in the forearm and hand.

- Volkmann's ischemic contracture, an acute compartment syndrome obstructing arterial blood flow, results from antecubital swelling or damage to the brachial artery. The patient is unable to extend the fingers, describes severe pain at the elbow, and increasing tenseness of the forearm with signs of diminished circulation to the hand.

NURSING ALERT
Absence of a radial pulse is a critical finding that warrants emergency notification of the provider.

HAND

- Trauma to the hand often requires extensive reconstructive surgery.
- For an undisplaced fracture of the phalanx (finger bone), the finger is splinted for 3 to 4 weeks to relieve pain and to protect the finger from further trauma.
- Displaced fractures and open fractures may require ORIF, using wires or pins.

ARM

- The most frequently broken arm bone is the radius, and the site most commonly affected is the distal radius.
- Fractures of the distal radius that may involve the distal ulna, termed a Colles' fracture, are usually the result of a fall on an open, dorsiflexed hand; this is frequently seen in elderly women with osteoporosis or in younger people, resulting from sports injuries.
- The patient presents with a deformed wrist, radial deviation, pain, swelling, weakness, limited finger ROM, and numbness.
- Treatment usually consists of closed reduction and immobilization with a short-arm cast. For excessive comminuted

fracture or impaction, ORIF, arthroscopic percutaneous pinning, or external fixation is used to achieve and maintain reduction and to allow for early functional rehabilitation.

- The wrist and forearm are elevated for 48 hours after reduction to control swelling, and active motion of the fingers and shoulder begins promptly. The nurse monitors for signs of neurovascular compromise, comparing findings on affected limb to unaffected limb.

TIBIA AND FIBULA

- The most common fractures below the knee are tibia and fibula fractures, which tend to result from a direct blow, falls with the foot in a flexed position, or a violent twisting motion.
- The patient presents with pain, deformity, obvious hematoma, and considerable edema. Frequently, these fractures are open and involve severe soft tissue damage because there is little subcutaneous tissue in the area.
- The peroneal nerve is assessed for damage that may result in foot drop; this is done by checking for sensation in the web between the great and second toes and increased sensitivity of the dorsal surfaces of the foot (top). If nerve function is impaired, the patient cannot dorsiflex the great toe and has diminished sensation in the first web space (between first metatarsal and hallux [big toe]).
- The patient is observed for signs of neurovascular complications, including acute compartment syndrome.
- Other complications include delayed union, infection, impaired wound edge healing due to limited soft tissue, and loosening of the internal fixation hardware (if ORIF is performed to repair fracture).
- Most closed tibial fractures are treated with closed reduction and initial immobilization in a long-leg walking cast or a patellar tendon–bearing cast.
- Comminuted fractures may be treated with skeletal traction; internal fixation with intramedullary nails, plates, and screws; or external fixation.

PELVIS

- Falls, motor vehicle crashes, and crush injuries can cause pelvic fractures.
- Pelvic fractures are serious because at least two-thirds of affected patients have significant and multiple injuries. Hemorrhage and thoracic, intra-abdominal, and cranial injuries have priority over treatment of fractures.
- There is a high mortality rate associated with pelvic fractures related to hemorrhage, pulmonary complications, fat emboli, thromboembolic complications, and infection.
- Signs and symptoms of pelvic fracture include ecchymosis; tenderness over the symphysis pubis, anterior iliac spines, iliac crest, sacrum, or coccyx (Fig. 42-7); local edema; numbness or tingling of the pubis, genitals, and proximal thighs; and inability to bear weight without discomfort.
- Hemorrhage and shock are two of the most serious consequences. Peritoneal lavage or abdominal computed tomography (CT) may be performed to detect intra-abdominal hemorrhage. The patient is handled gently to minimize further bleeding and shock. Neurovascular assessment of the lower extremities may demonstrate absence of a peripheral pulse, indicating a tear in the iliac artery or one of its branches.
- Injuries to the bladder, rectum, intestines, other abdominal organs, and pelvic vessels and nerves are associated with pelvic fracture. Observe for hematuria or blood at the introitus; for men, observe for scrotal hematoma. Ecchymosis of the anterior abdominal wall, flank, sacral, or gluteal region is suggestive of significant internal bleeding. Diffuse and intense abdominal pain, hyperactive or absent bowel sounds, and abdominal rigidity and hyperresonance (free air), or dullness to percussion (blood) suggest injury to the intestines or abdominal bleeding.
- Loss of dullness over the liver (normally percusses a dull sound) indicates the presence of free air, and dullness over regions normally tympanic may indicate the presence of blood or fluid.
- Long-term complications of pelvic fractures include malunion, nonunion, residual gait disturbances, and back pain from ligament injury.

F

Stable Pelvic Fractures

- Stable fractures of the pelvis heal rapidly due to its rich blood supply.
- Bed rest for a few days and symptom management until the pain and discomfort are controlled is prescribed.
- If the sacrum is fractured, the patient is at risk for paralytic ileus; the nurse monitors bowel sounds.

Unstable Pelvic Fractures

- Unstable fractures of the pelvis may result in rotational instability (eg, the "open book" type, in which a separation occurs at the symphysis pubis with sacral ligament disruption), vertical instability (eg, the vertical shear type, with superior–inferior displacement), or a combination of both.
- Emergent treatment includes stabilizing the pelvic bones and tamponading or compressing bleeding vessels. Tying a sheet around the hips at the level of the greater trochanters may be done to temporarily close the "open book" fracture and control bleeding.
- Laceration of major vessels may require interventional radiologic technique to provide emergent embolization prior to surgery.
- Patients with pelvic fractures can lose up to 4 to 5 L of blood and therefore are at risk for exsanguination. Mortality rates for patients presenting with hypotension associated with pelvic fractures is approximately 50%.
- Once the patient is hemodynamically stable, treatment generally involves external fixation or ORIF.

ACETABULAR FRACTURES

- Drivers and passengers sitting in the right front seat in motor vehicle crashes whose knees are forcibly propelled into the dashboard typically cause fractures of the acetabulum.
- Stable, nondisplaced fractures may be managed with traction and protective (toe-touch) weight-bearing so that the affected foot is only placed on the floor for balance.
- Displaced and unstable acetabular fractures are treated with open reduction, joint débridement, and internal fixation or

arthroplasty, which replaces all or part of the joint surfaces. Internal fixation permits early non–weight-bearing ambulation and ROM exercise.
- Complications seen with acetabular fractures include nerve palsy, heterotopic ossification, and posttraumatic arthritis.

FEMORAL SHAFT

- Most femoral fractures occur in young adults involved in a motor vehicle crash or who have fallen from a high place. Frequently, these patients have associated multiple injuries.
- Symptoms include an enlarged, deformed, painful thigh, and the patient cannot move the hip or the knee. Frequently, the patient develops shock, because the loss of 2 to 3 units of blood into the tissues is common with these fractures. An expanding diameter of the thigh may indicate continued bleeding.
- The fracture is immobilized so that additional soft-tissue damage does not occur. Generally, skeletal traction or splinting is used to immobilize fracture fragments until the patient is physiologically stable and ready for ORIF procedures.
- Internal fixation with intramedullary locking nail devices or screw plate fixation may be used, which permits early mobilization. A thigh cuff orthosis may be used for external support.
- The patient is instructed to exercise the hip and the lower leg, foot, and toes on a regular basis to preserve muscle strength, by increasing blood supply and electrical potentials at the fracture site.
- Prescribed weight-bearing limits are based on the type of fracture. Physical therapy includes ROM and strengthening exercises, safe use of ambulatory aids, and gait training. Healing time is 4 to 6 months.
- A common complication is restriction of knee motion; active and passive knee exercises should begin as soon as possible.

FEMUR

- Hip fracture refers to a break in the proximal femur, including the femoral head, femoral neck between the greater and lesser trochanter (termed an intertrochanteric fracture), and the

shaft of the femur below the lesser trochanter (termed a subtro-
chanteric fracture).

- Fractures of the neck of the femur may damage the vascular
  system that supplies blood to the head and the neck of the
  femur, and the bone may become ischemic, causing avascular
  necrosis (AVN).
- The elderly are particularly vulnerable to intertrochanteric fractures
  and generally have a much worse prognosis than younger patients.
- Hip fractures are associated with a high incidence of DVT and
  PE, and an increased mortality rate the year after surgery.

Clinical Manifestations and Assessment of Femur Fractures

- With fractures of the femoral neck, the leg is shortened and
  externally rotated. The patient complains of pain in the hip and
  groin or knee.
- Severe pain increases with movement.
- Impacted intracapsular femoral neck fractures cause moderate
  discomfort, may allow the patient to bear weight, and may not
  demonstrate obvious shortening or rotational changes.
- Extracapsular femoral fractures of the trochanteric or subtro-
  chanteric regions cause a significantly shortened extremity that
  is externally rotated, exhibit muscle spasm that resists positioning of the extremity in a neutral position, and has an associated
  large hematoma or area of ecchymosis.
- The diagnosis of fractured hip is confirmed with an X-ray.

Gerontologic Considerations

- Elderly people (particularly women) with osteoporosis and who
  tend to fall frequently have a high incidence of hip fracture.
- Weak quadriceps muscles, general frailty due to age, and
  comorbidities that produce decreased cerebral arterial perfusion (transient ischemic attacks, anemia, emboli, cardiovascular disease, and medication effects) contribute to the incidence of falls.
- Many elderly people hospitalized with hip fractures exhibit delirium as a result of the stress of the trauma, unfamiliar surroundings, sleep deprivation, hypoxemia, anesthesia, and medications.

- Assess elderly patients as described above and for polypharmacy, dehydration, and hemoconcentration, which predisposes the patient to venous thromboemboli, and for poor nutrition.
- Muscle weakness and wasting that may have initially contributed to the fall and fracture will be further compromised by bed rest and immobility. Encourage the patient to move all unaffected joints; strengthening of the arms and shoulders will facilitate walking with assistive devices.

NURSING ALERT

When a patient presents with altered level of consciousness (LOC), the nurse uses the mnemonic DOG: Drugs are reviewed to evaluate their effect on altered sensorium; Oxygen saturation level via oximeter assesses for hypoxemia; and Glucose level by fingerstick is obtained to evaluate for hypoglycemia/hyperglycemia.

Medical Management of Femur Fractures

- Skin or skeletal traction (pins or wires inserted into bones) may be used until the patient is stable for surgical treatment. Continued neurovascular monitoring and assessment of the skin is performed.
- Skin traction, such as Buck's extension traction, is an example of straight or running traction used to reduce muscle spasm, immobilize the extremity, and relieve pain. Balanced suspension traction "floats" or suspends the affected extremity in the traction apparatus through use of balanced weights.
- Skeletal traction is used more frequently to immobilize fracture fragments until the patient is physiologically stable and ready for surgical treatment. However, skeletal traction can increase the risk of infection since sterile pin(s) are drilled or wires are placed into the bone.

Surgical Management of Femur Fractures

Surgical intervention is carried out promptly after hip fracture to provide early mobility and prevent complications. Surgical treatment consists of one of the following:

- Open or closed reduction of the fracture and internal fixation; a thigh cuff orthosis may be used for external support

- Replacement of the femoral head with prosthesis (hemiarthroplasty). This is usually reserved for fractures that cannot be satisfactorily reduced or securely nailed or to avoid complications of nonunion and AVN of the head of the femur. Closed reduction with percutaneous stabilization is used for an intracapsular fracture.

Nursing Management of Femur Fractures

The immediate postoperative care for a patient with a hip fracture is similar to that for other patients undergoing major surgery.

Encouraging Activity

- The patient is encouraged to use the overbed trapeze for exercise and to strengthen the arms and shoulders in preparation for ambulation.
- Active and passive knee exercises begin as soon as possible.
- The patient is instructed to exercise the noninjured hip and the lower leg, foot, and toes on a regular basis.
- The surgeon prescribes the degree of weight bearing: On the first postoperative day, generally, the patient transfers to a chair with assistance and begins assisted ambulation. Typically, hip flexion and internal rotation restrictions apply *only* if the patient has had a hemiarthroplasty (replacement of the ball of the hip).
- The patient can anticipate discharge to home or to an extended care facility with the use of an ambulatory aid. Some modifications in the home may be needed, such as installation of elevated toilet seats and grab bars.

Monitoring and Managing Potential Complications

Attention is given to pain management and to prevention of secondary medical problems, such as hemorrhagic shock, atelectasis, pneumonia, DVT, heart failure, constipation, pressure ulcer development, and bladder control problems.

- Early mobilization of the patient is important, so that independent functioning can be restored.
- Observe for shock related to loss of 2 to 3 units of blood into the tissues.

- Observe the wound for drainage; assess laboratory results and physical assessment findings, as well as collaborative management, including adjustment of therapeutic interventions as indicated.
- Check neurovascular status of the affected extremity, especially popliteal, posterior tibial, and pedal pulses; toe capillary refill time; color; temperature; sensation; and movement. A Doppler ultrasound device may be needed to assess blood flow.
- Excessive swelling due to bleeding into tissues further impairs the neurovascular status. Patients may complain of increased pain at the site, and swelling may be noted in the thigh and buttock due to hematoma formation. Ice may be applied to decrease the swelling.
- Mark the extent of drainage on the dressing by circling the extent and noting initials, date, and time.
- Encourage intake of fluids, and ankle and foot exercises to prevent DVT. Assess for signs of DVT, including unilateral calf tenderness, warmth, redness, swelling, and low-grade fever, malaise, elevated white blood cell (WBC) count and sedimentation rate.
- Administer anticoagulant and mechanical-based prophylaxis (eg, elastic compression stockings, sequential compression devices, and prophylactic anticoagulant therapy) as prescribed.
- Encourage deep-breathing exercises, change of position at least every 2 hours, and the use of an incentive spirometer to prevent respiratory complications.
- Assess breath sounds for adventitious or diminished sounds every 4 hours.
- Assess oxygen saturation; provide supplemental oxygen to maintain saturation greater than 95%.
- Administer analgesics, typically opioids. Encourage coughing and deep breathing.
- Observe for signs and symptoms associated with left-sided heart failure, including shortness of breath, cough, dyspnea on exertion (DOE), crackles, S_3, orthopnea, and paroxysmal nocturnal dyspnea. Right ventricular failure presents with peripheral edema (may be pitting) or sacral edema in dependent areas, jugular vein distention, and abdominal distention. Monitor intake and output (I & O), noting oliguria and vital signs,

decreasing blood pressure, tachycardia, and tachypnea; fluid restriction or diuretics may be needed.

- Skin breakdown is often seen in elderly patients with hip fracture. Blisters caused by tape and damage caused by resisting position changes may cause pressure ulcers. Special mattress may provide protection by distributing pressure evenly.

- Reduced gastrointestinal motility, immobility, and the effects of anesthesia may result in constipation. Assess bowel sounds and note distention of the abdomen. Encourage a diet high in fiber and fluids. Encourage ambulation to improve peristalsis. Stool softeners, laxatives, suppositories, and enemas are used to relieve constipation.

- Incontinence or urinary retention may occur. Routine use of indwelling catheters is avoided due to high risk for urinary tract infection; if inserted, remove as soon as possible, often on the first postoperative day. Observe for bladder distention and frequently voiding small amounts of urine (<100 mL).

- Monitor for infection, including complaints of persistent, moderate discomfort in the hip, chills or malaise, and an elevated WBC count and erythrocyte sedimentation rate. The nurse observes the surgical incision for erythema, warmth, tenderness and notes color, amount and consistency of wound drainage. In the elderly, symptoms of infection may be nonspecific and marked by a decline in functional status and/or the presence of confusion.

- Delayed complications include malunion, delayed union, or nonunion; AVN of the femoral head; and fixation device problems. Healing time is 4 to 6 months.

Promoting Health

- Patient education regarding dietary requirements, lifestyle changes, and weight-bearing exercise to promote bone health for patients with osteoporosis is needed to prevent future fractures.

- Prevention of falls through exercises to improve muscle tone and balance and through the elimination of environmental hazards (such as throw rugs) is provided. Other environmental considerations are the use of hand rails on the stairs, nonskid surfaces in the bathroom, grab bars in the shower, raised toilet seats, well-fitting shoes with nonskid soles, and adequate home lighting.

Patient Education

Cast Care
- Move about as normally as possible, but avoid excessive use of the injured extremity, and avoid walking on wet, slippery floors or sidewalks:
  - If the cast is on an upper extremity, you may use a sling when you ambulate. To prevent pressure on the cervical spinal nerves, the sling should distribute the supported weight over a large area and not onto the back of the neck. Remove the arm from the sling and elevate it frequently.
- Perform prescribed exercises regularly, as prescribed.
- Elevate the casted extremity to heart level frequently to prevent swelling. For example: when lying down, elevate the arm so that each joint is positioned higher than the preceding proximal joint (eg, elbow higher than the shoulder, hand higher than the elbow).
- Do not attempt to scratch the skin under the cast. This may cause a break in the skin and result in the formation of a skin ulcer. Cool air from a hair dryer may alleviate an itch. Do not insert objects such as coat hangers inside the cast to scratch itching skin. If itching persists, contact your provider.
- Cushion rough edges of the cast with tape.
- Keep the cast dry but do not cover it with plastic or rubber, because this causes condensation, which dampens the cast and skin. Moisture softens a plaster cast (a wet fiberglass cast must be dried thoroughly with a hair dryer on a cool setting to avoid skin burns).
- Report any of the following to the provider: persistent pain, swelling that does not respond to elevation, changes in sensation, decreased ability to move exposed fingers or toes, or changes in capillary refill, skin color, and temperature.
- Note odors around the cast, stained areas, warm spots, and pressure areas. Report them to the physician.
- Report a broken cast to the provider; do not attempt to fix it yourself.

CASTS

- A cast is a rigid external immobilizing device that permits mobilization of the patient, while restricting movement of a body part.
- Casts may be made of fiberglass, which is lightweight, strong, water-resistant, and durable, or of plaster, which give off heat as it dries. Patients should be taught that the increasing warmth lasts about 15 minutes; the cast needs to remain uncovered, until completely dry (24 to 72 hours).
- See Box F-2 for cast care.

NURSING MANAGEMENT

Teaching Patient Self-Care

The nurse encourages the patient to participate actively in personal care and to use assistive devices safely. The nurse assists the patient in identifying areas of need and in developing strategies to achieve independence in activities of daily living (ADLs).

Providing Continuing Care

- Explain the procedure for cast removal or change, especially that the cast cutter vibrates, but does not penetrate deeply enough to hurt the patient's skin.
- Provide support when the cast is removed as the affected extremity is weak from disuse, stiff, and atrophied. The skin, if dry and scaly, should be washed gently and lubricated with an emollient lotion.
- The nurse and physical therapist teach the patient to resume activities gradually; the muscles are weak from disuse, the body part that has been casted cannot withstand normal stresses immediately. If swelling of the affected extremity occurs, continue to elevate the extremity until normal muscle tone and use are reestablished.

MONITORING AND MANAGING POTENTIAL COMPLICATIONS

Compartment Syndrome

Compartment syndrome results when fascia, a tough connective tissue surrounding muscle groups, organs, nerves, and blood vessels, limits swelling in the area of the muscle. Swelling causes the pressure in the area to rise, compromising circulation and nerve and motor function to the point where the limb may need to be amputated.

- Risk factors for this complication include trauma from accidents, surgery, or crushing injuries, in which massive edema and bleeding is expected; casts and tight bandages; or individuals taking anticoagulants or who have bleeding dyscrasias.
- Acute compartment syndrome occurs when there is increased pressure in a limited space (eg, cast or muscle compartment) that compresses the blood vessels and nerves in the area. Without prompt intervention, decreases in blood flow to the tissues distal to the injury result in ischemic necrosis; permanent damage and threat to the limb result.
- Chronic compartment syndrome develops when a muscle or muscle group has been subjected to inordinate stress or exercise. It is characterized by pain, aching, and tightness in the muscle as muscle volume increases in a short time, the fascia stretches, and inflammation occurs.
- Crush compartment syndrome is caused by massive external compression or crushing of a compartment; this type of massive injury results in systemic effects that include rhabdomyolysis that causes acute renal failure and that may eventually lead to multiple organ dysfunction syndrome (MODS).
- Volkmann's contracture, discussed earlier in the chapter, is a specific type of compartment syndrome associated with supracondylar fractures of the humerus.
- Prompt detection is through assessment for pain intensifying with passive ROM, paleness of limb, cool skin temperature, delayed capillary refill, weak pulsations, paresthesia, tingling/ burning sensation in the involved muscle, decreased sensation and mobility, tight and full muscle, and pain (unrelenting pain not relieved by position changes, ice, or analgesia, or pain that is disproportional to the injury).

NURSING ALERT

It is important to note that *late signs* of compartment syndrome are pulselessness and pallor. The presence of a pulse does not rule out compartment syndrome

Nursing Interventions

- Nursing interventions include assisting the physician in loosening the bandage or bivalving the cast (cutting the cast in half longitudinally) to release the constriction.
- Monitoring intracompartmental pressure may be necessary. Normal intracompartmental pressure at rest is less than 10 mm Hg.
- Pressures exceeding 30 mm Hg suggest the need to consider a fasciotomy, a surgical procedure in which the skin and affected compartments fascia are opened, allowing the pressure to be relieved and circulation restored. This may be surgically repaired or grafted when swelling subsides.
- Observe for a pressure ulcer developing under a cast or dressing when pain and tightness are reported in a defined casted area. Inspect for drainage on the cast and odor, note increasing warmth, suggesting underlying tissue erythema. The cast may be bivalved or have a window cut into it to allow inspection and treatment of the affected area.
- Disuse syndrome, the nursing diagnosis associated with musculoskeletal inactivity, refers to muscle that has been inactive and loses its strength and size. Teach the patient to tense or contract muscles (isometric muscle contraction) hourly.
- During positioning, use sufficient personnel to support the cast with palms of the hands at vulnerable points to prevent cracking. If a body cast is applied, turn the patient as a unit toward the uninjured side every 2 hours to relieve pressure and allow the cast to dry.

TRACTION

- Skin traction, including Buck's extension traction, is discussed on page 326.
- The nurse maintains alignment of the patient's body in traction to promote an effective line of pull. Position the patient's foot to avoid footdrop (plantar flexion), inward rotation (inversion), and outward rotation (eversion).
- Skeletal traction is applied directly to the bone occasionally to treat fractures of the femur, tibia, and cervical spine. Metal pin or wire (eg, Steinmann pin, Kirschner wire) is inserted through the bone distal to the fracture or tongs are fixed to the skull to apply traction that immobilizes cervical fractures.

F

- Local anesthesia is applied, the surgeon uses surgical asepsis to make a small skin incision, and sterile pins are drilled or wire is placed through the bone. The patient feels pressure during this procedure and possibly some pain when the periosteum is penetrated.
- After insertion, the pin or wire is attached to the traction bow or caliper, then weights are attached.
- Often, skeletal traction is balanced traction, which supports the affected extremity, allows for some patient movement, and facilitates patient independence and nursing care. The Thomas splint with a Pearson attachment is frequently used with skeletal traction for fractures of the femur. Because upward traction is required, an overbed frame is used.
- When discontinuing skeletal traction, gently support the extremity while the weights are removed. The pin is removed by the physician and internal fixation, casts, or splints are then applied.
- External fixators are used to maintain the position of unstable fractures when use of a cast is prohibited or the patient is unstable. They can also be used to manage open fractures or severe comminuted fractures while permitting active treatment of damaged soft tissues. Complicated fractures of the humerus, forearm, femur, tibia, and pelvis are often managed with external skeletal fixators. The fracture is reduced, aligned, and immobilized by a series of pins or screws inserted directly into the bone above and below the fracture and secured with the use of a metal frame. Complications due to disuse and immobility are minimized.
- Provide pin care according to institutional protocol to prevent infection and osteomyelitis. Current recommendations include performing the procedure on a daily or weekly basis, applying chlorhexidine solution, teaching the patient pin care, and observing redemonstration prior to discharge. Patients and families should receive written instructions, including signs and symptoms of infection.
- Monitor pin sites daily for fever and reactions, including redness, warmth, and serous or slightly sanguinous drainage at the site; this should subside after 72 hours

☀ NURSING ALERT

The nurse *never* adjusts the clamps on the external fixator frame. It is the physician's responsibility to do so.

- Prevent skin breakdown by protecting the heel of the unaffected leg and the elbows, ischial tuberosity, popliteal space, and Achilles tendon. Obtain a trapeze to encourage movement. Provide back care and to keep the bed dry and free of crumbs and wrinkles. A pressure-relieving air-filled or high-density foam mattress overlay may reduce the risk of pressure ulcers.
- Change bed linens top to bottom rather than side to side. Sheets and blankets are placed over the patient in such a way that the traction is not disrupted.

JOINT REPLACEMENT SURGERY

- Joint replacement may be elected over an ORIF for fractures that disrupt the blood supply or if AVN develops. Joint disease, disability, or deformity may also require joint replacement to relieve pain, improve stability, and improve function.
- Total hip arthroplasty or surgical replacement of the hip joint with an artificial prosthesis, is indicated for idiopathic osteoarthritis, acetabular dysplasia, rheumatoid arthritis, avascular necrosis, posttraumatic injury, and other causes.
- The nurse teaches the patient to prevent dislocation of the prosthesis through abduction using abduction pillows or splints.

N u r s i n g   A l e r t

For total hip replacement surgery, the legs should be slightly *abducted*. Prevent hip flexion beyond 90 degrees to avoid dislocation of the hip after joint replacement surgery.

- Prevent infection by administering preoperative or perioperative antibiotics.

INTRAOPERATIVE MANAGEMENT

- Blood is conserved during surgery to minimize loss via a pneumatic tourniquet that produces a "bloodless field." Blood salvage with reinfusion is used when a large volume of blood loss is anticipated, and salvage has shown to substantially reduce the need for allogeneic transfusions
- Strict aseptic principles and a controlled environment in the operating area are adhered to.

- Culture of the joint during surgery may be important in identifying and treating subsequent infections.

POSTOPERATIVE MANAGEMENT

Repositioning the Patient and Preventing Dislocation

- Position the patient onto the affected or unaffected extremity as prescribed by the surgeon. Maintain the abductor pillow between the legs when in a supine or side-lying position and when turning. The patient's hip is never flexed more than 90 degrees. Avoid elevating the head by greater than 60 degrees. When out of bed, an abduction splint or pillows are kept between the legs, encourage the patient to keep the affected hip in extension and instruct the patient to pivot on the unaffected leg.
- Use a fracture bedpan and use the trapeze to lift the pelvis onto the pan. Instruct the patient not to cross the legs. Use of elevated toilet seats and chairs are suggested, as well as "reaching devices" that will limit hip flexion to less than 90 degrees.
- A cradle boot may be used to prevent leg rotation and to support the heel off the bed, thus preventing development of a pressure ulcer. The nurse instructs the patient not to sleep on the operative side without consulting the surgeon. Hip precautions should be enforced for 4 or more months after surgery.
- Dislocation may occur with positioning that exceeds the limits of the prosthesis. Indicators are as follows:
  - Increased pain at the surgical site, swelling, and immobilization
  - Acute groin pain in the affected hip or increased discomfort
  - Shortening of the leg
  - Abnormal external or internal rotation
  - Restricted ability or inability to move the leg
  - Reported "popping" sensation in the hip
- If a prosthesis becomes dislocated, the nurse (or the patient, if at home) immediately notifies the surgeon, to prevent circulatory and nerve damage.

Promoting Ambulation

- Patients with total hip replacement begin ambulation with a physical therapist, generally within a day after surgery.

- Observe for orthostatic hypotension, an abnormal drop in blood pressure and dizziness when changing from lying to standing.

NURSING ALERT

Orthostasis occurs if the systolic pressure drops 20 mm Hg or the diastolic drops more than 10 mm Hg. It may be related to hypovolemia, dehydration, drug-induced hypotension, or prolonged bed rest. Patients should be encouraged to rise slowly and move their legs prior to rising to facilitate venous return from the extremities.

- Monitor for additional complications, including wound drainage via suction devices of more than 200 to 500 mL in the first day, DVT (usually occurring 2 to 7 days postoperatively), and infection of wound or urinary tract.

Teaching the Patient Self-Care

- Teach the patient of the importance of the daily exercise program in maintaining the functional motion of the hip joint and strengthening the abductor muscles of the hip.
- Assistive devices (crutches, walker, or cane) are used for about 3 months; the patient can resume routine ADLs. Stair climbing is permitted as prescribed but is kept to a minimum for 3 to 6 months. Frequent walks, swimming, and use of a high rocking chair are excellent for hip exercise.
- Sexual intercourse can be resumed based upon surgeon recommendation (typically 3 to 6 months postoperatively) and should be carried out with the patient in the dependent position.
- At no time during the first 4 months should the patient cross the legs or flex the hip more than 90 degrees; the patient should avoid low chairs and sitting for longer than 45 minutes at a time. Assistance in putting on shoes and socks may be needed. Traveling long distances should be avoided unless frequent position changes are possible. Other activities to avoid include tub baths, jogging, lifting heavy loads, and excessive bending and twisting (eg, lifting, shoveling snow, forceful turning).

For more information, see Chapter 42 in Pellico, L.H. (2013). *Focus on adult health. Medical-surgical nursing.* Philadelphia: Wolters Kluwer Health | Lippincott Williams & Wilkins.

G

Gastritis

Gastritis is inflammation of the stomach mucosa, which may be acute or chronic.

PATHOPHYSIOLOGY

In gastritis, the gastric mucous membrane becomes edematous and hyperemic (congested with fluid and blood) and undergoes superficial erosion. It secretes a scanty amount of gastric juice, containing very little acid but much mucus. Superficial ulceration may occur.

RISK FACTORS

- Acute gastritis: Acute illnesses, especially with major traumatic injuries, burns, severe infection, hepatic, renal, or respiratory failure, or major surgery
- Chronic gastritis: Infections such as with *Helicobacter pylori,* and ulcer-causing organism, or infected food
- Benign or malignant ulcers
- Nonsteroidal anti-inflammatory drugs (NSAIDs), aspirin, or bisphosphonates
- Alcohol or caffeine
- Chronic reflux of pancreatic secretions and bile into stomach
- Autoimmune diseases, such as pernicious anemia
- Smoking

CLINICAL MANIFESTATIONS AND ASSESSMENT

Acute Gastritis

May have rapid onset of symptoms: Abdominal discomfort, headache, lassitude, nausea, anorexia, vomiting, and hiccupping lasting a few hours to a few days.

Chronic Gastritis

- May complain of anorexia, heartburn after eating, belching, a sour taste in the mouth, or nausea and vomiting. Some patients may have only mild epigastric discomfort or report intolerance to spicy or fatty foods, or slight pain that is relieved by eating.
- Patients with chronic gastritis from vitamin deficiency usually have evidence of malabsorption of vitamin B_{12}.

DIAGNOSTIC METHODS

- Gastritis is sometimes associated with achlorhydria or hypochlorhydria (absence or low levels of hydrochloric acid) or with high acid levels.
- Upper gastrointestinal (GI) X-ray series, endoscopy with biopsy
- *H. pylori* infection present

MEDICAL AND NURSING MANAGEMENT

The gastric mucosa is capable of repairing itself after an episode of gastritis. As a rule, the patient recovers in about 1 day, although the appetite may be diminished for an additional 2 or 3 days.

Acute Gastritis

- Refrain from alcohol and eating until symptoms subside, then progress to a nonirritating diet. If symptoms persist, IV fluids may be necessary. If bleeding is present, management is similar to that of upper GI tract hemorrhage.

- Ingestion of strong acids or alkali: Dilute and neutralize the acid with common antacids (eg, aluminum hydroxide); neutralize alkali with diluted lemon juice or diluted vinegar. If corrosion is extensive or severe, avoid emetics and lavage because of danger of perforation and damage to esophagus.
- Supportive therapy may include nasogastric intubation, analgesic agents and sedatives, antacids, and IV fluids.
- Fiberoptic endoscopy may be necessary; emergency surgery may be required to remove gangrenous or perforated tissue; gastric resection (gastrojejunostomy) may be necessary to treat pyloric obstruction.

Chronic Gastritis

Diet modification, rest, stress reduction, avoidance of alcohol and NSAIDs, and pharmacotherapy are key treatment measures. Gastritis related to *H. pylori* infection is treated with selected drug combinations.

G

For more information, see Chapter 23 in Pellico, L.H. (2013). *Focus on adult health. Medical-surgical nursing.* Philadelphia: Wolters Kluwer Health | Lippincott Williams & Wilkins.

Glaucoma

Glaucoma is a group of ocular conditions characterized by optic nerve damage. The optic nerve damage is related to increased intraocular pressure (IOP), caused by congestion of aqueous humor in the eye.

PATHOPHYSIOLOGY

Glaucoma is one of the leading causes of irreversible blindness in the world and is the leading cause of blindness among adults in the United States. This problem develops when outflow of aqueous fluid through the canal of Schlemm is impeded or when a narrow angle develops between the iris and the cornea. Normal IOP is between 10 and 21 mm Hg. Increased IOP is theorized to mechanically damage the retina or compress the microcirculation, causing cell injury and death. Typically, most cases are a combination of both.

Classification of glaucoma includes open-angle glaucoma, angle-closure glaucoma (also called pupillary block), congenital glaucoma, and glaucoma associated with other conditions, such as developmental anomalies or corticosteroid use. Glaucoma can be primary or secondary, depending on whether associated factors contribute to the rise in IOP.

RISK FACTORS

- Age greater than 40 and increases with age
- More prevalent in men, African Americans, and Asian populations
- Corticosteroid use

CLASSIFICATION OF GLAUCOMAS

There are several types of glaucoma. Current clinical forms of glaucoma are identified as open-angle glaucoma, angle-closure glaucoma (also called pupillary block), congenital glaucoma, and glaucoma associated with other conditions. Glaucoma can be primary or secondary, depending on whether associated factors contribute to the rise in IOP. The two common clinical forms of glaucoma encountered in adults are primary open-angle glaucoma (POAG) and angle-closure glaucoma, which are differentiated by the mechanisms that cause impaired aqueous outflow.

CLINICAL MANIFESTATIONS AND ASSESSMENT

- Often called the "silent thief of sight" because most patients are unaware that they have the disease until they have experienced visual changes and vision loss

- Blurred vision or "halos" around lights, difficulty focusing, difficulty adjusting eyes in low lighting, loss of peripheral vision, aching or discomfort around the eyes, and headache
- Changes in the optic nerve related to glaucoma are pallor and cupping of the optic nerve disc.

DIAGNOSTIC METHODS

- Ocular and medical history (to investigate predisposing factors)
- Major diagnostic tests include tonometry (measures IOP), ophthalmoscopy to inspect the optic nerve, gonioscopy (to examine the filtration angle of the anterior chamber), and perimetry (visual fields assessment).

MEDICAL AND NURSING MANAGEMENT

The goal of glaucoma treatment is to prevent optic nerve damage and prevent further damage. Treatment focuses on pharmacologic therapy, laser procedures, surgery, or a combination of these approaches. The objective is to achieve the greatest benefit at the least risk, cost, and inconvenience to the patient, while maintaining IOP within an acceptable range.

Pharmacologic Therapy

Medical management of glaucoma relies on systemic and topical ocular medications that lower IOP. Periodic follow-up examinations are essential to monitor IOP, the appearance of the optic nerve, the visual fields, and side effects of medications.

- Patient is usually started on the lowest dose of topical medication and then advanced to increased concentrations until the desired IOP level is reached and maintained.
- Topical beta blocker to decrease production of aqueous humor and IOP are usually chosen as initial therapy.
- One eye is treated first, with the other eye used as a control in determining the efficacy of the medication. When successful,

the other eye is treated; if treatment is not successful, a new medication is substituted.

- Miotics and sympathomimetics decrease the size of the pupil, thus facilitating the outflow of aqueous humor, which decreases the IOP, alpha$_2$-agonists (ie, adrenergic agents), carbonic anhydrase inhibitors, and prostaglandins.

Surgical Management

- Laser trabeculoplasty or iridotomy is indicated when IOP is inadequately controlled by medications.
- Filtering procedures with trabeculectomy create an opening or a fistula in the trabecular meshwork.

Nursing Management

- Emphasize glaucoma management is life-long and strict adherence to the medication regimen is needed.
- When using drops, teach the patient to wash his hands, pull the lower lid down, and instill the drops in the conjunctival sac. After drops are instilled, the patient applies gentile pressure on the inner canthus.
- The patient should avoid touching the tip of the medication container to the eye and should wait 5 minutes before instilling another medication.
- Explain that miotics and sympathomimetics may result in altered focus; therefore, patients need to be cautious in navigating their surroundings.
- Refer patients to services for assistance with activities of daily living (ADLs) or rehabilitation services; patients who meet the criteria for legal blindness should be offered referrals to agencies that can assist them in obtaining federal assistance.
- Provide emotional support due to possible loss of sight; include family in the plan of care.
- As the disease has a familial tendency, encourage family members to undergo examinations at least every 2 years to detect glaucoma early.

For more information, see Chapter 49 in Pellico, L.H. (2013). *Focus on adult health. Medical-surgical nursing.* Philadelphia: Wolters Kluwer Health | Lippincott Williams & Wilkins.

Glomerulonephritis, Acute

Glomerulonephritis is an inflammation of the glomerular capillaries. Acute glomerulonephritis is more common in children older than 2 years of age, but it can occur at any age.

PATHOPHYSIOLOGY

Acute glomerulonephritis is an inflammatory disease of the glomeruli associated with an antigen–antibody response to infection. Typically, group A beta-hemolytic streptococcal infection of the throat or other strep or viral infections precedes the onset of glomerulonephritis by 2 to 3 weeks.

The kidneys become large, edematous, and congested, resulting in a buildup of nitrogenous wastes (BUN) and proteinuria.

RISK FACTORS

- Exposure to streptococcal infection or other infectious diseases, such as hepatitis, mumps, and varicella
- Goodpasture's syndrome, Wegener's granulomatosis, systemic lupus erythematosus (SLE), subacute bacterial endocarditis, and sepsis have been implicated as risk factors.
- Family history of glomerulonephritis

CLINICAL MANIFESTATIONS AND ASSESSMENT

- Edema, proteinuria (>3.5 g daily), and azotemia
- Hematuria, which may be microscopic or macroscopic

- Cola-colored urine due to red blood cell (RBC) protein or casts
- Headache, malaise, flank pain
- May present incidentally through routine urinalysis or present as acute renal failure with oliguria
- Atypical symptoms include confusion, somnolence, and seizures, which are often confused with the symptoms of a primary neurologic disorder.
- Elderly patients may experience circulatory overload with dyspnea, engorged neck veins, cardiomegaly, and pulmonary edema.

DIAGNOSTIC METHODS

- Elevated BUN and creatinine
- Proteinuria
- Urinalysis reveals gross or microscopic hematuria.

MEDICAL AND NURSING MANAGEMENT

G

Management consists primarily of treating symptoms, attempting to preserve kidney function, and treating complications promptly.

- Sodium is restricted when the patient has hypertension, edema, or heart failure.
- Intake and output (I & O) is monitored carefully with fluid replacement based on fluid loss and daily weights
- Dietary protein is restricted when renal insufficiency and nitrogen retention (elevated BUN) develop.
- High-carbohydrate diet is given to provide energy and reduce protein catabolism.
- Diuresis usually begins about 1 week after the onset of symptoms with a decrease in edema and blood pressure. Proteinuria and microscopic hematuria may persist for many months.
- Instruct the patient to notify the health care provider for symptoms of renal failure: Fatigue, nausea, vomiting, diminishing urine output, or at the first sign of any infection.
- Information is given verbally and in writing.

Pharmacologic Therapy

- Penicillin is given for residual streptococcal infection.
- Corticosteroids and immunosuppressant medications may be prescribed for patients with rapidly progressive acute glomerulonephritis.
- Loop diuretic and antihypertensive medications may be prescribed to control hypertension.

COMPLICATIONS

- Chronic glomerulonephritis
- Hypertensive encephalopathy
- Rapidly progressive glomerulonephritis may lead to end-stage renal disease (ESRD), requiring plasmapheresis, corticosteroids, and cytotoxic agents.

> For more information, see Chapter 27 in Pellico, L.H. (2013). *Focus on adult health. Medical-surgical nursing.* Philadelphia: Wolters Kluwer Health | Lippincott Williams & Wilkins.

G

Glomerulonephritis, Chronic

Glomerulonephritis is an inflammation of the glomerular capillaries leading to severe glomerular damage.

PATHOPHYSIOLOGY

Chronic glomerulonephritis is characterized by proteinuria, usually caused by repeated episodes of glomerular injury that results in renal destruction. The kidneys are reduced to as little as one-fifth their normal size, consisting largely of fibrous tissue. The glomeruli and their tubules become scarred, and the branches of the renal artery are thickened. The result is severe glomerular damage that can progress to ESRD.

RISK FACTORS

- Acute glomerulonephritis
- Diabetes
- Hypertensive nephrosclerosis
- Hyperlipidemia
- Chronic tubulointerstitial injury
- Hemodynamically mediated glomerular sclerosis
- Secondary glomerular diseases that can have systemic effects include lupus erythematosus and Goodpasture's syndrome (autoimmune diseases), diabetic glomerulosclerosis, and amyloidosis.

CLINICAL MANIFESTATIONS AND ASSESSMENT

The symptoms of chronic glomerulonephritis vary. Some patients with severe disease are asymptomatic for many years and may present with the following:

- Hypertension or elevated BUN and serum creatinine levels
- Retinal vascular changes or retinal hemorrhages
- General symptoms: Weight loss, decreasing strength, increasing irritability, nocturia, headaches, dizziness, and digestive disturbances are also common.
- The disease may progress, with the patient developing signs and symptoms of renal failure: Periorbital and peripheral edema, pallor, yellow-gray skin color, crackles and symptoms of heart failure, and neurologic changes including decreased attention span and confusion.

DIAGNOSTIC METHODS

On laboratory analysis, the following abnormalities may be found:

- Urinalysis: Fixed specific gravity of 1.010, variable proteinuria, and urinary casts

- Blood studies: Hyperkalemia, metabolic acidosis, anemia, hypoalbuminemia, decreased serum calcium and increased serum phosphorus, and hypermagnesemia
- Impaired nerve conduction; mental status changes
- Chest X-rays: Cardiac enlargement and pulmonary edema
- Electrocardiogram (ECG): Normal or may reflect left ventricular hypertrophy, tall tented T waves, or arrhythmias indicative of hyperkalemia.
- Computed tomography (CT) and magnetic resonance imaging (MRI) scans show a decrease in the size of the renal cortex

NURSING AND MEDICAL MANAGEMENT

Treatment is directed toward reversing the renal impairment and eliminating the underlying cause where possible.

- Hypertension is treated by restricting fluid and sodium and administering antihypertensive medications as ordered.
- Fluid volume excess manifested by acute weight gain, edema, crackles, SOB is treated with fluid and sodium restriction, diuretics, and dialysis when indicated.
- Potassium excess is treated with dietary restriction, IV glucose and insulin, sodium polystyrene resin (Kayexalate), and dialysis.
- Dialysis is considered for progression to renal failure.

Nursing Management

- Monitor BUN, creatinine, potassium, and symptoms of fluid volume excess such as periorbital and peripheral edema.
- Observe for metabolic acidosis, anemia, and hypoalbuminemia.
- Observe for hyperphosphatemia and hypocalcemia.
- Observe for mental status changes due to build-up of nitrogenous waste products.
- Provide emotional support, providing opportunities for patient and family to verbalize concerns. Encourage patient to explore treatment options should kidney failure develop.
- Educate patient and family about need for follow-up evaluations of blood pressure, urinalysis for protein and casts, blood for BUN, and creatinine.

- Educate the patient of the need to contact the health care provider for worsening signs and symptoms of renal failure, such as nausea, vomiting, and diminished urine output.
- Refer to community health or home care nurse for assessment of patient progress and continued education about problems to report to health care provider.
- Instruct the patient to inform all health care providers about the diagnosis of glomerulonephritis to ensure medical management and pharmacologic therapy is based on altered renal function.

COMPLICATIONS

- Chronic renal failure
- ESRD

For more information, see Chapter 27 in Pellico, L.H. (2013). *Focus on adult health. Medical-surgical nursing.* Philadelphia: Wolters Kluwer Health | Lippincott Williams & Wilkins.

G

Gout

Gout, one of the most common of the inflammatory arthritides, is a metabolic disorder marked by the deposition of monosodium urate crystals within joints and other tissues. Primary gout is characterized by hyperuricemia caused by an overproduction of uric acid or a decreased urate excretion in the kidney.

PATHOPHYSIOLOGY

Hyperuricemia denotes an elevated level of uric acid (urate) in the blood and, in recent years, it has been recognized that the reference ranges are quite wide. Thus, it is more clinically relevant to use the biologic value of 6.8 mg/dL or 408 μmol/L, a level of serum uric acid above the saturation point for crystals. Asymptomatic hyperuricemia is a laboratory finding, not a disease, but it can lead to gout pathogenesis. Attacks of gout appear to be related to sudden increases or decreases of serum uric acid levels. When the uric acid precipitates and then deposits within a joint as urate crystals, an inflammatory response occurs, and an attack of gout begins. With repeated attacks, accumulations of sodium urate crystals, called *tophi,* are deposited in peripheral areas of the body, such as the great toe, the hands, and the ear (lower-temperature areas). Renal urate lithiasis (kidney stones), with chronic renal disease secondary to urate deposition, may develop.

RISK FACTORS

- First attack 40 to 60 years in men and after 60 in women
- Primary gout: Inherited disorder in purine metabolism
- Secondary gout:
  - Diabetic ketoacidosis (DKA), severe dieting, starvation, metabolic syndrome
  - Multiple myeloma and leukemia
  - Diuretics such as thiazides and furosemide, salicylates, or ethanol
  - High-purine diet (shellfish, organ meats) in susceptible persons

CLINICAL MANIFESTATIONS AND ASSESSMENT

Manifestations of the gout syndrome include acute gouty arthritis (recurrent attacks of severe articular and periarticular inflammation), tophi (crystalline deposits accumulating in articular tissue, osseous tissue, soft tissue, and cartilage), gouty nephropathy (renal impairment), and uric acid urinary calculi.

Four stages of gout can be identified: Asymptomatic hyperuricemia, acute gouty arthritis, intercritical gout, and chronic tophaceous gout.

- Acute arthritis of gout is the most common early sign.
- Excruciating pain and inflammation in one or more small joints; metatarsophalangeal (MTP) joint of the big toe is most commonly affected; the tarsal area, ankle, or knee may also be affected.

G

- Abrupt onset occurs at night, causing severe pain, redness, swelling, and warmth over the affected joint.
- Early attacks tend to subside spontaneously over 3 to 10 days without treatment.
- The next attack may not come for months or years; in time, attacks tend to occur more frequently, involve more joints, last longer, and lead to long-term sequelae.
- Tophi are generally associated with frequent and severe inflammatory episodes.
- Higher serum concentrations of uric acid are associated with tophus formation.
- Tophi occur in the synovium, olecranon bursa, subchondral bone, infrapatellar and Achilles' tendons, subcutaneous tissue, and overlying joints.
- Tophi have also been found in aortic walls, heart valves, nasal and ear cartilage, eyelids, cornea, and sclerae.
- Joint enlargement may cause loss of joint motion.
- Uric acid deposits may cause renal stones and kidney damage.

MEDICAL AND NURSING MANAGEMENT

Treatment of gout is managed into two major phases: management of acute gouty inflammation and long-term management to prevent flares and to control hyperuricemia.

- NSAIDs, such as indomethacin or ibuprofen are first-choice agents, with colchicine as an alternative. Low-dose colchicine has been used for prophylaxis after resolution of attacks, but does not prevent accumulation of urate in joints and tophi.
- A corticosteroid or adrenocorticotropic hormones (ACTH) may be used because of their anti-inflammatory properties.
- Allopurinol (Zyloprim), a xanthine oxidase inhibitor, is considered the drug of choice for preventing an attack and tophi formation, and for promoting the regression of existing tophi.
- Uricosuric agents, such as probenecid (Benemid), correct hyperuricemia and dissolve deposited urate. Sulfinpyrazone (Anturane) is very similar to probenecid but it is more potent. Severe blood dyscrasias may occur with use, so it is generally reserved for patients with symptoms resistant to other agents.

- Target goal of therapy is a serum uric acid level of less than 6 mg/dL, a level below the saturation point of 6.8 mg/dL at which urate crystals precipitate from solution.
- Newer urate-lowering agents, such as uricase, are currently under investigation and show promise for successful gout treatment.
- Corticosteroids may be used in patients who have no response to other therapy.
- Prophylactic treatment considered if patient experiences several acute episodes or there is evidence of tophi formation.

Nursing Management

- Pain management is the primary concern during the acute phase of an attack. The joint should be rested and application of ice, not heat, may help with reducing discomfort.
- Teach self-care measures to decrease the risk of attacks (eg, avoidance of aspirin [because doses below 2 to 3 g/day impair renal excretion of uric acid, and higher doses are associated with high renal excretion of uric acids], trauma, stress, alcohol) and to avoid long-term complications (eg, importance of medication compliance).
- Dietary modifications are controversial; some providers recommend patients restrict foods high in purines, especially organ meats and shellfish; others believe limiting protein or trigger foods is sufficient.
- Limit alcohol intake and avoid fad starvation diets.
- Drink at least 2,000 mL of fluid daily to prevent renal involvement and urinary stones.
- Dietary restriction of sodium, fat, and cholesterol may reduce gout symptoms and decrease effects associated with coexisting metabolic syndrome. Although research is limited, first acute gout attacks may precede the diagnosis of metabolic abnormalities and associated diseases.

For more information, see Chapter 39 in Pellico, L.H. (2013). *Focus on adult health. Medical-surgical nursing.* Philadelphia: Wolters Kluwer Health | Lippincott Williams & Wilkins.

Guillain-Barré Syndrome

Guillain-Barré syndrome (GBS) is an autoimmune attack on the peripheral nerve myelin, producing ascending weakness and dyskinesia.

PATHOPHYSIOLOGY

Guillain-Barré syndrome is the result of a cell-mediated and humoral immune attack on peripheral nerve myelin proteins that causes inflammatory demyelination. The immune system cannot distinguish between the two proteins and attacks and destroys peripheral nerve myelin. Symptoms usually occur/ develop about 2 weeks after an acute viral infection or immunization. The result is acute, rapid segmental demyelination of peripheral nerves and some cranial nerves, producing ascending weakness, dyskinesia, hyporeflexia, and paresthesia. In GBS, the Schwann cell that produces myelin is spared, allowing for remyelination in the recovery phase of the disease. In North America, there are approximately 1.5 to 2.0 cases of GBS for every 100,000 people each year. GBS affects males and females of all ages and races.

G

CLINICAL MANIFESTATIONS AND ASSESSMENT

- Guillain-Barré syndrome typically begins with muscle weakness and diminished reflexes of the lower extremities.
- Hyporeflexia and weakness may progress to tetraplegia. Demyelination of the nerves that innervate the diaphragm and intercostal muscles results in neuromuscular respiratory failure.
- Sensory symptoms include paresthesias of the hands and feet and pain related to the demyelination of sensory fibers.
- Cranial nerve demyelination can result in a variety of clinical manifestations.
- Optic nerve demyelination may result in blindness.

- Bulbar muscle weakness related to demyelination of the glossopharyngeal and vagus nerves results in the inability to swallow or clear secretions.
- Vagus nerve demyelination results in autonomic dysfunction, causing instability of the cardiovascular system manifested by tachycardia, bradycardia, hypertension, or orthostatic hypotension.

DIAGNOSTIC METHODS

- Decreased vital capacity and negative inspiratory force are assessed to identify impending neuromuscular respiratory failure.
- Elevated protein levels are detected in cerebrospinal fluid (CSF) evaluation, without an increase in other cells.
- Evoked potential studies demonstrate a progressive loss of nerve conduction velocity.

MEDICAL AND NURSING MANAGEMENT

- Because of the possibility of rapid progression and neuromuscular respiratory failure, GBS is a medical emergency, requiring management in an intensive care unit.
- Respiratory support with mechanical ventilation may be necessary for extended periods.
- Elective intubation may be suggested before the onset of extreme respiratory muscle fatigue.
- Complications of immobility are prevented with anticoagulants and antiembolism stockings, or sequential compression boots may be used to prevent thrombosis and pulmonary emboli (PE).

Pharmacologic Therapy

- Plasmapheresis and IV immunoglobulin (IVIG) are used to decrease antibody levels and reduce time of immobilization; IVIG is associated with fewer side effects.
- Labile autonomic dysfunction requires continuous ECG monitoring to detect tachycardia. Tachycardia and hypertension are treated with short-acting medications such as alpha-adrenergic blocking agents.

- Hypotension is managed by increasing the amount of IV fluid administered.

NURSING MANAGEMENT

- Monitor for respiratory failure, cardiac arrhythmias, autonomic dysfunction, deep vein thrombosis (DVT), and skin integrity.
- Assess swallowing, for paralytic ileus and nutritional status.
- Assess for fear and anxiety, as well as isolation, loneliness, and lack of control.

Nursing Diagnoses

- Impaired gas exchange
- Risk for aspiration
- Risk for anxiety and social isolation
- Impaired mobility
- Risk for altered nutrition less than body requirement
- Impaired communication

Planning and Goals

Major goals include improved respiratory function, increased mobility, improved nutritional status, effective communication, decreased fear and anxiety, and absence of complications.

Nursing Interventions

Maintaining Respiratory Function

- Encourage use of incentive spirometry and provide chest physiotherapy.
- Monitor for changes in vital capacity and negative inspiratory force; vital capacity of less than 15 mL/kg indicates need for mechanical ventilation.
- Suction to maintain a clear airway.

Enhancing Physical Mobility

- Support the paralyzed extremities in a functional position, and perform passive range-of-motion exercises at least twice daily.
- Pad bony prominences and change patient's position at least every 2 hours.

- Administer prescribed anticoagulant regimen to prevent DVT and PE; provide antiembolism stockings or sequential compression boots, as well as adequate hydration.

Providing Adequate Nutrition

- Collaborate with health care provider and dietitian to meet patient's nutritional and hydration needs.
- Evaluate laboratory test results that may indicate malnutrition or dehydration.
- If paralytic ileus is present, provide IV fluids and parenteral nutrition as prescribed, and monitor for return of bowel sounds.
- Provide gastrostomy tube feedings if patient cannot swallow.
- Assess the return of the gag reflex and bowel sounds before resuming oral nutrition.

Improving Communication

- Establish communication through lip reading, use of picture cards, or eye blinking.
- Collaborate with speech therapist, as indicated.

Decreasing Fear and Anxiety

- Refer patient and family to a support group.
- Provide instruction and support for family members to participate in physical care.
- Teach patient and family about the disorder and its generally favorable prognosis.
- Encourage relaxation exercises and distraction techniques.
- Create a positive attitude and atmosphere.
- Encourage diversional activities to decrease loneliness and isolation. Encourage visitors, engage visitors or volunteers to read to the patient; suggest that the patient may listen to music or books on tape, and watch TV.

COMPLICATIONS

- Assess for respiratory failure, which can develop quickly.
- Symptoms of respiratory failure include for breathlessness while talking, shallow and irregular breathing, use of accessory

muscles, tachycardia, weak cough, and changes in respiratory pattern.
• Cardiac arrhythmias, transient hypertension, orthostatic hypotension, DVT, PE, urinary retention are complications of immobility.

For more information, see Chapter 46 in Pellico, L.H. (2013). *Focus on adult health. Medical-surgical nursing.* Philadelphia: Wolters Kluwer Health | Lippincott Williams & Wilkins.

Head Injury (Brain Injury)

Injuries to the head involve trauma to the scalp, skull, and brain. Head injury is the most common cause of death from trauma in the United States with approximately 1.5 million people receiving treatment yearly.

PATHOPHYSIOLOGY

Research has shown that not all brain damage occurs at the moment of impact. Damage to the brain from traumatic injury takes two forms: Primary injury and secondary injury. Primary injury is the initial damage to the brain that results from the traumatic event. This may include contusions, lacerations, and torn blood vessels due to impact, acceleration/deceleration, or foreign object penetration. Secondary injury evolves over the ensuing hours and days after the initial injury and can be due to cerebral edema, ischemia, seizures, infection, hyperthermia, hypovolemia, and hypoxia.

Brain injury is different from other injured body areas because the brain resides within the skull, which is a rigid, closed compartment. The confines of the skull do not allow for the expansion of cranial contents; therefore, bleeding or swelling within the skull increases the volume of contents and can cause increased intracranial pressure (ICP). If the increased pressure is high enough, it can cause herniation of the brain through or against the rigid structures of the skull, restricting blood flow to the brain, ischemia, infarction, irreversible brain damage, and brain death. Traumatic brain injury (TBI) is the most serious form of head injury. The most common causes of TBI are falls (28%), motor vehicle accidents (20%), collisions with stationary or moving objects (17%), and assaults (11%). Despite advances in care, only 40% of patients with severe TBI have good outcomes; the best treatment is prevention.

RISK FACTORS

- Male between 15 and 24 years old
- Very young (<5 years) and very old (>75 years)

SKULL FRACTURES

- A skull fracture is a break in the continuity of the skull caused by forceful trauma, occurring with or without damage to the brain.
- Skull fractures can be classified as simple, comminuted, depressed, or basilar:
  - A simple (linear) fracture is a break in the continuity of the bone.
  - A comminuted skull fracture refers to a splintered fracture line.
  - When bone fragments are embedded into brain tissue, the fracture is depressed. A fracture of the base of the skull is called a basilar or basal skull fracture.

CLINICAL MANIFESTATIONS AND ASSESSMENT OF SKULL FACTURE

- The symptoms, apart from those of the local injury, depend on the severity and the distribution of the underlying brain injury; swelling in the area may not be present. Persistent, localized pain suggests that a fracture is present.
- Skull fractures frequently produce hemorrhage from the nose, pharynx, or ears, and blood may appear under the conjunctiva.
- Battle's sign, an area of ecchymosis (bruising) may be seen over the mastoid.

- Otorrhea (cerebrospinal fluid [CSF] leaking from ears) and rhinorrhea (CSF leaking from nose) should cause the examiner to suspect basilar skull fracture.
- Halo sign, suggestive of CSF leak, may be present on dressings or bed linens (a blood stain surrounded by a yellowish stain).
- Drainage of CSF is serious because meningeal infection can occur in the cranium via the nose, ear, or sinus, through a tear in the dura.

DIAGNOSTIC METHODS FOR SKULL FRACTURE

- Radiologic examination confirms the presence and extent of a skull fracture
- Computed tomography (CT) scan to detect less apparent abnormalities
- Magnetic resonance imaging (MRI) to evaluate patients with head injury when a more accurate picture of the anatomic nature of the injury is warranted and when the patient is stable

MEDICAL AND NURSING MANAGEMENT OF SKULL FRACTURE

- Nondepressed skull fractures generally do not require surgical treatment; however, close observation of the patient is essential. Nurses may observe the patient in the hospital, but if no underlying brain injury is present, the patient may return home. If the patient is discharged, specific instructions must be given to the family.
- Depressed skull fractures usually require surgery, particularly if contaminated or deformed fractures are present. Large defects can be repaired immediately with bone or artificial grafts; if significant cerebral edema is present, repair of the defect may be delayed for 3 to 6 months. Penetrating wounds require surgical débridement to remove foreign bodies and devitalized brain tissue and to control hemorrhage. Intravenous antibiotic treatment is instituted immediately, particularly with a dural laceration, and blood products are administered if indicated.

- Clear fluid draining from nose or ears is checked for glucose; CSF is positive for glucose. Positive findings must be reported to the provider. Early CSF rhinorrhea (resolving within 3 to 5 days) usually does not require surgery. Late onset (7 or more days after the initial injury) and persistent CSF rhinorrhea usually requires surgical intervention to prevent development of meningitis.
- Care of patient with a CSF leak:
  - Caution patient not to blow nose as this may worsen the leak.
  - Elevate head of bed 30 degrees to reduce ICP and promote spontaneous closure of leak.
  - Early detection may help avoid meningitis.

☀ N U R S I N G   A L E R T

Any patient with extensive facial fractures or suspected basilar skull fracture may also have a fracture of the cribriform plate (portion of the ethmoid bone that separates the roof of the nose from the cranial cavity). Attempted intubation with a nasogastric (NG) tube or nasotracheal tube or suctioning is prohibited to avoid intracranial penetration of the brain with the tube or catheter.

H

BRAIN INJURY

The most important consideration in any head injury is whether or not the brain is injured. Even seemingly minor injury can cause significant brain damage secondary to obstructed blood flow and decreased tissue perfusion. The brain cannot store oxygen or glucose to any significant degree. Because neurons need an uninterrupted blood supply to obtain these nutrients, irreversible brain damage and cell death occur if the blood supply is interrupted for even a few minutes.

- Closed (blunt) brain injury occurs when the head accelerates and then rapidly decelerates or collides with another object (ie, a wall, the dashboard of a car); brain tissue is damaged but there is no opening through the skull and dura.

- Open brain injury occurs when an object penetrates the skull, enters the brain, and damages the soft brain tissue in its path (penetrating injury), or when blunt trauma to the head is so severe that it opens the scalp, skull, and dura to expose the brain.

TYPES OF BRAIN INJURY

Concussion (Brain Injury)

- Concussion, also referred to as a mild TBI, involves an alteration in mental status that results from trauma; it may or may not involve loss of consciousness. Symptoms typically last no longer than 24 hours and may include headache, nausea, vomiting, photophobia (sensitivity to light), amnesia, and blurred vision.
- Treatment involves observing the patient for symptoms including headache, dizziness, lethargy, irritability, anxiety, photophobia, phonophobia, difficulty concentrating, and memory difficulties. The occurrence of these symptoms after the injury is referred to as *postconcussive syndrome.*
- Giving the patient information, explanations, and encouragement may reduce some of the problems associated with postconcussive syndrome. The patient is advised to resume normal activities slowly; the exact recovery time is not known.
- Once the patient is discharged, he or she should be closely observed for the next 24 hours, and awakened every 2 hours in order to detect any changes in mental status. Neuroimaging (CT and MRI) is generally not indicated in concussion.

Contusion

- Cerebral contusion is more severe than concussion, involving bruising of the brain, with possible surface hemorrhage. The patient is unconscious for more than a few seconds or minutes.
- Clinical signs and symptoms depend on the size of the contusion and the amount of associated swelling of the brain (cerebral edema).

- The patient may lie motionless, with a faint pulse, shallow respirations, and cool, pale skin. The patient may be aroused with effort but soon slips back into unconsciousness. Blood pressure and temperature are subnormal, and the clinical picture is somewhat similar to that of shock.
- Patients may recover consciousness but pass into a stage of cerebral irritability. In this stage, the patient is conscious and easily disturbed by any form of stimulation, such as noises, light, and voices; he or she may become hyperactive at times.

> ⚡ **N U R S I N G   A L E R T**
> When the patient begins to emerge from unconsciousness, every measure that is available and appropriate for calming and quieting the patient should be used. Any form of restraint is likely to be countered with resistance leading to self-injury or to a dangerous increase in ICP. Therefore, physical restraints should be avoided, if possible.

- Gradually, the pulse, respirations, temperature, and other body functions return to normal, but full recovery can be delayed for months. Residual headache and vertigo are common, and impaired mental function or seizures may occur as a result of irreparable cerebral damage.

Diffuse Axonal Injury

- Diffuse axonal injury involves widespread damage to axons in the cerebral hemispheres, corpus callosum, and brainstem. It can be seen with mild, moderate, or severe head trauma. The patient experiences immediate coma, global cerebral edema, decorticate and decerebrate rigidity, or "posturing." Decorticate posturing involves abnormal flexion of the upper extremities and extension of the lower extremities and indicates damage to the upper midbrain; decerebrate posturing involves extreme extension of the upper and lower extremities and indicates severe damage to the brain at the lower midbrain and upper pons.
- Diagnosis of diffuse axonal injury is made by clinical signs in conjunction with a CT or MRI scan. These tests are usually normal;

a definitive diagnosis can only be made at autopsy. Recovery depends on the severity of the axonal injury.

Intracranial Hemorrhage

Hematomas (collections of blood) that develop within the cranial vault are the most serious type of brain injury. Major symptoms are frequently delayed until the hematoma is large enough to cause distortion of the brain and increased ICP.

Epidural Hematoma (Extradural Hematoma or Hemorrhage)

- After a head injury, blood may collect in the epidural (extradural) space between the skull and the dura.
- Typically, this results from a skull fracture causing a rupture or laceration of the middle meningeal artery. Resulting hemorrhage causes a rapid increase in ICP.
- Symptoms include momentary loss of consciousness at the time of injury, followed by an interval of apparent recovery (lucid interval). Although a lucid interval is a classic characteristic, its absence does not rule out the diagnosis. After the lucid interval, rapid signs of deterioration appear (usually deterioration of consciousness and signs of focal neurologic deficits, such as dilation and fixation of a pupil or paralysis of an extremity).
- Considered an extreme emergency, marked neurologic deficit and respiratory arrest can occur within minutes. Treatment consists of making openings through the skull (burr holes) to decrease ICP emergently, remove the clot, and control the bleeding. A craniotomy (surgical procedure that removes part of the skull to gain access to the brain) may be required to remove the clot and control the bleeding. A drain may be inserted after creation of burr holes or a craniotomy to prevent reaccumulation of blood.

Subdural Hematoma

A subdural hematoma (SDH) is a collection of blood between the dura and the brain, a space normally occupied by a thin cushion of

CSF. The most common cause of subdural hematoma is trauma, but it can also occur as a result of coagulopathies (bleeding disorders) or rupture of an aneurysm. The elderly are at increased risk for subdural hemorrhage secondary to whole-brain atrophy. Subdural hematomas can be acute, subacute, or chronic, depending on when the bleed occurred.

Acute and Subacute Subdural Hematoma

Acute subdural hematomas are associated with major head injury involving contusion or laceration. Clinical symptoms develop over 24 to 48 hours. Signs and symptoms include changes in the level of consciousness (LOC), changes in the reactivity of the pupils, and hemiparesis (weakness on one side of the body). There may be minor or even no symptoms with small collections of blood. Coma, increasing blood pressure, decreasing heart rate, and slowing respiratory rate are all signs of a rapidly expanding mass requiring immediate intervention.

Subacute subdural hematomas are the result of less severe contusions and head trauma. Clinical manifestations usually appear between 48 hours and 2 weeks after the injury. Signs and symptoms are similar to those of an acute subdural hematoma. Immediate surgery may be performed to open the dura, allowing the subdural clot to be evacuated. Successful outcome also depends on the control of ICP and careful monitoring of respiratory function. The mortality rate for patients with acute or subacute subdural hematoma is high because of associated brain damage.

Chronic Subdural Hematoma

- Chronic subdural hematomas can develop from seemingly minor head injuries and are seen most frequently in the elderly. The time between injury and onset of symptoms can be lengthy (ie, 3 weeks to many months), so the actual injury may be forgotten.
- The treatment of a chronic subdural hematoma typically consists of surgical evacuation of the clot if the patient is symptomatic and the bleed is at least 1 cm in size. Smaller bleeds are monitored until the blood reabsorbs.

Intracerebral Hemorrhage and Hematoma

- Intracerebral hemorrhage (ICH) is bleeding into the parenchyma of the brain secondary to head injury when force is exerted to the head over a small area (eg, bullet wounds and stab injuries). May also result from:
  - Systemic hypertension (HTN), which causes degeneration and rupture of a vessel
  - Rupture of a saccular aneurysm
  - Vascular anomalies
  - Intracranial tumors
  - Bleeding disorders such as leukemia, hemophilia, aplastic anemia, and thrombocytopenia
  - Complications of anticoagulant therapy
- Onset may be insidious, beginning with the development of neurologic deficits followed by headache. Management includes supportive care, control of ICP, and careful administration of fluids, electrolytes, and antihypertensive medications. Craniotomy allows removal of the blood clot and control of hemorrhage but may not be possible because of the inaccessible location of the bleeding or the lack of a clearly circumscribed area of blood that can be removed. Decompressive craniectomies that are performed up to 24 hours after the initial injury have been shown to improve outcomes. These procedures are performed to allow for swelling of the brain, which decreases ICP. The earlier the craniectomy can be done, the greater benefit it can have for the patient

MANAGEMENT OF BRAIN INJURIES

Assessment and diagnosis of the extent of injury are accomplished by the initial physical and neurologic examinations. Computed tomography and MRI are the primary neuroimaging diagnostic tools of choice and are useful in evaluating the brain structure.

- Patient is transported from the scene on a board with the head and neck maintained in alignment, a hard cervical collar is applied and maintained until cervical spine X-rays document absence of C-spine injury.

☀ **N U R S I N G A L E R T**

Any patient with a head injury is presumed to have a cervical spine injury until ruled out therefore immobilization of the spine via cervical collar or spinal backboard and the avoidance of movement is essential.

- All therapy is directed toward preserving brain homeostasis and preventing secondary brain injury through stabilization of cardiovascular and respiratory function to maintain adequate cerebral perfusion, control of hemorrhage, and hypovolemia, and maintenance of optimal blood gas values.

See "Medical and Nursing Management" under "Increased Intracranial Pressure" on pages 424–431 for additional information.

For more information, see Chapter 45 in Pellico, L.H. (2013). *Focus on adult health: Medical-surgical nursing.* Philadelphia: Wolters Kluwer Health | Lippincott Williams & Wilkins.

H

Heart Failure

Heart failure (HF) is the inability of the heart to pump sufficient blood to meet the needs of the tissues for oxygen and nutrients. In the past, HF was often referred to as congestive HF (CHF), because many patients experience pulmonary or peripheral congestion.

PATHOPHYSIOLOGY

Heart failure results when the heart cannot generate cardiac output (CO) sufficient to meet the body's demands. The myocardium has either impaired systolic function (impaired contraction) or impaired filing (diastolic dysfunction). Fluid overload and decreased tissue perfusion result when the heart cannot generate a cardiac output (CO) sufficient to meet the body's demands Pulmonary or systemic congestion may result. Although some cases of HF are reversible, generally HF is progressive and requires life-long management. Heart failure is the most common reason for hospitalization of people older than 65 years of age and the second most common reason for visits to a health care provider.

TYPES AND CLASSIFICATION

The most common type of HF is systolic HF characterized by a weakened heart muscle. Less common is diastolic HF, characterized by a stiff and noncompliant myocardium, making it difficult to fill. The ejection fraction (EF), normally 55% to 65%, remains normal in diastolic HF but severely reduced in systolic HF.

Heart failure can be classified as left-sided or right-sided. Left-sided HF causes pulmonary congestion and impaired gas exchange. Right-sided HF leads to congestion in peripheral tissues and viscera; jugular vein distention (JVD) and peripheral edema result.

RISK FACTORS

- Age over 65, male sex
- Hypertension or diabetes
- Coronary artery disease (CAD), myocardial infarction (MI), and high cholesterol
- Valvular disease
- Pulmonary embolus
- Hypoxemia
- Arrhythmias
- Fever, infection, or thyrotoxicosis
- Alcohol consumption
- Sleep-disordered breathing
- Psychological stress, sedentary lifestyle, genetics

- Several systemic conditions, including progressive renal failure and uncontrolled HTN, can contribute to the development and severity of cardiac failure.

CLINICAL MANIFESTATIONS AND ASSESSMENT

Significant myocardial dysfunction most often occurs before the patient experiences signs and symptoms of HF; systolic and diastolic failure share similar findings.

- Overt signs of HF, include resting dyspnea, cyanosis, and cachexia (physical wasting) result from longstanding heart disease.
- Weight gain and dependent edema
- Tachycardia, a weak and thready pulse, or pulsus alternans (regular pulse with varying force of amplitude)
- Crackles or wheezes
- S_3 and apical impulse displace downwardly; S_4 with increased stiffness of the myocardium; murmurs may be present.
- Skin cool, pale, or cyanotic
- Changes in sensorium and LOC, dizziness or lightheadedness
- Jugular vein distension, hepatomegaly, and hepatojugular reflux in right-sided HF

H

DIAGNOSTIC METHODS

- Chest X-ray to determine cardiac enlargement or cardiomegaly. Normal-sized heart suggests diastolic dysfunction
- Electrocardiogram (ECG)
- 2-D echocardiogram with Doppler flow and assessment of EJ; an EJ of less than 40% indicates systolic dysfunction; an EF of 40% with impaired ventricular relaxation and signs and symptoms of HF indicates diastolic dysfunction.
- B-type natriuretic peptide (BNP) of over 100 pg/mL
- Complete blood cell count, electrolyte levels (including calcium and magnesium), blood urea nitrogen (BUN), creatinine, serum

glucose, serum albumin, liver function tests, thyroid-stimulating hormone
- Cardiac stress testing, cardiac catheterization

MEDICAL AND NURSING MANAGEMENT

Identifying patients at risk and interventions for prevention are the first steps in the care and treatment of HF. The overall goals of management of HF are to relieve patient symptoms, improve functional status and quality of life, and extend survival.

- Eliminate or reduce contributory factors, especially those that may be reversible (eg, atrial fibrillation, excessive alcohol ingestion, uncontrolled HTN).
- Reduce the workload on the heart by reducing afterload and preload.
- Optimize all therapeutic regimens.
- Prevent exacerbations of HF.
- Ultrafiltration may be used to remove excess fluid.

Treatment options vary according to the severity of the patient's condition.

Lifestyle Changes

- Sodium restriction and avoidance of excess fluid, alcohol, and smoking
- Weight reduction when indicated, and regular exercise
- Education on signs and symptoms to report to health care professional, including weight gain, increasing shortness of breath (SOB), fatigue, and edema

Pharmacologic Therapy

- Alone or in combination: Vasodilator therapy (angiotensin-converting enzyme [ACE] inhibitors), angiotensin II receptor blockers (ARBs), selected beta blockers, therapy, and digitalis
- Loop diuretics and aldosterone receptor antagonists
- Inotropic agents including dobutamine, dopamine, and milrinone

- Vasodilators including nitrates and arterial vasodilators, such as hydralazine
- Management of associated problems with anticoagulants, antilipemics (statins)

Surgical Management

- Coronary bypass surgery, percutaneous transluminal coronary angioplasty (PTCA)
- Other therapies as indicated: Ventricular assist devices, heart transplant, cardiac resynchronization with biventricular pacemaker, implantable cardiac defibrillator (ICD),

Nursing Management

The nursing assessment for the patient with HF focuses on observing for effectiveness of therapy and for the patient's ability to understand and implement self-management strategies. Assess the patient's understanding of HF, self-management strategies, and the desire to adhere to those strategies.

- Observe for symptoms of HF including SOB, DOE, and cough
- Question the patient about interrupted sleep due to SOB, called *paroxysmal nocturnal dyspnea* (PND) and an inability to breathe while lying flat, called *orthopnea*. Ask how many pillows the patient uses for sleep.
- Assess for edema, abdominal symptoms, altered mental status, ability to perform activities of daily living, and activities that cause fatigue.
- Monitor intake and output (I & O), correlate positive fluid balance to weight gain. Observe for oliguria or anuria. Weigh patient daily wearing same type of clothes and on same scale.
- Auscultate lungs to detect crackles and wheezes. Note rate and depth of respirations.
- Auscultate for S_3; monitor heart rate and rhythm.
- Assess sensorium and LOC.
- Assess dependent parts of body for perfusion and edema and the liver for hepatojugular reflux; assess JVD.
- Report symptoms of HF or worsening symptoms to health care provider immediately.

H

COMPLICATIONS

- Hypotension, poor perfusion, and cardiogenic shock
- Arrhythmias
- Thromboembolism
- Pericardial effusion and cardiac tamponade

For more information, see Chapter 15 in Pellico, L.H. (2013). *Focus on adult health: Medical-surgical nursing.* Philadelphia: Wolters Kluwer Health | Lippincott Williams & Wilkins.

Hepatic Encephalopathy and Hepatic Coma

Hepatic encephalopathy and hepatic coma are complications of liver failure caused by accumulation of ammonia and toxic metabolites in the bloodstream.

PATHOPHYSIOLOGY

Ammonia is produced in the liver as a by-product of protein and amino acid breakdown including intestinal ammonia production resulting from bacterial action. The liver converts ammonia into urea, which is then excreted into the urine. In normal liver function, this process prevents the toxic buildup of ammonia in the blood. Damaged liver cells fail to detoxify and convert the ammonia to urea, and the elevated ammonia enters the bloodstream. The increased ammonia concentration in the blood causes brain dysfunction and damage, resulting in hepatic encephalopathy.

RISK FACTORS

- Digestion of dietary and blood proteins, ingestion of ammonium salts

- High-protein diet
- Uremia
- Excessive diuresis, dehydration, and hypokalemia
- Constipation
- Surgery
- Fever
- Medications (sedatives, tranquilizers, analgesics, and diuretics that promote potassium loss)

CLINICAL MANIFESTATIONS AND ASSESSMENT

- Earliest symptoms of hepatic encephalopathy include minor mental changes and motor disturbances; slight confusion and unkept appearance with alterations in mood and sleep pattern.
- With progression, patient may be difficult to awaken and progress to coma.
- Asterixis, flapping tremor of the hands, may occur. A handwriting or drawing sample (eg, star figure), taken daily, may provide graphic evidence of progression or reversal of hepatic encephalopathy
- In early stages, patient's reflexes are hyperactive; with worsening encephalopathy, reflexes disappear and extremities become flaccid.
- Occasionally fetor hepaticus, a sweet, slightly fecal odor of the breath, described as freshly mowed grass, acetone, or old wine, may be noticed.
- In a more advanced stage, there are gross disturbances of consciousness and the patient is completely disoriented with respect to time and place.

DIAGNOSTIC FINDINGS

- Elevated serum ammonia levels
- Electroencephalogram (EEG) shows generalized slowing, an increase in the amplitude of brain waves, and characteristic triphasic waves.

MEDICAL AND NURSING MANAGEMENT

Medical management of hepatic encephalopathy focuses on identifying and correcting the precipitating cause if possible.

- Lactulose (Cephulac) is administered orally, by NG tube or enema, to reduce serum ammonia levels. Side effects include intestinal bloating and cramps, which usually disappear within a week. Monitor for hypokalemia.

> **NURSING ALERT**
> The patient receiving lactulose is monitored closely for the development of watery diarrheal stools, because they indicate a medication overdose.

- Administer IV glucose to minimize protein breakdown and vitamins to correct deficiencies, correct electrolyte imbalances (especially potassium).
- Assess mental and neurologic status frequently.
- Monitor I & O.
- Evaluate vital signs every 4 hours.
- Potential sites of infection (peritoneum, lungs) are assessed frequently, and abnormal findings are reported promptly.
- Monitor serum ammonia levels.
- Restrict protein intake in patients who are comatose or who have encephalopathy that is refractory to lactulose and antibiotic therapy.
- Give enemas to reduce ammonia absorption from the gastrointestinal (GI) tract.
- Administer antibiotics and electrolytes when needed.
- Stop all sedation, tranquilizers, and analgesics. Benzodiazepine antagonists such as flumazenil (Romazicon) may be administered to improve encephalopathy, whether or not the patient has previously taken benzodiazepines.

Nursing Management

- Maintain a safe environment to prevent bleeding, injury, and infection.

- Recognize rehabilitation is likely to be prolonged; communicate to patient about status and assist them to understand the cause of this process and likelihood of recurrence.
- Explain to patient and family the consequences of vitamin deficiencies, especially clotting factors secondary to inability to use vitamin K to manufacture prothrombin due to underlying condition. Other deficiencies include vitamin A, thiamine, riboflavin, pyridoxine, vitamin C, and folic acid.
- Patient with encephalopathy and liver disease is chronically ill and at risk for thrombocytopenia, anemia, and decreased white cells causing bruising, bleeding, and increased susceptibility to infection.
- Monitor for hypoglycemia.
- Assess patients with hepatic disease for gynecomastia, testicular atrophy, decreased libido, and impotence in men. Women may have irregular or absent menstrual cycles, and decreased sexual function as well.

For more information, see Chapter 25 in Pellico, L.H. (2013). *Focus on adult health: Medical-surgical nursing.* Philadelphia: Wolters Kluwer Health | Lippincott Williams & Wilkins.

H

Hepatic Failure, Fulminant

Fulminant hepatic failure is the clinical syndrome of sudden and severely impaired liver function in a previously healthy person.

PATHOPHYSIOLOGY

Fulminant liver failure is caused by many different etiologies. Viral hepatitis caused by A, B, and E is a common culprit worldwide. Acetaminophen overdoses accounts for over 50% of fulminant liver failure cases in the United States and is the leading cause for acute liver failure (ALF) in Great Britain and parts of Europe.

Other causes of fulminant liver failure include drug overdoses or reactions, viruses such as herpes simplex and varicella zoster, toxins, metabolic diseases such as Wilson's, mushroom ingestion, and obstruction to hepatic blood flow (Budd-Chiari syndrome).

CLINICAL MANIFESTATIONS AND ASSESSMENT

- Hepatic encephalopathy, jaundice, nausea, anorexia, vomiting, and coagulopathy in a patient with no history of prior liver disease
- Jaundice and profound anorexia
- Onset is abrupt; the patient or family may or may not be able to identify the precipitating event.

MEDICAL AND NURSING MANAGEMENT

The clinical decision of whether a patient will recover from acute liver injury with intense medical management or require liver transplantation is made on a case-by-case basis.

- The United Network for Organ Sharing (UNOS) has identified those patients qualifying for urgent transplant listing as those with life expectancy of less than 7 days without liver transplant.
- Coagulation defects, renal failure, electrolyte disturbances, cardiovascular abnormalities, infection, hypoglycemia, encephalopathy, and cerebral edema require early recognition and treatment.
- Patients with stage 3 (somnolent but can be aroused) or 4 (coma) encephalopathy, or elevated serum ammonia, are at high risk for cerebral edema. Intracranial pressure monitoring may be used, although its use remains controversial. Promote adequate cerebral perfusion with careful fluid balance, hemodynamic assessments, a quiet environment, diuresis with mannitol, barbiturate anesthesia or pharmacologic paralysis, and sedation to prevent surges in ICP related to agitation.
- Other supportive measures include monitoring for and treating hypoglycemia, coagulopathy, renal impairment, and infection.

For more information, see Chapter 25 in Pellico, L.H. (2013). *Focus on adult health: Medical-surgical nursing.* Philadelphia: Wolters Kluwer Health | Lippincott Williams & Wilkins.

Hepatitis, Viral: Types A, B, C, D, E, and G

Viral hepatitis is a systemic, viral infection in which necrosis and inflammation of liver cells produce a characteristic cluster of clinical, biochemical, and cellular changes. To date, six types of viral hepatitis have been identified: A, B, C, D, E, and G. These viruses infect the liver and can result in either acute or chronic liver dysfunction and disease. Patients may have nonspecific symptoms of malaise, GI distress, or present with frank jaundice and elevations of aminotransferases.

HEPATITIS A VIRUS

PATHOPHYSIOLOGY

The mode of transmission of hepatitis A virus (HAV) occurs through fecal–oral route, primarily through person-to-person contact and/or ingestion of fecally contaminated food or water. Uncooked or poor food handling practices is a common method of transmission of HAV.

HAV replicates in the liver, is excreted in bile, and shed in the stool. Incubation averages 28 days, with signs and symptoms typically lasting less than 2 months (although in some patients, this can extend up to 6 months). The peak period for transmission of HAV from one person to another occurs in the 2-week period prior to development of jaundice or symptoms, when the concentration of virus in the stool is highest. Typically, persons infected with HAV spontaneously recover; however, adults over 50 years of age or with chronic liver disease may progress to fulminant liver failure

CLINICAL MANIFESTATIONS AND ASSESSMENT

- Many patients are asymptomatic.
- May present with acute symptoms such as fever, malaise, anorexia, nausea, diarrhea, vomiting, abdominal pain. Jaundice is present in over 70% of adults.

DIAGNOSTIC METHODS

- Serologic testing is required for accurate diagnosis of HAV infection.
- A positive Anti-HAV (IgM) signifies serum IgM antibodies that are reactive to HAV and confirms an acute infection.
- Anti-HAV (IgG) becomes positive shortly after onset of infection, and remains positive throughout the person's life, conferring immunity.
- Total anti-HAV positivity and negative anti-HAV (IgM) indicates immunity to HAV infection either through exposure or vaccination.

PREVENTION

- Current recommendations are to routinely vaccinate all children, to identify and vaccinate persons at high risk for contracting HAV, and to vaccinate any person who wishes to prevent HAV.
- Two doses of hepatitis A antigen are given intramuscularly in the deltoid; passive immunization is achieved with immunoglobulin containing HAV antibodies given to persons for prophylaxis after exposure to the virus. Its use is indicated for patients with no evidence of immunity.
- Proper personal hygiene, community, and home sanitation are crucial to prevention.
- Effective health supervision of schools, dormitories, extended-care facilities, barracks, and camps is essential.

MEDICAL AND NURSING MANAGEMENT

Acute HAV infection in most patients is managed with supportive care.

- Prevent dehydration, using IV fluids if necessary.
- Encourage physical activity as tolerated.
- Promptly identify signs and symptoms indicating possible fulminant liver failure, such as altered mental status or severe vomiting, with referral to a liver transplant center.

Nursing Management

- Assist patient and family in coping with the temporary disability and fatigue that are common in hepatitis and instruct them to seek additional health care if the symptoms persist or worsen.
- Educate about diet, rest, follow-up blood work, and the importance of avoiding alcohol, as well as sanitation and hygiene measures (particularly hand washing after bowel movements and before eating).
- Review environmental sanitation (safe food and water supply, effective sewage disposal) and proper food storage and thorough cooking of foods to recommended temperatures.

HEPATITIS B VIRUS

Hepatitis B virus (HBV) infection is an important public health problem, with as many as 350 million people worldwide with chronic infection. HBV is highly prevalent in Asia, Africa, the Middle East, parts of Europe, the Caribbean, and Central and South America.

PATHOPHYSIOLOGY

HBV is transmitted primarily through blood, saliva, and semen; it may be transmitted through mucous membranes and breaks in the skin. HBV is also transferred from carrier mothers to their babies, especially in areas with a high incidence. HBV is primarily transmitted by perinatal, percutaneous, sexual exposure, and close person-to-person contact via contact with open cuts or sores, shared

H

razors or toothbrushes, and contaminated surfaces. HBV has a long incubation period. Acute HBV infection can result in fulminant liver failure or progress to chronic infection. Patients with chronic HBV infection may eventually develop cirrhosis, end-stage liver disease, and cancer of the liver.

RISK FACTORS

- Individuals born in areas with high rates of HBV infection
- Exposure to blood, blood products, or other body fluids; health care workers
- Hemodialysis
- Male homosexual and bisexual activity
- Intravenous/injection drug use
- Close contact with carrier of HBV
- Travel to or residence in area with uncertain sanitary conditions
- Multiple sexual partners
- Recent history of sexually transmitted disease
- Receipt of blood or blood products (eg, clotting factor concentrate)

CLINICAL MANIFESTATIONS AND ASSESSMENT

Symptoms may be insidious and variable.

- Anorexia, fevers, dyspepsia, abdominal pain, generalized aching, malaise, and weakness may occur. Jaundice may be evident or absent.
- Skin rashes and arthralgias (pain in the joints) may occur.
- May remain asymptomatic until development of cirrhosis and signs of hepatic decompensation.

DIAGNOSTIC METHODS

Complete blood counts (CBC with platelets), hepatic function panel, and prothrombin time and International normalized ratio

(INR). Lab tests to detect hepatitis B replication and other viral co-infections (HAV, HCV, HIV) should be included in the assessment.

PREVENTION

The goals of prevention are to interrupt the chain of transmission, to protect those at high risk by active immunization with hepatitis B vaccine, and to use passive immunization for unprotected people exposed to HBV.

- Vaccinate sexual contacts of individuals with chronic hepatitis B, use barrier protection during intercourse.
- Avoid sharing toothbrushes or razors with others, and cover open sores or skin lesions. Blood spills should be cleaned with a solution of 1 part bleach to 10 parts water. Persons with HBV infection should be advised to avoid donation of blood, organs, or sperm.
- Administer HBV vaccine at birth and to those unvaccinated: Three doses intramuscularly at 0, 1-month, and 6-month intervals for adults.

NURSING ALERT

The FDA has approved a combined hepatitis A and B vaccine (Twinrix) for vaccination of people 18 years of age and older with indications for both hepatitis A and B vaccination. Vaccination consists of three doses, on the same schedule as that used for single-antigen hepatitis B vaccine (ACIP, 2010).

- Hepatitis B immune globulin (HBIG) provides passive immunity; it is indicated for people exposed to HBV who are unvaccinated or never had hepatitis B.

MEDICAL MANAGEMENT

The goals of treatment for hepatitis B are to prevent replication of active HBV (viral suppression) and reduce the effects of chronic liver inflammation.

H

- Antiviral therapies are available to treat hepatitis B; of these pegylated interferon alfa, adefovir and entecavir, and telbivudine and tenofovir are the preferred medications singly or in combination.
- Periodic laboratory testing is used to assess elevations in hepatic function and replication of HBV DNA.
- Patients at high risk for hepatocellular carcinoma (patients with cirrhosis) should receive ultrasound screening every 6 months

NURSING MANAGEMENT

- Management of the symptoms of malaise, anorexia, nausea, vomiting and fever are primarily supportive to maintain nutrition, fluid intake, and adequate rest during recovery.
- Observe for signs of progression to fulminant liver failure (discussed later in the chapter); however, alterations in mental status, severe vomiting, and increasing jaundice should initiate referral to a tertiary care center or liver transplant center.
- Educate patient and family patient in the prevention of transmission and on the avoidance of lifestyle factors that may exacerbate existing liver disease.

HEPATITIS C VIRUS

Hepatitis C virus (HCV) infection is the leading cause of liver disease and the primary indication for liver transplantation.

PATHOPHYSIOLOGY

HCV is a blood-borne RNA virus and is avidly replicated in the liver. Transmission of HCV occurs primarily through injection of drugs and through transfusion of blood products prior to 1992. Its route is through parenteral contact with blood. Sexual transmission may also occur, with high risk associated with multiple sex partners. Other less common modes of transmission include via hemodialysis, health care workers exposure to needlestick injury or contaminated blood, and tattooing.

The acute infection clears in only 15% of cases; the majority of individuals will develop chronic infection with evidence of hepatitis C RNA viremia. Unlike other hepatitis viruses, the acute stage of hepatitis C often is asymptomatic for decades. Hepatitis C infection with progression to cirrhosis occurs in up to 20% of patients over 20 years or longer. Factors contributing to the severity of liver disease include increased alcohol use, male gender, older age at infection, HIV or HBV coinfection, and obesity. Individuals with HCV cirrhosis are at higher risk of developing hepatic decompensation and hepatocellular carcinoma.

CLINICAL MANIFESTATIONS AND ASSESSMENT

Most patients with acute or chronic hepatitis C are asymptomatic. Some patients will develop jaundice, nausea, vomiting, and malaise during the acute stage. Patients may be diagnosed incidentally during routine lab testing, or when cirrhosis develops. Extrahepatic signs such as skin rashes, joint aches, and purpura (small blood vessels that rupture under the skin and leak, causing purple bruising) are common.

DIAGNOSTIC METHODS

The diagnosis of HCV infection is confirmed by serology with anti-HCV antibodies present and measurement of viremia through HCV RNA. Genotype testing and liver biopsy will provide information to assist in the management and treatment of hepatitis C, and stage the severity of disease. Other tests to assess the extent of liver disease include laboratory tests (ie, bilirubin, albumin, aminotransferases, prothrombin time, and INR). Ultrasound or other imaging may be used to assess for cirrhosis or presence of lesions.

MEDICAL AND NURSING MANAGEMENT

Treatment of hepatitis C is to prevent the progression of fibrosis and evolution to cirrhosis by reducing HCV RNA levels to nondetectable; nondetectable viral load or HCV RNA 6 months after completion of therapy is considered curative. Antiviral therapy consists of pegylated interferon alfa injected subcutaneously once weekly and ribavirin taken orally daily; most patients undergo therapy for 48 weeks or longer. Antiviral therapy has significant side effects and commonly causes patients to stop treatment. Side effects include moderate to severe flu-like symptoms, skin rashes, pruritus, insomnia, irritability, decreased concentration, and depression. The patient requires close monitoring of hematological function for evidence of anemia, neutropenia, and/or thrombocytopenia. Ribavirin is highly teratogenic; females of childbearing age should be advised to use reliable contraception; female partners of men undergoing therapy should also use contraception.

HEPATITIS D VIRUS

Hepatitis D (delta agent) occurs in some cases of hepatitis B. Because the virus requires hepatitis B surface antigen for its replication, only patients with hepatitis B are at risk. Anti-HDV antibodies (IGg) in patients with chronic hepatitis B confirms the diagnosis The symptoms are similar to those of hepatitis B, except that patients are more likely to have fulminant hepatitis and cirrhosis. Current treatment for hepatitis D is the use of interferon or pegylated interferon alfa for 12 months.

HEPATITIS E VIRUS

It is believed that hepatitis E virus (HEV) is transmitted by the fecal–oral route, principally through contaminated water in endemic areas with poor sanitation. This form of hepatitis usually is self-limiting, with acute onset and subsequent recovery with no chronicity. HEV is responsible for most cases of fulminant hepatitis in India. Pregnant women infected with hepatitis E infection have a high mortality rate (up to 25%); this is increased during the last trimester. Currently, there is no vaccine or specific treatment for HEV; however, research in vaccine development may be promising in the near future.

Prevention of transmission is focused on improvement of sanitation, development of clean water supplies in endemic countries, and safe food handling practices.

HEPATITIS G VIRUS

The hepatitis G virus (HGV) is an RNA virus that has recently been identified; however, controversy exists as to its role in the pathogenesis of liver disease.

For more information, see Chapter 25 in Pellico, L.H. (2013). *Focus on adult health: Medical-surgical nursing.* Philadelphia: Wolters Kluwer Health | Lippincott Williams & Wilkins.

Hiatal Hernia

H

Hiatal (hiatus) hernia occurs when the opening in the diaphragm through which the esophagus passes becomes enlarged and the upper stomach moves up into the lower portion of the thorax.

PATHOPHYSIOLOGY

There are two types of hernias: Sliding and paraesophageal. Sliding, or type I, hiatal hernia occurs when the upper stomach and the gastroesophageal junction are displaced upward and slide in and out of the thorax; this occurs in about 90% of patients with esophageal hiatal hernias. A paraesophageal hernia is classified by extent of herniation (type II, III, or IV) and occurs when all or part of the stomach pushes through the diaphragm beside the esophagus.

RISK FACTORS

Hiatal hernia occurs more often in women than men.

CLINICAL MANIFESTATIONS AND ASSESSMENT

Hemorrhage, obstruction, and strangulation are possible with any type of hernia.

Sliding Hernia

- Heartburn, regurgitation, and dysphagia; at least half of cases are asymptomatic.
- Often implicated in reflux.

Paraesophageal Hernia

- Sense of fullness or chest pain after eating or may be asymptomatic.
- Reflux does not usually occur.

DIAGNOSTIC METHODS

Diagnosis is confirmed by X-ray studies, barium swallow, and fluoroscopy.

MEDICAL AND NURSING MANAGEMENT

- Frequent, small feedings that easily pass through the esophagus are given.
- Advise patient not to recline for 1 hour after eating (prevents reflux or hernia movement).
- Elevate the head of bed on 4- to 8-inch blocks to prevent hernia from sliding upward.

- Surgery is indicated when a patient has significant esophageal injury, or when he or she does not respond to medical management.
- Medical and surgical management of paraesophageal hernias is similar to that for gastroesophageal reflux; patients may require emergency surgery to correct torsion (twisting) of the stomach or other organs that leads to restriction of blood flow to that area.

For more information, see Chapter 22 in Pellico, L.H. (2013). *Focus on adult health: Medical-surgical nursing.* Philadelphia: Wolters Kluwer Health | Lippincott Williams & Wilkins.

Hodgkin's Lymphoma

Refer to Lymphoma, Hodgkin's on pages 448–451 and Chapter 20 in Pellico, L.H. (2013). *Focus on adult health: Medical-surgical nursing.* Philadelphia: Wolters Kluwer Health | Lippincott Williams & Wilkins.

H

Hyperglycemic Hyperosmolar Nonketotic Syndrome

Hyperglycemic hyperosmolar nonketotic syndrome (HHNS) is a life-threatening condition characterized by hyperosmolality and hyperglycemia with alterations in LOC. Ketosis is minimal or absent.

PATHOPHYSIOLOGY

Persistent hyperglycemia causes osmotic diuresis, resulting in water and electrolyte losses. In HHNS, the insulin level is too low to prevent hyperglycemia and subsequent osmotic diuresis, but it is high enough to prevent fat breakdown and ketoacidosis. Polydipsia, polyuria, and severe dehydration develop.

RISK FACTORS

- Ages between 50 and 70
- Infection, acute or chronic illness
- Medications that exacerbate hyperglycemia, such as thiazides
- Therapeutic procedures, such as surgery or dialysis

CLINICAL MANIFESTATIONS AND ASSESSMENT

- History of days to weeks of polyuria with adequate fluid intake
- Hypotension, tachycardia
- Profound dehydration (dry mucous membranes, poor skin turgor)
- Variable neurologic signs (alterations of sensorium, seizures, hemiparesis)

DIAGNOSTIC METHODS

- Severe hyperglycemia of 600 mg/dL or more; serum osmolality of 340 mOsm/L or more
- Electrolytes and BUN consistent with dehydration

MEDICAL AND NURSING MANAGEMENT

The overall treatment of HHNS is similar to that of diabetic ketoacidosis (DKA): Fluids, correction of electrolyte imbalance, and insulin.

- Administer 0.9% or 0.45% normal saline, depending on sodium level and severity of volume depletion.

- Central venous or hemodynamic pressure monitoring may be necessary to guide fluid replacement.
- Add potassium to replacement fluids when urinary output is adequate; guided by continuous ECG monitoring and laboratory determinations of potassium.
- Insulin is usually given at a continuous low rate to treat hyperglycemia; perform frequent glucose monitoring.
- Intravenous fluids with dextrose are administered after the glucose level has decreased to the range of 250 to 300 mg/dL.
- Other therapeutic modalities are determined by the underlying illness and results of continuing clinical and laboratory evaluation.
- It may take 3 to 5 days for neurologic symptoms to clear; treatment of HHNS usually continues well after metabolic abnormalities are resolved.
- After recovery from HHNS, patients can control their diabetes with diet, oral antidiabetic medications, or insulin as needed.

Nursing Management

See "Nursing Management" under "Diabetes Mellitus" on pages 265–270 and "Diabetic Ketoacidosis" on pages 272–275 for additional information.

- Closely monitor vital signs, fluid status, and laboratory values.
- Maintain safety and prevent injury due to changes in sensorium.
- Fluid status and urine output are closely monitored due to high risk of renal failure secondary to severe dehydration.
- Because HHNS tends to occur in older patients, the physiologic changes that occur with aging should be considered.
- Careful assessment of cardiovascular, pulmonary, and renal function throughout the acute and recovery phases of HHNS is important.

H

For more information, see Chapter 30 in Pellico, L.H. (2013). *Focus on adult health: Medical-surgical nursing.* Philadelphia: Wolters Kluwer Health | Lippincott Williams & Wilkins.

Hyperparathyroidism

Hyperparathyroidism is characterized by excess parathormone (PTH) levels leading to a markedly increased level of serum calcium that can present as a potentially life-threatening situation.

PATHOPHYSIOLOGY

The actions of PTH are increased by the presence of vitamin D. The serum level of ionized calcium regulates the output of parathormone. Increased serum calcium leads to a decreased parathormone secretion, based on a negative feedback system. When the product of serum calcium and serum phosphorus rises, calcium phosphate may precipitate and calcify in various organs of the body such as the kidneys.

RISK FACTORS

- Increases tenfold between 15 and 65 years
- Tumor or hyperplasia of the parathyroids occurs two to four times more often in women.
- Secondary hyperparathyroidism occurs in chronic renal failure.

CLINICAL MANIFESTATIONS AND ASSESSMENT

- Half of individuals are asymptomatic.
- Main symptoms are related to hypercalcemia:
  - Apathy, fatigue, muscle weakness, nausea, vomiting, constipation
- Direct effect of calcium on the brain and nervous system: Psychological manifestations such as irritability, neurosis, or psychoses
- Cardiac responses include increased cardiac contractility and the development of ventricular arrhythmias. Digitalis accentuates the cardiac response of hypercalcemia.

- Kidneys stones develop in 55% of patients with primary hyperparathyroidism; may cause obstruction, pyelonephritis, and renal failure.
- Musculoskeletal symptoms include skeletal pain and tenderness, especially of the back and joints, pain on weight bearing, pathologic fractures, deformities, and shortening of body stature. Bone resorption, loss of calcium from the bone, or demineralization, causes kyphosis, compression fractures, and fragile bones, increasing the risk for fracture.
- Gastric secretions may increase, causing peptic ulcer and abdominal pain. Pancreatitis may develop as a result of stones in the pancreatic ducts.

DIAGNOSTIC METHODS

- Elevation of serum calcium levels and an elevated concentration of PTH is noted.
- Radioimmunoassay for PTH is sensitive and differentiates primary hyperparathyroidism from other causes of hypercalcemia; an elevated serum calcium level alone is nonspecific as serum levels may be altered by diet, medications, and renal and bone changes.
- Bone changes on X-ray or bone scans indicate advanced disease.
- The double-antibody parathyroid hormone test distinguishes between primary hyperparathyroidism and malignancy as a cause of hypercalcemia.
- Ultrasound, MRI, thallium scan, and fine-needle biopsy evaluate the parathyroid functions and localize parathyroid cysts, adenomas, or hyperplasia.

MEDICAL AND NURSING MANAGEMENT

The recommended treatment of primary hyperparathyroidism is surgical removal of abnormal parathyroid tissue (parathyroidectomy). In patients without symptoms, mildly elevated serum calcium levels, and normal renal function, surgery may be delayed and the patient monitored closely for complications.

Providing Hydration Therapy

- Patients with hyperparathyroidism are at risk for renal failure.
- Strict I & O is monitored in hospitalized patients. Encourage a daily fluid intake of 2,000 mL or more to prevent calculus formation; cranberry juice or cranberry extract tablets are suggested to lower the urinary pH. Instruct patient to report symptoms of renal calculi, such as abdominal pain and hematuria.
- Thiazide diuretics are avoided because they decrease the renal excretion of calcium and further elevate serum calcium levels.
- Instruct the patient to avoid dehydration and to seek immediate health care for conditions that commonly produce dehydration (eg, vomiting and diarrhea).

Encouraging Mobility

- Encourage ambulation using a walker. For limited mobility, a rocking chair is useful; bones that are subjected to stress give up less calcium. Bed rest increases calcium excretion and the risk for renal calculi.
- Oral phosphates lower the serum calcium level in some patients; however, long-term use is not recommended due to the risk of ectopic calcium phosphate deposits into soft tissues.

Administering Nutrition and Medication

- Dietary calcium will be restricted or increased, depending on the patient's serum calcium level.
- If peptic ulcer is present, antacids and protein feedings are necessary.
- Prevent constipation, offering prune juice and stool softeners (eg, Colace or Senna), increasing physical activity, and increasing fluid intake.

Providing Emotional Support

Diverse and vague symptoms may lead to depression and frustration. Educate family that patient's illness is not psychosomatic; discuss course of the disorder to help the patient and family deal with their reactions and feelings.

Managing Hypercalcemic Crisis

- Acute hypercalcemic crisis can occur with extreme elevation of serum calcium levels.
- Serum calcium levels greater than 15 mg/dL (3.7 mmol/L) result in neurologic, cardiovascular, and renal symptoms that can be life-threatening.
- Rehydration uses large volumes of IV fluids (normal saline expands volume and inhibits calcium resorption), diuretics to promote renal excretion of excess calcium, and phosphate therapy which corrects calcium.
- Cytotoxic agents (eg, mithramycin), calcitonin, and dialysis may be used in emergency situations to decrease serum calcium levels quickly. Effective results occur within 24 hours but last only about 1 to 2 weeks.
- Calcitonin and corticosteroids have been administered in emergencies to reduce the serum calcium level by increasing calcium deposition in bone.
- Other agents that may be administered to decrease serum calcium levels include bisphosphonates (eg, etidronate [Didronel], pamidronate [Aredia]).
- Careful assessment and care are required to minimize life-threatening complications; attention to cardiac function is advised since death from hypercalcemic crisis is often caused by cardiac arrest.

H

> For more information, see Chapter 30 in Pellico, L.H. (2013). *Focus on adult health: Medical-surgical nursing.* Philadelphia: Wolters Kluwer Health | Lippincott Williams & Wilkins.

Hypertension and Hypertensive Crisis

Hypertension is defined as a systolic blood pressure greater than 140 mm Hg and a diastolic pressure greater than 90 mm Hg, based on two or more measurements. Hypertension can be classified as follows:

- Normal: Systolic less than 120 mm Hg; diastolic less than 80 mm Hg
- Prehypertension: Systolic 120 to 139 mm Hg; diastolic 80 to 89 mm Hg
- Stage 1: Systolic 140 to 159 mm Hg; diastolic 90 to 99 mm Hg or higher
- Stage 2: Systolic 160 mm Hg or higher; diastolic 100 mm Hg or higher
- Hypertensive crisis: Systolic blood pressure higher than 180 mm Hg or a diastolic blood pressure of higher than 120 mm Hg

Hypertension is a major risk factor for atherosclerotic disease, HF, stroke, and kidney failure, as well as for damage to the eyes. Hypertension carries the risk for premature morbidity or mortality, which increases as systolic and diastolic pressures rise. Some 30% of individuals are unaware they have HTN and of those already diagnosed, 70% do not achieve adequate blood pressure control.

PATHOPHYSIOLOGY

Blood pressure is the product of cardiac output multiplied by peripheral resistance. Cardiac output is the volume of blood being pumped by the heart per minute and is the product of the heart rate (HR) multiplied by the stroke volume (SV), which is the amount of blood pumped out from the ventricles per beat. Peripheral vascular resistance (PVR) is related to the diameter of the blood vessel and the viscosity of the blood. For HTN to develop, there must be a change in one or more factors affecting peripheral vascular resistance or cardiac output, as well as a problem with the body's control systems that monitor or regulate pressure. Hypertensive emergencies and urgencies may occur in patients whose HTN has been poorly controlled, whose HTN has been undiagnosed, or in those who have abruptly discontinued their medications.

RISK FACTORS

- Primary or essential HTN from unidentified causes
- Aging

- More common in younger men than women
- Obesity
- African American
- Secondary HTN from narrowing of the renal arteries or renal artery stenosis, renal disease, hyperaldosteronism (mineralocorticoid HTN), medications, pregnancy, and coarctation of the aorta
- "White-coat HTN" exhibits normal ambulatory blood pressure readings but elevated pressures (>140/90) in office or clinic.
- Masked HTN presents as a normal pressure reading in provider settings but elevated blood pressures at home or work.

CLINICAL MANIFESTATIONS AND ASSESSMENT

- Physical examination may reveal no abnormality other than high blood pressure.
- Question the patient about signs and symptoms of target organ damage including anginal pain; SOB; alterations in speech, vision, or balance; epistaxis (nosebleeds); headaches; dizziness; or nocturia.
- Assess for personal, social, and financial factors or unacceptable pharmaceutical side effects that may interfere with the patient's ability to adhere to the medication regimen.
- Asymptomatic for many years until vascular damage related to organ systems served by involved vessels lead to MI, HF, kidney damage or disease, transient ischemic attack (TIA), cerebrovascular accident (CVA), or changes in the retinas with hemorrhages, exudates, narrowed arterioles, and cotton-wool spots (small infarctions).

DIAGNOSTIC METHODS

- Laboratory tests include urinalysis, evaluation for microalbuminuria or proteinuria
- Blood chemistry for analysis of sodium, potassium, BUN and creatinine, fasting glucose, and total and high-density lipoprotein

- Twelve-lead ECG and echocardiography to assess left ventricular hypertrophy
- Additional studies, such as creatinine clearance, renin level, urine tests, and 24-hour urine protein, may be performed.

MEDICAL AND NURSING MANAGEMENT

The treatment goal for individuals with HTN without complicating features is less than 140/90 mm Hg; for patients with diabetes or chronic kidney disease, the goal is under 130/80. The aim for individuals with prehypertension without complicating conditions is to lower blood pressure to normal and to delay progression to HTN with lifestyle modifications.

- Nonpharmacologic approaches include weight reduction, restriction of alcohol and sodium, regular exercise and relaxation, and smoking cessation.
- The DASH (Dietary Approaches to Stop Hypertension) diet, which is high in fruits, vegetables, whole grains and low-fat dairy products, can decrease blood pressure.
- Complementary and alternative medicine and mind–body interventions including relaxation, meditation, guided imagery, hypnosis, and yoga are potentially effective in reducing blood pressure.
- The nurse emphasizes the concept of life-long blood pressure control rather than cure.

Pharmacologic Therapy

- The goal is to prescribe medication that is most effective with fewest side effects, and with the best chance of acceptance by patient.
- Thiazide diuretics are recommended as initial treatment for uncomplicated HTN.
- Angiotensin-converting enzyme (ACE) inhibitor or angiotensin receptor blocker (ARB) is recommended for patients with diabetes, HF, or cardiovascular disease.
- Beta blockers may be used with heart disease or HF.

- Additional medications used include calcium channel blockers, alpha-2 stimulating agents, and alpha-beta blockers.
- Treatment of other risk factors related to HTN are instituted, including statins to lower cholesterol and ASA to prevent cardiovascular complications.
- Caution patients not to abruptly stop antihypertensive medications because rebound HTN may occur.
- Caution patients to avoid over-the-counter medications, especially nasal decongestants containing vasoconstrictors, which can further elevate blood pressure.

NURSING ALERT

Frequent use of nonsteroidal anti-inflammatory drugs (NSAIDs) with ACE inhibitors and ARBs may decrease the antihypertensive effects.

NURSING PROCESS

The Patient With Hypertension

Assessment

- Assess blood pressure at frequent intervals; know baseline level.
- Assess for patient use of home blood pressure monitor.
- Assess for signs and symptoms that indicate target organ damage.
- Note the apical and peripheral pulse rate, rhythm, and character.
- Assess for use of medications, herbal preparation, or nutritional supplements that may increase blood pressure, including caffeine, ephedra, licorice, oral contraceptives, acetaminophen, and NSAIDs.

Diagnosis

Nursing Diagnoses

- Deficient knowledge related to relationship of blood pressure control and disease progression
- Noncompliance with therapeutic regimen related to side effects of prescribed therapy

(continues on page 398)

Planning

The major goals for the patient include understanding relationship of HTN to sodium restriction, prevention of complications, treatment, and adherence.

Nursing Interventions

Increasing Knowledge

- Emphasize control of HTN rather than cure.
- Encourage self-monitoring of blood pressure.
- Assist patient in reduction of sodium, weight loss, and increased physical activity as indicated; may consult dietician, suggest support groups.
- Advise patient to limit alcohol intake and avoid use of tobacco.
- Take patient's culture and perspectives into account.

Gerontologic Considerations

Compliance may be more difficult for the elderly. The medication regimen can be difficult to remember, and the expense can be a problem. Monotherapy (treatment with a single agent), if appropriate, may simplify the medication regimen and make it less expensive.

- Ensure that the elderly patient understands the regimen and can see and read instructions, open the medication container, and get the prescription refilled.
- Include family members or caregivers in the teaching program so that they understand the patient's needs, can encourage adherence to the treatment plan, and know when and whom to call if problems arise or information is needed.

Evaluation

Expected Patient Outcomes

- Blood pressure in target range
- Adheres to self-care program
- Free from complications

H

COMPLICATIONS

- Left ventricular hypertrophy and/or HF
- MI
- TIA/CVA
- Renal insufficiency or failure
- Retinal hemorrhage
- Hypertensive crisis

HYPERTENSIVE CRISIS

Hypertensive crisis is heralded by a systolic blood pressure of over 180 mm Hg or a diastolic blood pressure of over 120 mm Hg.

RISK FACTORS

- Patients with poorly controlled HTN or in those who have discontinued their medications
- Head injury
- Pheochromocytoma
- Food–drug interactions (such as tyramine combined with a monamine oxidase [MAO] inhibitor)
- Eclampsia or preeclampsia
- Substance abuse (eg, cocaine intoxication)
- Renal disease

CLASSIFICATION OF HYPERTENSIVE CRISIS

Hypertensive Emergency

Hypertensive emergency is a situation in which blood pressure is higher than 180/120 mm Hg and must be lowered quickly to halt or prevent damage to the target organs

- The therapeutic goals are reduction of the mean blood pressure by up to 25% within the first hour of treatment, a further reduction to a goal pressure of about 160/100 mm Hg over a period of 2 to 6 hours, and then a more gradual reduction in pressure to the target goal over a period of days
- Too rapid reduction may cause decreased tissue perfusion with resulting MI or CVA; exception is aortic dissection, in which systolic pressure should be reduced to less than 100 mm Hg.

Hypertensive Urgency

- Blood pressure is severely elevated but there is no evidence of impending or progressive target organ damage; associated severe headache, epistaxis, or anxiety are classified as urgencies.
- The goal is to reduce blood pressure to 160/110 over several hours to several days. This can be accomplished by keeping the patient several hours in the emergency department followed by outpatient management using oral medications.

PHARMACOLOGIC THERAPY

- Hypertensive emergencies are best managed with continuous IV infusion of a short-acting titratable antihypertensive agent.
- The nurse avoids the sublingual and IM routes as their absorption and dynamics are unpredictable.
- Medications may include labetalol, nicardipine, or clevidipine hydrochloride, fenoldopam mesylate, enalaprilat, esmolol, hydralazine, nitroglycerin, which have immediate, short-lived actions.
- The nurse follows-up with teaching about the hypertensive crisis and encourages the patient to take charge of managing HTN.

For more information, see Chapter 13 in Pellico, L.H. (2013). *Focus on adult health: Medical-surgical nursing.* Philadelphia: Wolters Kluwer Health | Lippincott Williams & Wilkins.

Hyperthyroidism (Graves' Disease)

Hyperthyroidism occurs as a result of the over production of thyroxine (T_3), triiodothyronine (T_4), or both from the thyroid gland.

PATHOPHYSIOLOGY

Oversecretion of thyroid hormones causes greatly increased metabolic rate and is usually associated with an enlarged thyroid gland (goiter). Graves' disease, an autoimmune disease in which antibodies are bound to thyroid-stimulating hormone (TSH), is a common cause of hyperthyroidism. Symptoms of hyperthyroidism may also occur with the release of excessive amounts of thyroid hormone as a result of inflammation after irradiation of the thyroid or destruction of thyroid tissue by tumor. Signs and symptoms are associated with hypermetabolism; if untreated, the disease may progress relentlessly, leading to the emaciation, nervousness, delirium, disorientation, and HF.

Thyrotoxicosis refers to *symptomatic* hyperthyroxinemia associated with thyroid gland inflammation or ingestion of thyroid hormone. An increase in release of stored thyroid hormone or increased exogenous hormone ingestion occurs, not accelerated synthesis. A life-threatening complication of hyperthyroidism in which profound hypermetabolism involves multiple systems is called *thyrotoxic crisis* or *thyroid storm.*

RISK FACTORS

- Women are eight times more likely to be affected than men, with onset usually between the second and fourth decades of life.
- Symptoms may appear after an emotional shock, stress, or an infection, but the exact significance of these relationships is not understood.
- Other less common causes of hyperthyroidism include thyroiditis, overmedication of synthetic thyroid hormone, and thyroid nodules.

CLINICAL MANIFESTATIONS AND ASSESSMENT

Hyperthyroidism presents a characteristic group of signs and symptoms (thyrotoxicosis).

- Nervousness, emotional hyperexcitability, irritability, apprehensiveness; inability to sit quietly; palpitations
- Palpitations, elevated resting heart rate manifested as sinus tachycardia or atrial fibrillation and elevation of systolic blood pressure
- Heat intolerance; excessive perspiration; skin is flushed, warm, soft, and moist.
- Fine tremor of the hands and tongue
- Exophthalmos (bulging eyes), causing startled facial expression
- Increased appetite and dietary intake, progressive weight loss, abnormal muscle fatigability, weakness, amenorrhea, decreased fertility, and changes in bowel function secondary to increased peristalsis
- Enlarged thyroid gland may feel soft and may pulsate; palpable thrill and bruit over thyroid arteries. Thyroid may enlarge enough to impinge on trachea or esophagus.
- Myocardial hypertrophy and HF if untreated or if elderly

DIAGNOSTIC FINDINGS

- Decreased TSH
- T_3 and T_4 increased
- Increased radioactive iodine uptake

Gerontologic Considerations

Patients older than 60 years account for 10% to 15% of the cases of hyperthyroidism. Elderly patients commonly present with vague and nonspecific signs and symptoms. The only presenting manifestations may be anorexia and weight loss or isolated atrial fibrillation with an absence of ocular signs.

New or worsening HF or angina is common in the elderly as is weakness. Spontaneous remission of hyperthyroidism is rare in the elderly. Measurement of TSH uptake is indicated in elderly patients with unexplained physical or mental deterioration. Use of radioactive iodine is generally recommended for treatment of thyrotoxicosis unless an enlarged thyroid gland is compressing the airway. Thyrotoxicosis is controlled by medications before radioactive iodine is administered because radiation may precipitate thyroid storm. Antithyroid medications are not recommended for the elderly due to resulting granulocytopenia, however beta-adrenergic blocking agents may be indicated.

MEDICAL AND NURSING MANAGEMENT

Treatment of hyperthyroidism depends on the underlying cause and consists of a combination of therapies, including radioactive iodine, antithyroid agents, and surgery. The goal of treatment is to reduce thyroid hyperactivity to relieve symptoms and prevent complications.

Radioisotope Iodine-131 (^{131}I) Therapy

- Radioactive iodine-131 to destroy the thyroid gland is most common; contraindicated during pregnancy.
- For patients who fear radioactive medication, antithyroid medication may be used.

Antithyroid Drug Therapy

- Antithyroid medications, including propylthiouracil (PTU) or methimazole (Tapazole), inhibit thyroid hormone synthesis or release but do not affect previously formed hormone. It may take several weeks to relieve symptoms.
- Side effects of antithyroid medications include fever, rash, urticaria, thrombocytopenia, or agranulocytosis; patients must notify the health care provider of any sign of infection

H

including fever, sore throat, or mouth ulcers as this may indicate agranulocytosis.

- Contraindicated in late pregnancy, because the fetus may develop fetal hypothyroidism, fetal bradycardia, goiter, and cretinism.
- Maintenance dose is established, followed by gradual withdrawal of the medication over the next several months.

Adjunctive Therapy

- Adjunctive treatment with iodine or iodide compounds such as potassium iodide (KI), Lugol's solution, and saturated solution of potassium iodide (SSKI) are no longer considered as sole treatment. These drugs reduce the activity of the thyroid hormone and the vascularity of the thyroid gland prior to surgery.
- Beta blockers control nervousness, tachycardia, tremor, anxiety, and heat intolerance; used until T_4 normalizes and TSH approaches normal.

Surgical Intervention

- Thyroidectomy or subtotal thyroidectomy is reserved for patients with nodular goiters with suspicion of malignancy, pregnant women with thyrotoxicosis not controlled with low doses of thioureas, children with Graves' disease, and patients who are allergic or unable to take antithyroid medications.
- Subtotal thyroidectomy is performed approximately 4 to 6 weeks after thyroid function has returned to normal; about five-sixths of the thyroid tissue is removed.
- Preoperatively, PTU is administered until signs of hyperthyroidism have disappeared.
- A beta-adrenergic blocking agent (propranolol) may be used to reduce the heart rate and other signs and symptoms of hyperthyroidism.
- Iodine (Lugol's solution or KI) may be prescribed in an effort to reduce blood loss; however, the effectiveness of this treatment is unknown.

NURSING PROCESS

The Patient With Hyperthyroidism

Assessment

The patient history and assessment focuses on symptoms related to accelerated or exaggerated metabolism.

- Note reports of irritability or increased emotional reaction and the impact of these changes in patient's interaction with family, friends, and coworkers.
- Additional symptoms include anxiety, sleep disturbances, apathy, and lethargy.
- The family can provide useful information about the recent changes in the patient's emotional status. Assess for other stressors and the patient's ability to cope with stress.
- Assess nutritional status by obtaining the typical dietary habit of patient; recording I & O, height and weight.
- Assess for changes in vision and appearance of eyes.
- Periodically assess cardiac status: Heart rate, blood pressure, heart sounds, and peripheral pulses.
- Assess emotional and psychological status and symptoms related to excessive nervous system activation.

Diagnosis

Nursing Diagnoses

- Altered nutrition: Less than body requirements related to exaggerated metabolic rate, excessive appetite, and increased GI activity
- Ineffective coping related to irritability, hyperexcitability, apprehension, and emotional instability
- Low self-esteem related to changes in appearance, excessive appetite, and weight loss
- Altered body temperature related to hypermetabolic status
- Discomfort related to eye changes secondary to hyperthyroidism

(continues on page 406)

Planning

Goals include improved nutritional status, improved coping ability, improved self-esteem, maintenance of normal body temperature, and absence of complications.

Nursing Interventions

Improving Nutritional Status

- Provide up to six small, well-balanced, high-calorie, high-protein meals based on increased appetite.
- Select food and fluids to replace losses from diarrhea and diaphoresis; to control diarrhea, suggest patient avoid highly seasoned foods and stimulants such as coffee, tea, cola, and alcohol.
- Provide quiet atmosphere during mealtime to aid digestion.

Enhancing Coping Measures

- Reassure the patient, family, and friends that the emotional reactions will be controlled with effective treatment.
- Maintain a calm, unhurried approach, and minimize stressful experiences.
- Minimize noises, such as loud music, conversation, and equipment alarms.
- Provide information regarding thyroidectomy and preparatory pharmacotherapy to alleviate anxiety; encourage adherence to the therapeutic regimen.
- Repeat information often, and provide written instructions as indicated due to short attention span.

Improving Self-Esteem

Reinforce that problems with appearance, appetite, weight, and emotions are a result of the disease, out of the patient's control, and will resolve with treatment.

Maintaining Normal Body Temperature

- Provide a cool, comfortable environment and fresh bedding and gown as needed.
- Give cool baths and provide cool or cold fluids; monitor body temperature.

- Avoid shivering as it increases metabolic rate and energy expenditure.

Providing Eye Care

- Provide eye care and protection for exposed cornea.
- Teach patient proper way to instill eye drops or ointments.

Monitoring and Managing Potential Complications: Thyrotoxicosis or Thyroid Storm

- Assess cardiac and respiratory function through vital signs, cardiac output, ECG monitoring, ABGs, pulse oximetry.
- Administer oxygen to prevent hypoxemia, to improve tissue oxygenation, and to meet the high metabolic demands.
- Administer IV fluids to maintain blood glucose levels and replace lost fluids.
- Administer antithyroid medications to reduce thyroid hormone levels; administer beta blockers and digitalis to treat cardiac symptoms.
- Treat shock as needed.
- Monitor for hypothyroidism, which may develop as a result of treatment.
- Instruct patient and family about the need to continue therapy indefinitely and consequences of nonadherence.

Evaluation

Expected Patient Outcomes

- Demonstrates improvement in nutritional status
- Demonstrates effective coping methods in dealing with family, friends, and coworkers
- Achieves increased self-esteem
- Maintains normal body temperature
- Displays relief of symptoms absence of complications
- States importance of regular follow-up and life-long mainte-nance of prescribed therapy

COMPLICATIONS

- Thyrotoxicosis or thyroid storm
- Hypothyroidism

H

For more information, see Chapter 31 in Pellico, L.H. (2013). *Focus on adult health: Medical-surgical nursing.* Philadelphia: Wolters Kluwer Health | Lippincott Williams & Wilkins.

Hypoglycemia

Hypoglycemia, low blood glucose level, occurs when the blood glucose falls below 50 to 60 mg/dL.

PATHOPHYSIOLOGY

Hypoglycemia can be caused by too much insulin or oral hypoglycemic agents, too little food, or excessive physical activity. Low blood glucose may occur at any time, often before meals, especially if meals are delayed or if snacks are omitted. Hypoglycemia may occur with peak activity of insulins or in the middle of the night for patients who have not eaten a bedtime snack. The clinical manifestations of hypoglycemia are related to autonomic nervous system (ANS) and central nervous system (CNS) activation. Initially, the parasympathetic system is activated, causing hunger, then the sympathetic nervous system is activated, resulting in a surge of epinephrine and norepinephrine.

RISK FACTORS

- Excessive antidiabetic medication
- Insufficient food or increased physical activity
- Peak time of insulin
- Alcohol intake

CLINICAL MANIFESTATIONS AND ASSESSMENT

- Initially, mild hypoglycemia causes the patient to feel hungry and develop sweating, tremors, tachycardia, palpitations, and anxiety.

- In moderate hypoglycemia, deprivation of glucose to the brain causes an inability to concentrate, headache, lightheadedness, confusion, memory lapses, numbness of the lips and tongue, slurred speech, impaired coordination, emotional changes, irrational or combative behavior, double vision, and drowsiness.

- Severe hypoglycemia results in disoriented behavior, seizures, difficulty arousing from sleep, or loss of consciousness. The patient needs the assistance of another for treatment.

- Hypoglycemic symptoms may occur suddenly and unexpectedly and vary from person to person or occur at varying blood glucose levels. One person may feel hypoglycemic symptoms when the blood glucose falls rapidly to 120 mg/dL, other patients who frequently have low normal glucose levels (eg, 80 to 100 mg/dL) may be asymptomatic when the blood glucose falls slowly to less than 50 mg/dL.

- Hypoglycemic unawareness results when the normal compensatory response to low blood sugar fails to cause symptoms; profound hypoglycemia may occur. This typically occurs in patients who have had diabetes for many years.

DIAGNOSTIC METHODS

Hypoglycemia is diagnosed through the measurement of serum glucose levels.

MEDICAL AND NURSING MANAGEMENT

Giving Carbohydrates

Immediate treatment is required when hypoglycemia occurs.

- The usual recommendation is 15 g of a fast-acting concentrated source of carbohydrate (CHO) orally. This may include three or four commercially prepared glucose tablets; 4 to 6 oz of fruit juice or regular soda, 6 to 10 hard candies, or 2 to 3 tsp of sugar or honey.

- Patient should avoid adding table sugar to juice, even "unsweetened" juice, which may cause a sharp increase in glucose, resulting in hyperglycemia hours later.

NURSING ALERT

Sugar should *not* be added to juice, even if it is labeled unsweetened. Adding table sugar to fruit juice may cause a sharp increase in the blood glucose level, causing prolonged hyperglycemia.

- Repeat blood glucose testing in 15 minutes and retreated with 15 g of CHO for blood glucose level of less than 70 to 75 mg/dL. If blood glucose testing is not possible and the patient is symptomatic, treatment is given and repeated as described.
- Once symptoms resolve, the patient should eat a snack containing protein and starch (milk, or cheese and crackers), unless a meal or snack is planned within the next 30 to 60 minutes.
- Glucagon injection or bolus of $D_{50}W$ via IV push is administered when the patient is unconscious rather than risking aspiration of oral carbohydrates. A concentrated source of CHO followed by a snack should be given when the patient regains consciousness.

Nursing Management

- Teach patient to prevent hypoglycemia by following a consistent, regular pattern for eating, administering insulin, and exercising. Advise patient to consume between-meal and bedtime snacks to counteract the maximum insulin effect.
- Reinforce the need for routine blood glucose tests.
- Encourage patients taking insulin to wear an identification bracelet or tag indicating they have diabetes.
- Instruct patient to notify health care provider after severe hypoglycemia has occurred.
- Instruct patients and family about symptoms of hypoglycemia and use of glucagon.
- Teach family that hypoglycemia can cause irrational and unintentional behavior.

- Teach patient the importance of performing self-monitoring of blood glucose on a frequent and regular basis.
- Teach patients with type 2 diabetes who take oral agents that symptoms of hypoglycemia may also develop.
- Patients with diabetes should carry a form of simple sugar with them at all times.

For more information, see Chapter 30 in Pellico, L.H. (2013). *Focus on adult health: Medical-surgical nursing.* Philadelphia: Wolters Kluwer Health | Lippincott Williams & Wilkins.

Hypoparathyroidism

Hypoparathyroidism results from hyposecretion of the parathyroid glands, leading to low levels of PTH that eventually results in hypocalcemia and hyperphosphatemia.

PATHOPHYSIOLOGY

In the absence of PTH, there is increased blood phosphate (hyperphosphatemia) and a resultant decreased blood calcium (hypocalcemia) level due to the inverse relationship between serum phosphorus and calcium. Without PTH, there is also decreased intestinal absorption of dietary calcium, as well as decreased resorption of calcium from bone and through the renal tubules, causing hypocalcemia.

RISK FACTORS

- Incidental parathyroidectomy during thyroid surgery
- Subtotal or total parathyroidectomy

- Genetic predisposition
- Heavy metal exposure
- Magnesium depletion

CLINICAL MANIFESTATIONS AND ASSESSMENT

- The chief symptom is *tetany,* a general muscle hypertonia, with tremor and spasmodic or uncoordinated contractions occurring with or without efforts to make voluntary movements.
- Latent tetany: Numbness, tingling, and cramps in the extremities; stiffness in the hands and feet. A positive Trousseau's sign or a positive Chvostek's sign on physical assessment suggests latent tetany.
- Overt tetany: Bronchospasm, laryngeal spasm, carpopedal spasm, dysphagia, photophobia, cardiac arrhythmias, and seizures
- Other symptoms: Anxiety, irritability, depression, and delirium. Electrocardiographic changes and hypotension may also occur.

DIAGNOSTIC FINDINGS

Diagnosis is difficult because of vague symptoms; laboratory studies show increased serum phosphate; X-rays of bone show increased density and calcification of the subcutaneous or paraspinal basal ganglia of the brain.

MEDICAL AND NURSING MANAGEMENT

The goal is to increase the serum calcium level to 9 to 10 mg/dL (2.2 to 2.5 mmol/L) and to eliminate the symptoms of hypoparathyroidism and hypocalcemia.

- When hypocalcemia and tetany occur after thyroidectomy, IV calcium gluconate is given immediately. Sedatives (pentobarbital) may be administered if calcium gluconate is ineffective in decreasing neuromuscular irritability and seizure. Parenteral parathormone may be given, watching for an allergic reaction and changes in serum calcium levels.

- Chronic hypoparathyroidism is treated with a diet high in calcium and low in phosphorus. Patient should avoid milk, milk products, egg yolks, and spinach.
- Oral calcium tablets and vitamin D preparations (to enhance calcium absorption) are administered. Vitamin D preparations include dihydrotachysterol (AT 10 or Hytakerol), ergocalciferol (vitamin D), or cholecalciferol (vitamin D).
- Aluminum hydroxide gel or aluminum carbonate (Gelusil, Amphojel) may be used after meals to bind phosphate and promote its excretion through the GI tract.
- Tracheostomy or mechanical ventilation and bronchodilating medications may become necessary if the patient develops respiratory distress.

Nursing Management

Care is directed toward detecting early signs of hypocalcemia and anticipating signs of tetany, seizures, and respiratory difficulties.

- Observe for early signs of hypocalcemia and anticipate signs of tetany, seizures, and respiratory difficulties.
- Keep calcium gluconate at the bedside; administer slowly if patient has a cardiac disorder, such as arrhythmias, or in those receiving digitalis.
- Provide continuous cardiac monitoring and careful assessment; calcium and digitalis increase systolic contraction and also potentiate each other; this can produce potentially fatal arrhythmias.
- Teach patient about medications and diet therapy, the reason for high calcium and low phosphate intake, and the symptoms of hypocalcemia and hypercalcemia.
- Direct patient to contact health care provider if symptoms occur.

H

For more information, see Chapter 31 in Pellico, L.H. (2013). *Focus on adult health: Medical-surgical nursing.* Philadelphia: Wolters Kluwer Health | Lippincott Williams & Wilkins.

Hypopituitarism

Undersecretion (hyposecretion) usually involves all of the anterior pituitary hormones and is termed *panhypopituitarism.*

PATHOPHYSIOLOGY

In this condition, the thyroid gland, the adrenal cortex, and the gonads atrophy because of loss of the trophic-stimulating (influencing the activity of a gland) hormones. Hypopituitarism can result from destruction of the anterior lobe of the pituitary gland. Too little antidiuretic hormone (ADH), secreted by the posterior lobe of the pituitary gland results in diabetes insipidus; too much results in syndrome of inappropriate ADH (SIADH).

RISK FACTORS

- Multiple endocrine neoplasia, type 1 (MEN1), a hereditary condition associated with developing pituitary tumors
- Hypophysectomy, removal of the pituitary gland (may be a cause of hypopituitarism or the treatment for tumors of pituitary)

For more information, see Chapter 31 in Pellico, L.H. (2013). *Focus on adult health: Medical-surgical nursing.* Philadelphia: Wolters Kluwer Health | Lippincott Williams & Wilkins.

Hypothyroidism and Myxedema

Hypothyroidism results from insufficient levels of thyroid hormone affecting all body functions and may range from mild to life-threatening myxedema coma.

PATHOPHYSIOLOGY

Types of hypothyroidism include primary, which refers to dysfunction of the thyroid gland (>95% of cases); central, due to failure of the pituitary gland; or tertiary, if the cause is related to the hypothalamus. If thyroid deficiency is present at birth, the term *cretinism* is used. In such instances, the mother may also have thyroid deficiency

In hypothyroidism, decreased thyroxine (T_4) production leads to the stimulation of TSH by the pituitary gland. Subsequently, TSH stimulates the secretion of triiodothyronine (T_3) to increase production of T_4, leading to hypertrophy of the thyroid gland. The term *myxedema* refers to the accumulation of mucopolysaccharides in subcutaneous and other interstitial tissue and is used only to describe the extreme symptoms of severe hypothyroidism.

RISK FACTORS

- Most common cause in adults is autoimmune thyroiditis (Hashimoto's disease)
- Treatment with radioiodine, antithyroid medication, or thyroidectomy
- Radiation therapy for head and neck malignancy
- Women between the ages of 30 to 60 years; women are affected five times more often than are men.
- Mild to moderate hypothyroidism is seen in the elderly, perhaps related to altered immune function with aging.

CLINICAL MANIFESTATIONS AND ASSESSMENT

- Early symptoms are nonspecific, including fatigue, somnolence, loss of libido, amenorrhea, apathy, mental and physical sluggishness, nonpitting edema, and pleural and pericardial effusions.
- Hair loss, brittle nails, dry skin, and paresthesias or numbness and tingling of fingers
- Constipation

- Husky voice and hoarseness
- Late symptoms include slow speech, subdued emotional responses, apathy, absence of sweating, cold intolerance, constipation, thickening of skin (due to accumulation of mucopolysaccharides in subcutaneous tissues), dyspnea, weight gain, thinning of hair, alopecia, and deafness.
- Swelling of eyelids, pitting edema, bradycardia, hypotension, and hypothermia may occur.
- Advanced hypothyroidism may produce personality and cognitive changes characteristic of dementia.
- Respiratory manifestations include pleural effusion, respiratory muscle weakness, inadequate ventilation, and sleep apnea.
- Severe hypothyroidism is associated with an elevated serum cholesterol level, atherosclerosis, CAD, poor left ventricular function, and pericardial effusion.
- Subnormal temperature and pulse rate; weight gain without corresponding increase in food intake; cachexia
- Thinning hair or alopecia; expressionless and mask-like facial features
- Hypothermia; sensation of cold in a warm environment
- Abnormal sensitivity to sedatives, opiates, and anesthetic agents (these drugs are given with extreme caution)
- Myxedema coma (rare)

MEDICAL AND NURSING MANAGEMENT

The primary objective is to restore a normal metabolic state by replacing thyroid hormone.

Pharmacologic Therapy

- Synthetic levothyroxine (Synthroid or Levothroid) is the preferred preparation.
- Dosage is based on serum TSH and disappearance of symptoms.
- Additional management: Maintain vital functions, monitor ABG values, and administer fluids cautiously because of the danger of water intoxication.

Interaction of Thyroid Hormones With Other Drugs

- Thyroid hormones increase blood glucose levels, which may necessitate use of insulin or oral hypoglycemic agents.
- Thyroid hormone may increase the pharmacologic effect of digitalis, glycosides, anticoagulants, and indomethacin, requiring careful assessment.
- The effects of thyroid hormone may be increased by phenytoin and tricyclic antidepressants.

> ☼ **N U R S I N G A L E R T**
> Sedatives and hypnotics may last far longer than anticipated, causing profound somnolence and fatal respiratory depression; the dose should be one-third to one-half of usual.

Cardiac Management

- Be aware that underlying CAD may exist; administration of thyroid hormone may increase myocardial oxygen demand without increasing supply.
- Monitor for chest pain, CHF, and arrhythmia; should these develop, hold the thyroid medication and notify the health care provider.

Providing Supportive Management

- Measure ABGs and pulse oximetry.
- Administer fluids cautiously because of the danger of water intoxication.
- Concentrated glucose may be given if hypoglycemia is evident; oral antidiabetic agents or insulin may be administered to reduce the effect of hyperglycemia resulting from thyroid replacement therapy.
- If myxedema coma is present, thyroid hormone is given intravenously until consciousness is restored.

Nursing Management

Encouraging Mobility

Assist the patient with care and hygiene, encouraging the patient to participate within his or her ability; the ability to perform activities is limited by the changes in cardiovascular and pulmonary status.

Promoting Comfort and Safety

Avoid heating pads and electric blankets because of the risk for peripheral vasodilatation, further loss of body heat, and vascular collapse. Be aware that burns from these items may occur without the patient's awareness due to delayed responses and decreased mental status.

Enhancing Coping Mechanisms

If depression and guilt occur, inform the patient and family that the symptoms and inability to recognize them are common.

COMPLICATIONS

- Myxedema: Accumulation of mucopolysaccharides in subcutaneous and other interstitial tissues causing nonpitting edema. The face develops a puffy appearance with periorbital edema. Pericardial and pleural effusions may develop.
- Myxedema coma: The most extreme, severe stage of hypothyroidism; the patient is hypothermic with lethargy that may progress to stupor and then coma secondary to alveolar hypoventilation. Cardiovascular collapse and shock may ensue.

For more information, see Chapter 31 in Pellico, L.H. (2013). *Focus on adult health: Medical-surgical nursing.* Philadelphia: Wolters Kluwer Health | Lippincott Williams & Wilkins.

Immune Thrombocytopenic Purpura

Immune thrombocytopenic purpura (ITP), formerly "idiopathic" thrombocytopenia purpura, is an autoimmune disorder resulting in platelet destruction. ITP may be acute or chronic.

PATHOPHYSIOLOGY

Although the precise cause of ITP remains unknown, the platelet count is decreased by a combination of autoantibody mediated platelet destruction and impaired platelet production secondary to autoantibody effects on the megakaryocyte. Additionally, there is a decrease in serum thrombopoietin, a hormone that stimulates platelet production. There are two forms: acute (primarily in children) and chronic.

RISK FACTORS

- More common in children and young women
- Viral infection sometimes precedes the disease in children.
- Systemic lupus erythematosus
- Pregnancy
- Medications (sulfa drugs)

CLINICAL MANIFESTATIONS AND ASSESSMENT

- Many patients have no symptoms with low platelet count an incidental finding.

- Easy bruising, heavy menses, petechiae on extremities or trunk are noted.
- Patients with petechiae (dry purpura) tend to have fewer bleeding complications than those with mucosal bleeding from mouth, gastrointestinal (GI) tract, and pulmonary system (wet purpura; carries high risk of intracranial bleeding).
- Platelet count is generally below 20,000/mm^3, although platelets are functional.

DIAGNOSTIC METHODS

- Diagnosis is based on the decreased platelet count and survival time, increased bleeding time, and ruling out other causes of thrombocytopenia.
- Bone marrow aspiration shows an increase in megakaryocytes (platelet precursors).
- Many patients are infected with *Helicobacter pylori*. To date, effectiveness of *H. pylori* treatment in relation to management of ITP is unknown.

MEDICAL AND NURSING MANAGEMENT

Primary goal of treatment is to achieve a safe platelet count.

- Treatment may not be initiated unless bleeding becomes severe or life-threatening, the platelet count is extremely low (<10,000/mm^3), or in those with risk factors for bleeding, such as uncontrolled hypertension or peptic ulcer disease.
- Sedentary individual will tolerate a low platelet count more safely than will someone with an active lifestyle.
- Medications known to cause ITP (eg, quinine, sulfa-containing medications) are stopped immediately.

Pharmacologic Therapy

- Immunosuppressive medications, such as corticosteroids, are the treatment of choice. These agents block the binding receptors on macrophages so that the platelets are not destroyed.

- Azathioprine, danazol, cyclosporine, or mycophenolate mofetil, immunosuppressive agents, may be used if steroids fail to induce a response.
- Intravenous gamma globulin (controversial and expensive) and the chemotherapy agent vincristine may also be used.
- Rituximab, a monoclonal antibody that targets the CD 20 marker on B cells, has been used successfully to treat ITP following treatment with steroids.
- Romiplostim (Nplate) and eltrombopag (Promacta), thrombopoietin-like agents, stimulate platelet production. Romiplostim is administered subcutaneously as weekly injection; eltrombopag is administered orally. Both have increased platelet counts to over 50,000/mm^3 within 2 weeks of initiation.
- Platelet infusions are usually avoided except to stop catastrophic bleeding, as these platelets are destroyed as well.

Surgical Therapy

- Splenectomy is sometimes performed (thrombocytopenia may return months or years later).
- Patients who have undergone splenectomy are permanently at risk for sepsis and should receive pneumonia and meningococcal vaccines prior to surgery.

Nursing Management

- Assess patient's lifestyle to determine the risk of bleeding from activity.
- Obtain history of medication use, including over-the-counter medications, herbs, and nutritional supplements; recent viral illness; or complaints of headache or visual disturbances (intracranial bleed).
- Be alert for sulfa-containing medications and medications that alter platelet function (eg, aspirin or other nonsteroidal anti-inflammatory drugs [NSAIDs]). Physical assessment should include a thorough search for signs of bleeding, neurologic assessment, and vital sign measurement.
- Report headache or visual disturbances to the provider immediately; can signal intracranial bleeding. Perform neurological assessment with vital sign measurements.

- Avoid injections, rectal temperatures and medications.
- Teach patient to recognize exacerbations of disease (petechiae, ecchymoses), how to contact health care personnel, the names of medications that induce ITP, and the current medical regimen, including tapering schedule for steroids.
- Instruct patient to avoid all agents that interfere with platelet function.
- Instruct patient to avoid constipation and the Valsalva maneuver.
- Encourage patient to use electric razor for shaving and soft-bristled toothbrushes instead of stiff-bristled brushes.
- Advise patient to refrain from sexual intercourse when platelet count is less than 50,000/mm^3.
- Patients who are receiving long-term corticosteroids are at risk for osteoporosis, proximal muscle wasting, cataract formation, and dental caries. Bone mineral density should be monitored, and these patients may benefit from calcium and vitamin D supplementation and bisphosphonate therapy to prevent significant bone disease.

For more information, see Chapter 20 in Pellico, L.H. (2013). *Focus on adult health: Medical-surgical nursing.* Philadelphia: Wolters Kluwer Health | Lippincott Williams & Wilkins.

Increased Intracranial Pressure

Increased intracranial pressure (ICP) refers to elevated pressures within the skull.

PATHOPHYSIOLOGY

The Monro-Kellie hypothesis states that because of the limited space for expansion within the skull, an increase in any one of the components in the cranium causes a change in the volume of the others. Because brain tissue has limited space to expand, compensation typically is accomplished by increasing absorption or diminishing production of cerebrospinal fluid (CSF) or decreasing cerebral blood volume. Without such changes, ICP will begin to rise. Normal ICP is 5 to 15 mm Hg. Increased ICP from any cause decreases cerebral perfusion, stimulates further swelling, and may shift brain tissue, resulting in herniation, a dire and frequently fatal event.

RISK FACTORS

- Most commonly associated with head injury
- Brain tumors
- Intracranial hemorrhage (ie, subarachnoid hemorrhage)
- Toxic and viral encephalopathies

CLINICAL MANIFESTATIONS AND ASSESSMENT

Increased ICP is manifested by changes in level of consciousness and abnormal respiratory and vasomotor responses.

- Alterations in level of consciousness (LOC) with subtle behavioral changes, such as restlessness or anxiety; the patient may be disoriented or have decreased alertness.
- Assessment of motor response that demonstrates movement on only one side of the body suggests hemiparesis; withdrawal suggests purposeful behavior.
- Pupils become sluggish; as coma ensues, pupils become fixed.
- Verbal and motor responses are slow.
- Sudden onset of restlessness (without apparent cause), confusion, and increasing drowsiness is noted. As ICP increases, the patient becomes stuporous, reacting only to loud or painful stimuli.
- Bradycardia, hypertension, and bradypnea associated with this deterioration are known as Cushing's triad, a grave sign. At this point, herniation of the brainstem is imminent without immediate treatment.

- Evaluate the Glasgow Coma Scale (GCS), which includes eye opening (E), verbal response (V), and motor response (M). The severity of brain injury is rated on a scale from 3 to 15; a score of 13 to 15 is classified as mild traumatic brain injury (TBI), 9 to 12 is moderate TBI, and 3 to 8 is severe TBI.
- Posturing may be present: decorticate posture, flexion and internal rotation of forearms and hands, indicates damage to the upper midbrain; decorticate posture, flexion and internal rotation of forearms and hands, indicates deeper and more severe dysfunction and is a poor prognostic sign.

DIAGNOSTIC METHODS

- Computed tomography (CT) and magnetic resonance imaging (MRI)
- Intracranial pressure monitoring provides useful information (ventriculostomy, subarachnoid bolt/screw, epidural monitor, fiberoptic monitor).
- Toxic or metabolic disorders are ruled out.

MEDICAL AND NURSING MANAGEMENT

The first priority of treatment for the patient with altered LOC is to obtain and maintain a patent airway; intubation and mechanical ventilation may be used.

- Immediate management involves decreasing cerebral edema, lowering the volume of CSF, or decreasing cerebral blood volume to maintain cerebral perfusion. The nurse administers osmotic diuretics, restricts fluids, controls fever, maintains blood pressure and oxygenation, and reduces metabolic demands. ICP may be monitored.

Monitoring ICP

Nursing management focuses on detecting early signs of increasing ICP because medical interventions are usually ineffective once later signs develop.

- Perform frequent neurologic assessment and report any signs or symptoms of increasing ICP:
  - Disorientation, restlessness, increased respiratory effort, purposeless movements, and mental confusion that may deteriorate until coma has developed
  - Pupillary changes and impaired extraocular movements
  - Weakness in one extremity or on one side of the body
  - Headache that is constant, increasing in intensity, and aggravated by movement or straining

> ☀ **NURSING ALERT**
> The earliest sign of increasing ICP is a change in LOC. Any changes in LOC should be reported immediately.

- Late signs of increased ICP:
  - Respiratory rate decreases or becomes erratic, blood pressure and temperature increase. The pulse pressure widens and the pulse fluctuates rapidly, varying from bradycardia to tachycardia.
  - Cheyne-Stokes breathing (rhythmic waxing and waning of rate and depth of respirations alternating with brief periods of apnea) and ataxic breathing (irregular breathing with a random sequence of deep and shallow breaths)
  - Projectile vomiting may occur with increased pressure on the reflex center in the medulla.
  - Hemiplegia or decorticate or decerebrate posturing may develop as pressure on the brainstem increases; bilateral flaccidity occurs before death.
  - Loss of brainstem reflexes, including pupillary, corneal, gag, and swallowing reflexes, which is an ominous sign of impending death.

Invasive ICP Monitoring

Because clinical assessment is not always a reliable guide in recognizing increased ICP, especially in comatose patients, invasive ICP monitoring is frequently used in critically ill patients.

- Intraventricular catheter (ventriculostomy) involves insertion of a fine-bore catheter into a lateral ventricle, preferably in the nondominant hemisphere of the brain. This device allows for drainage of CSF during acute increases in pressure; excessive drainage may result in collapse of the ventricles and herniation. Complications associated with its use include infection, meningitis, ventricular collapse, occlusion of the catheter by brain tissue or blood, and problems with the monitoring system.

- Subarachnoid bolt or screw is a hollow device that is inserted through the skull and dura mater into the cranial subarachnoid space. Complications include infection and blockage of the bolt by clot or brain tissue, leading to a loss of pressure tracing and a decrease in accuracy at high ICP readings.
- Cerebrospinal fluid drainage may be carried out in the operating room, emergency room, or intensive care unit. A ventriculostomy without the ICP monitoring catheter is known as an external ventricular drain (EVD).
- Note trends in ICP measurements over time; assess vital signs when an increase in ICP is noted.

Monitoring and Managing Complications

- Assist with intubation and mechanical ventilation for airway protection or respiratory difficulty.
- Prevent complications of immobility such as pressure ulcers, venous stasis, musculoskeletal deterioration, and disturbed GI functioning.
- Prevent aspiration of gastric contents or feeding.
- Monitor for endocrine abnormalities:
  - Diabetes insipidus, the result of decreased secretion of antidiuretic hormone (ADH), causes excessive urine output, decreased urine osmolality, and serum hyperosmolarity; therapy consists of administration of fluids, electrolyte replacement, and vasopressin (desmopressin, DDAVP).
  - Syndrome of inappropriate antidiuretic hormone (SIADH) results from increased secretion of ADH. The patient becomes volume-overloaded, urine output diminishes, and hyponatremia develops. Treatment includes fluid restriction and administration of a 3% hypertonic saline solution.

- Observe for and promptly treat seizures related to underlying injury or hyponatremia.
- Provide skin care, protect the eyes, prevent and monitor for pressure ulcers as these patients are entirely dependent on nursing care.

Decreasing ICP and Cerebral Edema

Pharmacologic Therapy

- Osmotic diuretics, such as mannitol, may be administered to dehydrate the brain tissue and reduce cerebral edema. Serum osmolality should be determined to assess hydration status.

NURSING ALERT
Mannitol becomes ineffective when the serum osmolality exceeds 320 mOsm.

- Hypertonic saline may be used to reduce cerebral edema. Optimal concentration, dosing, timing, and duration of hypertonic saline has yet to be determined.
- Pharmacologic paralyzing agents such as pancuronium, vecuronium, and cisatracurium decrease metabolic oxygen demand. Because the patient cannot respond or report pain, sedation and analgesia must be provided.
- High doses of barbiturates are used if the patient is unresponsive to conventional treatment. The mechanism by which barbiturates decrease ICP and protect the brain is through inhibition of free radicals, alterations in vascular tone, and suppression of metabolism.

Fluid Restriction and Hypothermia

- Limit overall fluid intake to cause hemoconcentration, which draws fluid across the osmotic gradient and decreases cerebral edema.

NURSING ALERT
Hypotonic fluids should be avoided in patients with TBI as they can cause an increase in cerebral edema.

- Provide induced hypothermia to lower body metabolism; beneficial when maintained for at least 48 hours.

Controlling Fever

Fever must be controlled to reduce metabolic demands on the brain; persistent fevers in the first week of injury are associated with poor outcome and require aggressive treatment.

- Removing all bedding, except a light sheet or small drape.
- Administer acetaminophen as prescribed.
- Give cool sponge baths, allow a fan to blow over the patient to increase surface cooling.
- Use a hypothermia blanket.
- Monitor temperature frequently to assess the patient's response to treatment.
- Prevent an excessive decrease in temperature and shivering, which increases heat production.

Maintaining Blood Pressure, Oxygenation, and Hyperventilation

Patients with TBI may sustain a secondary insult if they become hypotensive or hypoxic.

- Maintain systolic blood pressure greater than 90 mm Hg and oxygen saturation greater than 90%
- Hyperventilation is an option for patients with ICP that is unresponsive to conventional therapies; use cautiously and avoid for the first 24 hours following the initial injury.

Reducing Metabolic Demands

- Provide continuous cardiac monitoring, endotracheal intubation, mechanical ventilation, ICP monitoring, and arterial pressure monitoring for patients receiving barbiturates or paralytics.
- Assess neurologic status with ICP, blood pressure, heart rate, respiratory rate, and response to ventilator therapy (eg, bucking or "fighting" the ventilator) for patients receiving barbiturates or paralytics, as sedation and neuromuscular blockade interfere with neurological assessments.

Seizure Prophylaxis

- Seizures that develop after head injury are known as posttraumatic seizures (PTS) and are classified according to when they occur.

Within 7 days of injury, they are known as early PTS; occurring after 7 days after the injury, they are known as late PTS.
- Prophylactic anticonvulsants are used only for early PTS.

Providing Mouth Care

- Inspect for dryness, inflammation, and crusting.
- Provide conscientious oral care to decrease risk of parotitis (inflammation of the salivary glands) when mouth not kept scrupulously clean.
- Moisten mucous membranes; a thin coating of petrolatum to lips prevents drying, cracking, and encrustations.
- If the patient has an endotracheal tube, move the tube to the opposite side of the mouth daily to prevent ulceration of the mouth and lips.

Maintaining Skin and Joint Integrity

- Prove a regular schedule of turning to avoid pressure ulcers, which can cause breakdown and necrosis of the skin.
- Be aware that turning provides kinesthetic (sensation of movement), proprioceptive (awareness of position), and vestibular (equilibrium) stimulation.
- Position carefully to prevent ischemic necrosis over pressure areas.

Preserving Corneal Integrity

- Monitor unconscious patients who have their eyes open and have inadequate or absent corneal reflexes; corneas may become irritated, dried out, or scratched, leading to ulceration.
- Cleanse eyes with cotton balls moistened with sterile normal saline to remove debris and discharge.
- Instill artificial tears every 2 hours.
- If postoperative periorbital edema occurs after cranial surgery, cold compresses may be applied, with care taken to avoid contact with the cornea.
- Use eye patches cautiously because of the potential for corneal abrasion from contact with the patch.

Managing Nutritional Needs

- Provide nasogastric tube or gastrostomy tube enteral feedings within 72 hours.

- Consult the nutritionist to determine caloric needs and for recommendations for the amount and type of tube feeding appropriate. Patients with TBI have high caloric needs due to increased metabolic expenditure.
- Monitor glucose as hyperglycemia is associated with worse outcomes.
- Record daily intake and output and daily weights to ensure the patient has adequate caloric intake.

Preventing Urinary Retention

- Palpate or scan the bladder at intervals to determine whether urinary retention is present; if the patient is not voiding, insert an indwelling urinary catheter and connect to a closed drainage system.
- Because catheters are a major factor in causing urinary tract infection (UTI), observe the patient for fever and cloudy urine.
- The urinary catheter is usually removed if the patient has a stable cardiovascular system and if no diuresis, sepsis, or voiding dysfunction existed before the onset of coma.
- An intermittent catheterization program may be initiated to ensure complete emptying of the bladder at intervals, if indicated.

Promoting Bowel Function

- Assess the abdomen for distention, auscultate for bowel sounds, and measure abdominal girth.
- Observe for diarrhea from infection, antibiotics, and hyperosmolar fluids.
- The nurse monitors the number and consistency of bowel movements and performs a rectal examination for signs of fecal impaction secondary to immobility and lack of dietary fiber.
- Administer stool softeners.
- To facilitate bowel emptying, a glycerin suppository may be indicated.
- The patient may require an enema every other day to empty the lower colon.

Protecting the Patient

- Prevent injury from invasive lines and equipment, restraints, tight dressings, environmental irritants, damp bedding or dressings, and tubes and drains.

- Ensure protection of the patient's dignity during altered LOC; provide privacy and speak to the patient during nursing care.
- Avoid speaking negatively about the patient's condition, because patients in a light coma may be able to hear.
- Be aware that the comatose patient has an increased need for advocacy, and the nurse is responsible for seeing that these advocacy needs are met.

New Therapies

- Current research has begun to focus more on novel treatments for TBI because as many as 30% of soldiers have suffered a TBI.
- The hormone progesterone, administered IV for 3 days, within 6 to 8 hours after the initial injury, showed a greater than 50% reduction in mortality when compared to controls at 30 days post-injury. Further clinical trials are currently under way.

Intracranial Surgery

- Decompressive craniectomy involves removal of a bone flap from the skull to allow expansion of the brain. The bone flap is implanted into the abdomen to remain viable.
- Once cerebral edema decreases, the bone flap is replaced. There are no randomized controlled trials investigating the utility of decompressive craniectomy; studies have suggested it is helpful.

COMPLICATIONS

- Brainstem herniation
- Diabetes insipidus
- SIADH

For more information, see Chapter 45 in Pellico, L.H. (2013). *Focus on adult health: Medical-surgical nursing.* Philadelphia: Wolters Kluwer Health | Lippincott Williams & Wilkins

K

Kaposi's Sarcoma

Kaposi's sarcoma (KS) is the most common HIV-related malignancy and involves the endothelial layer of blood and lymphatic vessels.

PATHOPHYSIOLOGY

Acquired KS occurs in patients who are treated with immunosuppressive agents and commonly in patients who have undergone organ transplantation. AIDS-related KS exhibits a more variable and aggressive course, ranging from localized cutaneous lesions to disseminated disease involving multiple organ systems. Cutaneous lesions develop in 90% of patients; the most common sites of visceral involvement are the lymph nodes, gastrointestinal tract, and lungs.

RISK FACTORS

- HIV
- Organ transplant recipients, use of immunosuppressive medication
- Male
- Homosexual or bisexual

CLINICAL MANIFESTATIONS AND ASSESSMENT

- Cutaneous lesions appear in 90% of HIV-infected patients and correlate to low CD4$^+$ counts.

- Cutaneous lesions may appear anywhere on the body and are usually brownish pink to deep purple. They may be flat or raised and surrounded by ecchymoses and edema.
- Rapid development of lesions involving large areas of skin is associated with extensive disfigurement.
- The location and size of the lesions can lead to venous stasis, lymphedema, and pain.
- Ulcerative lesions disrupt skin integrity and increase discomfort and susceptibility to infection.
- Involvement of internal organs may lead to infection, hemorrhage, and organ failure; death may result from tumor progression.

DIAGNOSTIC METHODS

- Biopsy confirms diagnosis.
- Prognosis depends on extent of tumor, presence of other symptoms of HIV infection, and the $CD4^+$ count.

MEDICAL AND NURSING MANAGEMENT

Management of KS is usually difficult because of the variability of symptoms and the organ systems involved.

- Treatment goals are to reduce symptoms by decreasing the size of the skin lesions, to reduce discomfort associated with edema and ulcerations, and to control symptoms associated with mucosal or visceral involvement.
- No one treatment has been shown to improve survival rates; surgical excision, application of liquid nitrogen, and local injection of intraoral lesions with dilute vinblastine may be used.
- Radiation therapy is effective as a palliative measure to relieve localized pain due to tumor mass (especially in the legs) and for KS lesions that are in sites such as the oral mucosa, conjunctiva, face, and soles of the feet.

K

Pharmacologic Therapy

- Alpha-interferon may cause tumor regression and improved immune system function in patients with cutaneous KS.
- Alpha-interferon is administered by the IV, intramuscular, or subcutaneous route. Patients may self-administer interferon at home or receive interferon in an outpatient setting.
- Nonsteroidal anti-inflammatory drugs (NSAIDs) and opioids may be used; monitor hepatic and hematologic status for patients taking NSAIDs and zidovudine.

Nursing Management

- Provide thorough and meticulous skin care, involving regular turning, cleansing, and application of medicated ointments and dressings.
- Avoid adhesive tape, and advise patients with foot lesions to wear cotton socks and shoes that do not cause perspiration.
- Provide antipruritic, antibiotic, and analgesic agents as prescribed.

For more information, see Chapter 37 in Pellico, L.H. (2013). *Focus on adult health: Medical-surgical nursing*. Philadelphia: Wolters Kluwer Health | Lippincott Williams & Wilkins.

K

L

Leukemia

Leukemia is a neoplastic disease causing unregulated, neoplastic proliferation of leukocytes in the bone marrow.

PATHOPHYSIOLOGY

Leukemia arises from a defect in myeloid or lymphoid hematopoietic stem cells. The bone marrow becomes packed with cells and prematurely releases these cells into the circulation. In acute forms or late stages of chronic forms, the proliferation of leukemic cells leaves little room for normal cell production, causing pancytopenia. Proliferation of cells in the liver and spleen (extramedullary hematopoiesis) may occur.

Acute leukemia is characterized by an abrupt onset, with death occurring within weeks to months without aggressive treatment. Leukocyte development is halted at the blast phase, resulting in the majority of leukocytes being released as undifferentiated, immature cells. In chronic leukemia, symptoms evolve over a period of months to years and progress more slowly, with a disease trajectory that can extend for years. Most of the leukocytes produced mature and retain some ability to function normally.

RISK FACTORS

- Not fully known
- Genetic influence and viral pathogenesis may be involved.

- Radiation exposure or chemicals such as benzene and alkylating agents may be a cause.

CLINICAL MANIFESTATIONS AND ASSESSMENT

Cardinal signs and symptoms include weakness and fatigue from anemia, bleeding tendencies, petechiae and ecchymoses from thrombocytopenia, pain, headache, vomiting, fever, and infection from immature leukocytes.

DIAGNOSTIC FINDINGS

- Complete blood count (CBC)
- Absolute neutrophil count
- Bone marrow studies confirm proliferation of white blood cells (WBCs, leukocytes) in the bone marrow.

ACUTE MYELOID LEUKEMIA

Acute myeloid leukemia (AML) results from a defect in the hematopoietic stem cell that differentiates into all myeloid cells: Monocytes, granulocytes (neutrophils, basophils, eosinophils), erythrocytes, and platelets. Prognosis is worse for those over 65 years, those developing leukemia stemming from preexisting myelodysplastic syndrome, or those who have received alkylating agents for cancers.

CLINICAL MANIFESTATIONS AND ASSESSMENT

- Fever and infection result from neutropenia, weakness and fatigue from anemia, and bleeding tendencies from thrombocytopenia.
- Develops without warning; symptoms occur over weeks to months.
- Ecchymosis, petechiae, spontaneous hemorrhage if platelet levels are below 10,000/mm^3.

- Additional symptoms: Pain from an enlarged liver or spleen, hyperplasia of the gums, and bone pain from expansion of the bone marrow
- Spontaneous hemorrhages also may develop when the platelet count drops to less than 10,000/mm^3.

DIAGNOSTIC METHODS

- Complete blood count with decrease in erythrocytes and platelets, low percentage of normal leukocytes regardless of overall WBC
- Bone marrow contains excess of immature blast cells.
- May have coagulopathy and disseminated intravascular coagulation (DIC), especially with acute promyelocytic leukemia

MEDICAL AND NURSING MANAGEMENT

The overall objective of treatment is to achieve complete remission, in which there is no evidence of residual leukemia in the bone marrow.

- Peripheral blood stem cell transplant (PBSCT) is considered for patients with high-risk leukemia or in those who have relapsed.
- Patients having PBSCT have a significant risk for infection, graft versus host disease (GVHD, in which the donor's lymphocytes [graft] recognize the patient's body as "foreign" and attack the "foreign" host), and other complications.

Pharmacologic Therapy

- Induction chemotherapy: Aggressive chemotherapy that may require hospitalization for several weeks
- Induction therapy typically involves IV administration of cytarabine (Cytosar, Ara-C) and an anthracycline such as idarubicin (Idamycin) based on patient status and previous treatment with antineoplastic drugs.

- Consolidation therapy is given after recovery from induction therapy with multiple cycles of chemotherapeutic drugs, usually with a form of cytarabine (Cytosar, Ara-C).
- Patients with low- or intermediate-risk leukemia may not require further treatment after they complete consolidation therapy.
- Patient and family may wish to consider supportive care if comorbidities exist.
- Hydroxyurea (Hydrea) may control number of blast cells when patients are not candidates for aggressive therapy.
- Granulocytic growth factors (GCSF or Filgrastim) to minimize the risk of infection has not demonstrated the same effects on survival in patients with AML compared to patients with nonhematologic malignancies; widespread use is not recommended.

Nursing Management

The priority nursing interventions for the patient with AML include infection prevention, bleeding prevention, comfort promotion, and patient education.

- Observe for severe neutropenia, anemia, and thrombocytopenia; treat with packed red blood cells (PRBCs) and platelets as indicated.
- Treat infections promptly.
- Alleviate anxiety by providing information tailored to the patient's readiness and educational level.
- PBSCT requires aggressive chemotherapy, then "rescue" with infusion of donor stem cells to reinitiate hematopoiesis.
- Assess for tumor lysis syndrome, elevation of uric acid levels, potassium, and phosphate secondary to cellular destruction from chemotherapy. Provide high fluid intake, alkalinization of the urine, and allopurinol to prevent crystallization of uric acid and stone formation.
- Observe for GI problems resulting from infiltration of abnormal leukocytes into the abdominal organs and from the toxicity of the chemotherapeutic agents. Anorexia, nausea, vomiting, diarrhea, and severe mucositis are common.
- Administer antimicrobials and transfusions as needed.
- Encourage fluids, alkalinization of the urine, and prophylaxis with allopurinol to prevent stone formation if tumor lysis syndrome develops.

L

CHRONIC MYELOID LEUKEMIA

Chronic myeloid leukemia (CML) arises from a mutation in the myeloid stem cell; normal myeloid cells continue to be produced; however, a pathologic increase in the production of blast cells occurs. A wide spectrum of cell types exists within the blood, from blast forms through mature neutrophils.

PATHOPHYSIOLOGY

Due to uncontrolled proliferation of cells, the marrow expands into the cavities of long bones. Cells are also formed in the liver and spleen (extramedullary hematopoiesis), resulting in enlargement of these organs, which is sometimes painful. Ninety to 95% of patients with CML, have the Philadelphia chromosome or philadelphia translocation, where a section of DNA from chromosome 9 is translocated onto chromosome 22.

There are three phases of the disease: the chronic phase, in which there are usually adequate numbers of healthy cells to fight infection; the accelerated phase, in which the numbers of abnormal cells are being produced at a faster rate; and the blast crisis, in which the predominant cell type is immature. Most patients are diagnosed in the chronic phase.

RISK FACTORS

- Uncommon in people younger than 20 years; incidence increases with age
- Median age in Caucasians is 75 years; African Americans have bimodal age distribution at 40 and 70 years

CLINICAL MANIFESTATIONS AND ASSESSMENT

The clinical picture of CML is based on the stage of the disease.

- Chronic phase may have few symptoms and complications; may be asymptomatic at time of diagnosis and discovered when CBC performed for other reasons.

- Common symptoms include fatigue, bleeding, or weight loss.
- Once the disease transforms to the acute phase (blast crisis), the overall survival rarely exceeds several months.
- With extremely high WBC levels, shortness of breath or slight confusion due to decreased capillary perfusion to the lungs and brain from leukostasis (increased leukocytes slows blood flow through capillaries) may occur.
- Hepatomegaly and enlarged, tender spleen may develop.
- Insidious symptoms, such as malaise, anorexia, and weight loss may occur; lymphadenopathy is rare.

DIAGNOSTIC FINDINGS

Leukocyte count is higher than $100,000/mm^3$.

MEDICAL AND NURSING MANAGEMENT

Pharmacologic Therapy

- Imatinib mesylate (Gleevec), dasatinib, and nilotinib, and tyrosine kinase inhibitors block signals within the leukemic cells expressing the BCR-ABL protein, preventing cell growth and division.
- Hydroxyurea (Hydrea) or busulfan (Myleran) may be used.

Medical Management

- Severe leukocytosis, with a leukocyte count of greater than $300,000/mm^3$, may be treated with leukapheresis (a process where the patient's blood is removed and separated, leukocytes withdrawn, and the remainder returned to the patient); this can temporarily reduce the number of leukocytes.
- For blast crisis, treatment may resemble induction therapy for acute leukemia, using the same medications as for AML or acute lymphocytic leukemia (ALL).
- Allogeneic stem cell transplantation remains the only curative treatment for CML.

Nursing Management

- Educate the patient that antacids and grapefruit juice may limit drug absorption.
- Teach the patient that large doses of acetaminophen can cause hepatotoxicity.

ACUTE LYMPHOCYTIC LEUKEMIA

Acute lymphocytic leukemia (ALL) results from an uncontrolled proliferation of immature cells (lymphoblasts) derived from the lymphoid stem cell.

PATHOPHYSIOLOGY

The cell of origin is the precursor to the B lymphocyte in approximately 75% of ALL cases; T-lymphocyte ALL occurs in approximately 25% of ALL cases. Immature lymphocytes proliferate in the marrow and impede the development of normal myeloid cells. As a result, normal hematopoiesis is inhibited, resulting in reduced numbers of leukocytes, erythrocytes, and platelets.

RISK FACTORS

- Most common in young children; peak incidence is 4 years of age; uncommon after age 15
- Boys affected more often than girls

CLINICAL MANIFESTATIONS AND ASSESSMENT

Manifestations of leukemic cell infiltration into other organs are more common with ALL than with other forms of leukemia.

- Pain from an enlarged liver or spleen and bone pain
- Testicular swelling or discomfort due to infiltration

- Headache, visual changes, vomiting, and neurologic deficits from central nervous system (CNS) invasion

DIAGNOSTIC FINDINGS

Leukocyte counts may be either low or high, but there is always a high proportion of immature cells.

MEDICAL AND NURSING MANAGEMENT

The expected outcome of treatment is complete remission.

- Chemotherapy uses vinca alkaloids and corticosteroids for induction therapy.
- Intracranial irradiation and chemotherapy with intrathecal methotrexate (methotrexate injected into the cerebrospinal fluid) may be used.
- PBSCT offers a chance for prolonged remission, or even cure, if the illness recurs after therapy.

Pharmacologic Therapy

Protocols for ALL tend to be complex, using a variety of chemo-therapeutic agents over a protracted period of time. Treatment includes an induction phase, followed by a consolidation phase, followed by a maintenance phase, when lower doses of medications are given for up to 3 years.

- Corticosteroids
- Vinca alkaloids
- Intrathecal injection of methotrexate
- Imatinib is used in those with Philadelphia chromosome, alone or in combination with other agents.
- Monoclonal antibodies, including alemtuzumab (Campath), may be used.
- Prophylactic antimicrobials are used to decrease the risk for infection.

- PBSCT offers a chance for prolonged remission, or even cure, if the illness recurs after therapy.

Nursing Management

Nursing management is similar to the care of patients with AML.

- Prevent infection and bleeding, and manage symptoms such as nausea and pain.
- As ALL is a disease that most commonly affects children and young adults, fertility preservation should be discussed prior to initiating treatment.

CHRONIC LYMPHOCYTIC LEUKEMIA

Chronic lymphocytic leukemia (CLL) is typically derived from a malignant clone of B lymphocytes and is a common malignancy of older adults. It is the most common form of leukemia in the United States and Europe, affecting more than 120,000 people.

PATHOPHYSIOLOGY

Most of the leukemia cells in CLL are fully mature; however, it appears that these cells can escape apoptosis (programmed cell death), resulting in excessive accumulation of cells in the marrow and circulation. Lymphadenopathy occurs as the lymphocytes are trapped within the lymph nodes; the nodes can become quite large and painful. Hepatomegaly and splenomegaly then develop.

Autoimmune complications can also occur at any stage, as either autoimmune hemolytic anemia or idiopathic thrombocytopenic purpura (ITP). Five percent to 10% of patients will experience a transformation from CLL to a more aggressive form of lymphoma.

RISK FACTORS

- Age older than 60 years
- Males twice as likely to develop CLL as females

CLINICAL MANIFESTATIONS AND ASSESSMENT

- Many patients are asymptomatic and are diagnosed incidentally during routine physical examinations or during treatment for another disease
- Lymphadenopathy with greatly enlarged, painful nodes; hepatomegaly, splenomegaly
- Anemia and thrombocytopenia in later stages when treatment is typically initiated
- Infections, including viral infections and herpes zoster, which may become widely disseminated.
- Anergy, absence or decreased reaction to skin sensitivity tests (eg, *Candida,* mumps)
- "B symptoms" comprise a constellation of symptoms including fevers, fatigue, drenching sweats (especially at night), and unintentional weight loss.

DIAGNOSTIC FINDINGS

- Increased lymphocyte count (lymphocytosis)
- Erythrocyte and platelet counts may be normal or, in later stages of the illness, decreased.

MEDICAL AND NURSING MANAGEMENT

In early stages, CLL may require no treatment. When symptoms are severe or when the disease progresses to later stages (with resultant anemia and thrombocytopenia), chemotherapy is often used.

Pharmacologic Therapy

- Fludarabine (Fludara), corticosteroids, and chlorambucil (Leukeran) are used when symptoms are severe.
- Monoclonal antibodies rituximab (Rituxan) and alemtuzumab (Campath) may be used with other chemotherapeutic medications.

- Prophylactic use of antiviral agents and antibiotics (eg, Acyclovir; trimethoprim/sulfamethoxazole [Bactrim, Septra]) for patients receiving alemtuzumab; treatment continues for 2 months after treatment.

Nursing Management

- Observe for weakness and fatigue secondary to disease and complications of treatment.
- Assess carefully for symptoms such as dry cough, mild dyspnea, and diminished breath sounds, which may indicate a pulmonary infection. Infection may not be evident initially on chest X-ray; the absence of neutrophils delays the inflammatory response that produces the X-ray changes.
- Monitor and trend the results of laboratory studies including leukocyte count, ANC, hematocrit, platelet, creatinine and electrolyte levels, and hepatic function tests. During initial treatment for acute leukemia, the ANC often drops below 100/mm^3, placing the patient at very high risk for infection.
- Plan to administer empiric antibiotics, which are used preemptively when the patient has a fever of 100.4°F or greater. Culture results need to be reported immediately so that antimicrobial therapy can be modified appropriately based on microbial sensitivity.

For more information, see Chapters 6, 19, and 20 in Pellico, L.H. (2013). *Focus on adult health: Medical-surgical nursing.* Philadelphia: Wolters Kluwer Health | Lippincott Williams & Wilkins.

L

Lymphedema and Elephantiasis

Lymphedema is swelling in the extremities due to an accumulation of lymph from blocked lymphatic vessels.

PATHOPHYSIOLOGY

Lymphedema is classified as primary (congenital malformations) or secondary (acquired obstruction). Tissues in the extremities swell because of an increased quantity of lymph that results from an obstruction of the lymphatic vessels. It is especially marked when the extremity is in a dependent position. Initially, the edema is soft and pitting. As the condition progresses, the edema becomes firm, nonpitting, and unresponsive to treatment. The most common type is congenital lymphedema (lymphedema praecox), caused by hypoplasia of the lymphatic system of the lower extremity.

The obstruction may be in both the lymph nodes and the lymphatic vessels. At times, it is seen in the arm after an axillary node dissection for breast cancer. It may also develop in the leg in association with varicose veins or a chronic thrombophlebitis (from lymphangitis). When chronic swelling is present, there may be frequent bouts of infection (high fever and chills) and increased residual edema after inflammation resolves. These lead to chronic fibrosis, thickening of the subcutaneous tissues, and hypertrophy of the skin. The condition in which chronic swelling of the extremity recedes only slightly with elevation is referred to as *elephantiasis.*

RISK FACTORS

• Congenital hypoplasia of lymph system
• Breast surgery with axillary node dissection
• Lymphangitis (an acute inflammation of the lymphatic channels most commonly from infection)
• Exposure to tropical parasite (filaria)

CLINICAL MANIFESTATIONS AND ASSESSMENT

Diagnosis of lymphedema is made by clinical evaluation and exclusion of other causes of edema.

- In early stages, the tissue is soft and pliable.
- In advanced lymphedema, the tissue is firm, thick, and may have overlapping folds of skin.

MEDICAL AND NURSING MANAGEMENT

Treatment is focused on reducing the edema and preventing increased edema, infections, and tissue damage; will vary depending on the stage and severity.

- External compression devices move the fluid proximally from the foot to the hip or from the hand to the axilla.
- Custom-fitted elastic compression stockings or sleeves are worn; those with the highest compression strength, exceeding 40 mm Hg, are required.
- Active and passive exercise assists in moving lymphatic fluid into the bloodstream.
- Elastic compression garments maintain edema reduction.
- Continuous bed rest with leg elevation helps mobilize fluids.
- Manual lymphatic drainage, a specialized massage technique, directs the lymph through lymph channels with preserved function.

Surgical Management

Surgery is performed if the edema is severe and uncontrolled by medical therapy, if mobility is severely compromised, or if infection persists.

- Excision of affected subcutaneous tissue and fascia with skin grafting to cover the defect
- Surgical relocation of superficial lymphatic vessels into the deep lymphatic system via buried dermal flap to provide a conduit for lymphatic drainage

Pharmacologic Therapy

- Diuretic therapy, initially with furosemide (Lasix) to prevent fluid overload when extracellular fluid is mobilized.

- Antibiotics for lymphangitis or cellulitis, or as prophylaxis where chronic infections exist

Nursing Management

- If the patient undergoes surgery, the management of skin grafts and flaps is the same as when these therapies are used for other conditions.
- Administer antibiotics postoperatively and as prescribed.
- Instruct patient or caregiver to inspect the dressing daily; unusual drainage or any inflammation around the wound margin should be reported to the surgeon.
- Inform patient that there may be a loss of sensation in the skin graft area.
- Instruct patient to avoid the application of heating pads or exposure to sun to prevent burns or trauma to the area.

For more information, see Chapter 18 in Pellico, L.H. (2013). *Focus on adult health: Medical-surgical nursing.* Philadelphia: Wolters Kluwer Health | Lippincott Williams & Wilkins.

Lymphoma, Hodgkin's

Hodgkin's lymphoma is a rare malignancy of the lymph nodes that initiates in a single lymph node (unicentric) and spreads continuously along the lymphatic system.

PATHOPHYSIOLOGY

The malignant cell of Hodgkin's lymphoma is the Reed-Sternberg cell, a large tumor cell that is morphologically unique and is thought to be of immature lymphoid origin. It is the pathologic hallmark and essential diagnostic criterion for Hodgkin's disease.

However, the tumor is very heterogeneous and may actually contain few Reed-Sternberg cells. Repeated biopsies may be required to establish the diagnosis.

RISK FACTORS

- Viral etiology suspected; Epstein-Barr virus is present in 20% to 50% of cases.
- Somewhat more common in men; peaks in early 20s and after 50 years of age.
- Familial pattern of low incidence but first-degree relatives have a higher-than-normal frequency of disease.
- Immunosuppressive therapy for transplant
- Woodworkers
- Exposure to Agent Orange

CLINICAL MANIFESTATIONS AND ASSESSMENT

- Painless enlargement of the lymph nodes above the diaphragm; 75% are cervical lymph nodes.
- Nodes are firm, painless, and rubbery; common sites are the cervical, supraclavicular, and mediastinal nodes.
- Mediastinal mass may be visible on chest X-ray; occasionally they are large enough to compress the trachea, causing dyspnea and cough.
- Pruritus is common and can be distressing; the cause is unknown.
- Pain at the site of the tumor after drinking alcohol is present in 10% of patients.
- All organs are vulnerable to invasion by Hodgkin's lymphoma. Symptoms may result from the tumor compressing other organs, causing cough and pulmonary effusion, jaundice from hepatic involvement or bile duct obstruction, abdominal pain (from splenomegaly or retroperitoneal adenopathy), or bone pain (from skeletal involvement).
- Herpes zoster infections are common.

- B symptoms or constitutional symptoms, including fever (without chills), drenching sweats (particularly at night), and unintentional weight loss of more than 10% of body weight, are found in 40% of patients and are more common in advanced disease.

DIAGNOSTIC METHODS

- Mild anemia develops.
- Leukocyte count may be elevated or decreased.
- Platelet count is typically normal unless the tumor has invaded the bone marrow, suppressing hematopoiesis.
- Impaired cellular immunity (evidenced by an absence of or decreased response to skin sensitivity tests such as candidal infection, mumps) may be noted.
- Elevated erythrocyte sedimentation rate (ESR) represents a poor prognostic indicator.
- Diagnostic studies are performed to rule out an infectious origin for the disease, as many manifestations are similar to those of infection.
- Excisional lymph node biopsy and the finding of the Reed–Sternberg cell confirms diagnosis.
- Laboratory tests: CBC count, platelet count, ESR, and liver and renal function studies.
- Bone marrow biopsy; bilateral biopsies may be performed occasionally.
- Bone scans may be performed.
- Chest X-ray, computed tomography (CT) scan of the chest, abdomen, and pelvis; positron emission tomography (PET) scan for staging the disease.

MEDICAL AND NURSING MANAGEMENT

Treatment is determined by the stage of the disease instead of the histologic type, with a goal of cure, regardless of stage.

- Chemotherapy followed by radiation therapy is used in early-stage disease.

- Combination chemotherapy with doxorubicin (Adriamycin), bleomycin (Blenoxane), vinblastine (Velban), and dacarbazine (DTIC), referred to as ABVD, is standard treatment for more advanced disease.
- Chemotherapy is often successful in obtaining remission even when relapse occurs.
- Autologous PBSCT can control the disease and extend survival time.

Long-Term Complications of Therapy

- Hypothyroidism, immune dysfunction, dental caries, cardiomyopathy, and secondary malignancies
- Long-term surveillance for cancer, especially lung or breast cancer in survivors is crucial.
- Encourage patients to reduce other factors that increase the risk of developing secondary cancers, such as use of tobacco and alcohol and exposure to environmental carcinogens.
- Revised treatment approaches are aimed at diminishing the risk for complications without sacrificing the potential for cure.

For more information, see Chapters 6 and 20 in Pellico, L.H. (2013). *Focus on adult health: Medical-surgical nursing.* Philadelphia: Wolters Kluwer Health | Lippincott Williams & Wilkins.

Lymphoma, Non-Hodgkin's

The non-Hodgkin lymphomas (NHLs) are a heterogeneous group of cancers that originate from the neoplastic growth of lymphoid tissue.

PATHOPHYSIOLOGY

Most NHLs involve malignant B lymphocytes; only 5% involve T lymphocytes. In contrast to Hodgkin's lymphoma, the lymphoid tissues involved are largely infiltrated with malignant cells. The spread of these malignant lymphoid cells occurs unpredictably, and true localized disease is uncommon. Lymph nodes from multiple sites may be infiltrated, as may sites outside the lymphoid system (extranodal tissue). It is the sixth most common type of cancer diagnosed in the United States, the eighth most common cause of cancer death in men, and the sixth most common cause of cancer death in women

RISK FACTORS

- Increases with each decade of life; average age at diagnosis is 50 to 60 years
- Immunodeficiencies, autoimmune disorders, prior treatment for cancer, organ transplant
- Viral infections including Epstein-Barr and HIV/AIDS
- Exposure to pesticides, solvents, dyes or defoliating agents including Agent Orange
- Men are affected more often than are women.

CLINICAL MANIFESTATIONS AND ASSESSMENT

Symptoms are highly variable, reflecting the diverse nature of the NHLs.

- Lymphadenopathy most common; may wax and wane. Lymphomatous masses may compromise organ function; for example, a mass in the mediastinum may cause respiratory distress.
- Often not diagnosed until the disease progresses to later stage.
- One-third of patients have B symptoms including recurrent fever, drenching night sweats, and unintentional weight loss of 10% or more.
- Abdominal masses can compromise the ureters, leading to renal dysfunction, and splenomegaly can cause abdominal discomfort, nausea, early satiety, anorexia, and weight loss.
- Central nervous system involvement occurs in fewer than 10% of patients at some point in their disease.

DIAGNOSTIC METHODS

Diagnosis of NHL is categorized into a highly complex classification system based on histopathology, immunophenotyping, and cytogenetic analyses of the malignant cells.

- Complete blood count, bone marrow aspiration, biopsy, needle biopsy
- Staging is based on data from CT and PET scans and occasionally CSF analysis.

MEDICAL AND NURSING MANAGEMENT

Treatment is based on the actual classification of disease, the stage of disease, prior treatment (if any), and the patient's ability to tolerate therapy.

- Low-grade lymphomas may not require treatment until the disease progresses to a later stage.
- Radiation therapy alone may be used for nonaggressive forms or palliation of symptoms.
- More aggressive types of NHL (eg, lymphoblastic lymphoma, Burkitt's lymphoma) require prompt initiation of chemotherapy; these types tend to be more responsive to treatment.

Pharmacologic Therapy

- Chemotherapy for aggressive types of NHL
- Rituximab with conventional chemotherapy (Cytoxan, doxorubicin, vincristine, and prednisone [CHOP]) is now considered standard treatment for common, aggressive B-cell lymphomas.
- Treatment for relapsed disease includes rituximab and combination chemotherapy followed by high-dose chemotherapy with stem cell support; intrathecal chemotherapy for CNS involvement

Nursing Management

- Monitor for side effects: Chemotherapy causes systemic side effects (eg, myelosuppression, nausea, hair loss, risk of infection), whereas radiation therapy causes site-specific effects.

L

- Observe for and respond to systemic side effects of myelosuppression: Nausea, hair loss, risk of infection
- Teach patients to minimize the risks of infection, to recognize signs of possible infection, and to contact the health care professional should such signs develop.
- Observe for and treat site-specific complications of radiation therapy.
- Protect patient from infection secondary to treatment-related myelosuppression but also from the defective immune response that results from the disease itself.
- Observe for complications related to the location of the lymphoma; focus assessment on the area/location of the lymphoma. For example: Assess patients with lymphomatous masses in the upper chest for superior vena cava obstruction, or for airway obstruction, if the mass is near the bronchus or trachea.

For more information, see Chapter 20 in Pellico, L.H. (2013). *Focus on adult health: Medical-surgical nursing.* Philadelphia: Wolters Kluwer Health | Lippincott Williams & Wilkins.

L

M

Ménière's Disease

Ménière's disease is a disorder of the inner ear which causes vertigo, tinnitus, a feeling of fullness or pressure in the ear, and fluctuating hearing loss.

PATHOPHYSIOLOGY

Ménière's disease is believed to be the result of fluctuating pressure within the inner ear or the mixing of inner ear fluids. The membranous labyrinth of the inner ear contains a fluid called *endolymph*. The membranes can become dilated because of malabsorption of the fluid in the endolymphatic sac or a blockage in the drainage of fluid in the endolymphatic duct within the labyrinth. This dilation is termed *endolymphatic hydrops* or a ballooning of the membranous labyrinth, which results in increased pressure in the system or rupture of the inner ear membrane, producing the symptoms of Ménière's disease.

RISK FACTORS

- More common in adults, with the average age of onset in the 40s
- Positive family history in about 50% of affected patients
- Recent viral illness, upper respiratory infection (URI), smokers, and allergy suffers
- Stress, fatigue, alcohol use, aspirin use

CLINICAL MANIFESTATIONS AND ASSESSMENT

- Symptoms range from mild to extreme disability
- There are two possible subsets of the disease: Cochlear and vestibular; patients may experience either; however, eventually all of the symptoms develop
- *Cochlear disease* is recognized as a fluctuating, progressive sensorineural hearing loss associated with tinnitus and aural pressure in the absence of vestibular symptoms or findings.
- *Vestibular disease* is characterized as the occurrence of episodic vertigo associated with aural pressure but no cochlear symptoms.

General Symptoms

- Fluctuating, progressive sensorineural hearing loss; tinnitus or a roaring sound; a feeling of pressure or fullness in the ear; and episodic, incapacitating vertigo, often accompanied by nausea and vomiting
- Vertigo is the most troublesome symptom, possibly accompanied by nausea or vomiting.
- Diaphoresis and persistent feeling of imbalance or disequilibrium may waken patients at night.
- Patient feels well between attacks; long remissions may occur.
- Hearing loss may fluctuate; tinnitus and aural pressure waxes and wanes.

DIAGNOSTIC METHODS

Physical examination findings are usually normal, with the exception of those of cranial nerve VIII.

- Sounds from a tuning fork (Weber test) may lateralize to the unaffected ear.
- Rinne's test; air conduction is greater than bone conduction.
- Audiogram typically reveals a sensorineural hearing loss in the affected ear.

- Sensorineural loss in the low frequencies occurs as the disease progresses.
- Electronystagmogram may be normal or may show reduced vestibular response.
- Magnetic resonance imaging (MRI) may also prove useful in diagnosis in which central nervous system (CNS) lesions are present.

MEDICAL AND NURSING MANAGEMENT

Most patients with Ménière's disease can be successfully treated with diet and medication.

- Avoidance of tobacco
- Stress reduction strategies
- Psychological evaluation due to comorbidity of vertigo and anxiety

Dietary Management

- Low-sodium diet (2,000 mg/day)
- Avoidance of alcohol and caffeine, monosodium glutamate (MSG), aspirin and aspirin-containing medications
- High-potassium diet is necessary if the patient takes a diuretic that causes potassium loss.

Pharmacologic Therapy

- Antihistamines and meclizine (Antivert) to suppress the vestibular system
- Tranquilizers such as diazepam (Valium) to help control vertigo in acute circumstances
- Antiemetics such as promethazine (Phenergan) suppositories to control the nausea, vomiting, and vertigo
- Betahistine hydrochloride and diuretic therapy may reduce the severity of symptoms by lowering the pressure in the endolymphatic system.
- Vasodilators are often used in conjunction with other therapies, despite lack of evidence to support their use.

M

Surgical Management

Surgical procedures for disabling attacks of vertigo to improve quality of life include endolymphatic sac procedures, middle and inner ear perfusion with ototoxic medications via intraotologic catheters, and vestibular nerve sectioning.

For more information, see Chapter 50 in Pellico, L.H. (2013). *Focus on adult health: Medical-surgical nursing.* Philadelphia: Wolters Kluwer Health | Lippincott Williams & Wilkins.

Meningitis

Meningitis is an inflammation of the meninges, the protective membranes covering the brain and spinal cord.

PATHOPHYSIOLOGY

Meningitis affects the pia mater, the arachnoid, the cerebrospinal fluid (CSF), subarachnoid space, and the dura mater. Meningitis is classified as septic or aseptic; septic meningitis is typically caused by bacteria; aseptic meningitis may be viral or secondary to lymphoma, leukemia, or HIV infection.

The causative organism enters the bloodstream, as a consequence of other infections or by direct spread after traumatic injury to the skull or spine or from sinusitis, otitis, brain abscess, or invasive procedures. The infection crosses the blood–brain barrier and proliferates in the CSF. Inflammation of the involved meninges and released neutrophils causes a thickening of the CSF, which may increase intracranial pressure (ICP). The prognosis for bacterial meningitis depends on the causative organism, the severity of the infection and illness, and the timeliness of treatment.

RISK FACTORS

- Bacterial meningitis risks include tobacco use, viral URI, otitis media, and mastoiditis.
- Diabetes
- Asplenia
- Alcohol abuse
- Immune deficiencies, including chemotherapy, immunosuppressive treatment, and AIDS

CLINICAL MANIFESTATIONS AND ASSESSMENT

- Severe headache and fever are frequently the initial symptoms; fever tends to remain high throughout the course of the illness; the headache is usually either steady or throbbing as a result of meningeal irritation.
- Altered level of consciousness (LOC); although normal LOC may occur in one-third of patients.
- Meningeal irritation results in a number of other well-recognized signs common to all types of meningitis:
  - Nuchal rigidity (stiff neck) seen in 30% to 70% of patients. Gentle forward flexion of the head while the patient is supine causes spasms in the neck.
  - Positive Kerning's sign: When lying with the hip flexed to a 90-degree angle, resistance to passive extension of the knee is a positive finding.
  - Positive Brudzinski's sign: After ruling out cervical trauma or injury, flexion of the patient's neck produces flexion of the knees and hips; when the lower extremity of one side is passively flexed, a similar movement is seen in the opposite extremity.
- Photophobia, extreme sensitivity to light, is common although the cause is unclear.
- Rash (*N. meningitidis*) or skin lesions may range from petechial rash with purpuric lesions to large areas of ecchymosis.
- Disorientation and memory impairment; as illness progresses, lethargy, unresponsiveness, and coma may develop.

M

- Seizures occur with bacterial meningitis within the first week as a result of areas of irritability in the brain.
- Intracranial pressure increases secondary to purulent exudate and cerebral edema. The initial signs of increased ICP include decreased LOC and focal motor deficits; brainstem herniation may occur from increased ICP. Vomiting may be associated with increased ICP.
- Acute fulminant infection occurs in about 10% of patients with meningococcal meningitis, producing signs of overwhelming septicemia: An abrupt onset of high fever, extensive purpuric lesions (over the face and extremities), shock, and signs of disseminated intravascular coagulation (DIC); death may occur within a few hours after onset of the infection.

DIAGNOSTIC METHODS

Bacterial culture and Gram staining of CSF and blood are key diagnostic tests.

MEDICAL AND NURSING MANAGEMENT

Successful outcomes depend on the early administration of antibiotics that cross the blood–brain barrier into the subarachnoid space in sufficient concentration to halt the multiplication of bacteria.

- A penicillin (eg, ampicillin, piperacillin) or a cephalosporin (eg, ceftriaxone sodium, cefotaxime sodium) may be used.
- Vancomycin hydrochloride alone or in combination with rifampin may be used if resistant strains of bacteria are identified.
- Dexamethasone (Decadron) has been used as adjunctive treatment; however, recent evidence suggests no significant reduction of death or neurological disability. Further research is needed.
- Dehydration and shock are treated with fluid volume expanders.

- Seizures, which may occur early in the course of the disease, are controlled with phenytoin (Dilantin).
- Increased ICP is treated as necessary.

Nursing Management

The patient with meningitis is critically ill; therefore, many of the nursing interventions are collaborative with the health care provider, respiratory therapist, and other members of the health care team:

- Assess neurologic status and vital signs continuously.
- Assess pulse oximetry and arterial blood gases (ABGs) to determine need for intubation and mechanical ventilation secondary to ICP compromising brainstem function.
- Assess blood pressure for incipient shock, which precedes cardiac or respiratory failure.
- Rapid IV fluid replacement may be prescribed; care is taken to avoid fluid overload contributing to cerebral edema.
- Reduce high fever to decrease cardiac workload and cerebral oxygen demands.
- Protect the patient from injury secondary to seizure activity or altered LOC.
- Monitor daily body weight; serum electrolytes; and urine output, specific gravity, and osmolality, especially if syndrome of inappropriate antidiuretic hormone (SIADH) is suspected.
- Prevent complications associated with immobility, such as pressure ulcers and pneumonia.
- Institute infection control precautions until 24 hours after initiation of antibiotic therapy (oral and nasal discharge is considered infectious).
- Facilitate family visits for coping and support of patient; assist family in identifying others who can offer them support during the crisis.

COMPLICATIONS

M

- Visual impairment
- Deafness
- Seizures

- Paralysis
- Hydrocephalus
- Septic shock
- Neuropsychological sequelae

For more information, see Chapter 46 in Pellico, L.H. (2013). *Focus on adult health: Medical-surgical nursing.* Philadelphia: Wolters Kluwer Health | Lippincott Williams & Wilkins.

Mitral Regurgitation (Mitral Insufficiency)

Mitral regurgitation (MR) occurs when the mitral valve fails to close completely, allowing blood to backflow from the left ventricle (LV) into the left atrium.

PATHOPHYSIOLOGY

When the mitral valve leaflets thicken, fibrose, and contract, they cannot close completely. With each systole, blood is forced backward into the left atrium; this regurgitation of blood causes the atrium to dilate and hypertrophy. Eventually, this leads to LV failure. Pulmonary congestion results, elevating pulmonary artery pressure and increasing workload of the right ventricle (RV). Right ventricular enlargement and RV failure ensue. Disease processes that alter valve leaflets, mitral annulus, chordae tendineae, and the papillary muscle may result in MR.

RISK FACTORS

- Papillary muscle rupture, a complication of myocardial infarction (MI)
- Prosthetic valve malfunction
- Rupture of chordae tendineae

CLINICAL MANIFESTATIONS AND ASSESSMENT

Chronic MR may be asymptomatic for years.

- Fatigue, tachycardia, and weakness
- Orthopnea, DOE, and paroxysmal nocturnal dyspnea (PND) secondary to pulmonary congestion
- Palpitations and/or atrial fibrillation
- Signs of left- and right-sided heart failure are seen in acute MR: Tachycardia, crackles, and hypotension, as well as peripheral edema, jugular venous distention, and ascites.
- Acute MR manifests as severe left-sided heart failure. Patients may report a sudden inability to breathe accompanied by chest pain.
- Hyperdynamic point of maximal impulse (PMI) is displaced leftward and downward due to ventricular hypertrophy.
- Holosystolic murmur (heard on S_1) is heard as a high-pitched, blowing sound at the apex; radiation to the axilla is possible.
- S_3 gallop may be present due to increased, rapid blood flow into the ventricle during diastole; S_4 may be present as well.

DIAGNOSTIC METHODS

- Chest X-ray may reveal LV and left atrial enlargement.
- Transthoracic echocardiogram (TTE) monitors severity and progression of MR, anatomy of the valve, LV size and function, left atrial size, and pulmonary artery pressures.
- Transesophageal echocardiogram (TEE) provides the best images of the mitral valve; performed if the TTE is inconclusive.

MEDICAL AND NURSING MANAGEMENT

M

Management is aimed at decreasing regurgitant volume into the left atrium, increasing cardiac output and reducing pulmonary congestion.

Pharmacologic Therapy

- Afterload reduction with angiotensin-converting enzyme (ACE) inhibitors, nitrates, or hydralazine
- Vasodilators, diuretics, and sodium restriction to reduce preload
- Digoxin may be used to increase contractility and slow rapid rates to allow for improved ventricular filling.
- Anticoagulation is initiated if indicated for atrial fibrillation.

Surgical Intervention

Valvuloplasty or mitral valve replacement is recommended for patients symptomatic with medical therapy prior to deterioration of LV function.

For more information, see Chapter 16 in Pellico, L.H. (2013). *Focus on adult health: Medical-surgical nursing.* Philadelphia: Wolters Kluwer Health | Lippincott Williams & Wilkins.

Mitral Stenosis

In mitral stenosis (MS), the valve orifice is narrowed, impairing blood flow from the left atrium into the LV.

PATHOPHYSIOLOGY

Left atrial pressure increases due to impaired blood flow into the LV through the narrowed valve orifice. Because there is no functional valve to protect the pulmonary veins from the backward flow of blood from the atrium, pulmonary venous pressure rises and circulation becomes congested. As a result, the RV must contract against an abnormally high pulmonary pressure and the RV and right atrium become enlarged. Eventually, the ventricle fails. Sluggish atrial blood flow can lead to clot formation and thromboembolism.

RISK FACTORS

- Rheumatic fever; MS occurs 20 to 40 years after rheumatic fever
- Radiation therapy to chest area

CLINICAL MANIFESTATIONS AND ASSESSMENT

Symptoms usually develop after the valve opening is reduced by one-third to one-half its usual size.

- Dyspnea on exertion due to pulmonary congestion, progressing to dyspnea at rest with severe MS
- Paroxysmal nocturnal dyspnea
- Cough, hemoptysis, hoarseness from dilated atrium impinging on the laryngeal nerve, orthopnea, and recurrent respiratory infections may be noted.
- Progressive fatigue as a result of low cardiac output
- Atrial fibrillation
- Symptoms of right-heart failure, including peripheral edema and ascites, occur.
- A loud S_1 due to abrupt closure of the mitral valve and early diastolic opening snap
- A low-pitched, rumbling, diastolic murmur, heard on S_2, at the apex.

DIAGNOSTIC METHODS

- Echocardiography is the most sensitive and specific noninvasive method to diagnose MS.
- Electrocardiography (ECG)
- Cardiac catheterization when clinical findings and echo results are discordant.

M

MEDICAL AND NURSING MANAGEMENT

Medical therapy is aimed at symptom management.

- Antidysrhythmics including digoxin, beta blockers, and calcium channel blockers for rate control with atrial fibrillation
- Anticoagulants if atrial fibrillation is present
- Diuretics to reduce pulmonary congestion
- Restriction of strenuous exercise and avoidance of competitive sports, which increase heart rate and forward blow of blood
- Symptoms worsen over time; percutaneous transluminal valvuloplasty or mitral valve replacement may be performed.

See "Medical and Nursing Management" under "Heart Failure" on pages 370–371 for additional information.

> For more information, see Chapter 16 in Pellico, L.H. (2013). *Focus on adult health: Medical-surgical nursing.* Philadelphia: Wolters Kluwer Health | Lippincott Williams & Wilkins.

Mitral Valve Prolapse

In mitral valve prolapse (MVP), a portion of one or both mitral valve leaflets bulges back into the left atrium during systole, usually with little or no mitral regurgitation.

PATHOPHYSIOLOGY

M

Myxomatous degeneration (pathological weakening of connective tissue) can cause enlargement of one or both of the valve leaflets with subsequent billowing into the left atrium during systole. Over time, the leaflet edges may not fully coapt, or close, resulting in mitral regurgitation.

RISK FACTORS

- Family history
- Female gender

CLINICAL MANIFESTATIONS AND ASSESSMENT

Mitral valve prolapse is commonly asymptomatic.

- Over time, fatigue, dyspnea, lightheadedness, palpitations, and chest pain may develop.
- Chest pain is not correlated to activity and may be caused by abnormal stress placed on the chordae tendineae and papillary muscles.
- Shortness of breath is not correlated with activity levels or pulmonary function.
- A mitral (systolic) click may be present, indicating the valve leaflet is ballooning into the left atrium.
- A late systolic murmur may be heard if progressive valve leaflet stretching and regurgitation have occurred.

DIAGNOSTIC METHODS

Echocardiography is used to diagnose and monitor the progression of MVP.

MEDICAL AND NURSING MANAGEMENT

No treatment is required for asymptomatic patients. If symptoms develop, management is aimed at symptom control.

- Dietary restrictions; avoidance of alcohol and caffeine; smoking cessation
- Beta blockers and calcium channel blockers may be used to relieve chest pain and palpitations.

M

- Over-the-counter products such as cough medicine are avoided; these products may contain alcohol, caffeine, ephedrine, and epinephrine, which may produce arrhythmias and other symptoms.

For information on the treatment of arrhythmias, heart failure, or other complications of MVP see Chapters 15 and 17, and for additional information on MVP see Chapter 16, in Pellico, L.H. (2013). *Focus on adult health: Medical-surgical nursing.* Philadelphia: Wolters Kluwer Health | Lippincott Williams & Wilkins.

Multiple Myeloma

Multiple myeloma is a malignant disease of the most mature form of B lymphocyte, the plasma cell.

PATHOPHYSIOLOGY

Plasma cells secrete immunoglobulins, proteins necessary for antibody production to fight infection. The malignant plasma cells produce monoclonal protein, or M protein, which is nonfunctional; functional immunoglobulins are still produced by nonmalignant plasma cells, but in lower-than-normal quantity. Malignant plasma cells also secrete substances to stimulate the creation of new blood vessels to enhance the growth of plasma cells; a process known as *angiogenesis.* Occasionally, the plasma cells infiltrate other tissue, in which case they are referred to as *plasmacytomas.* Plasmacytomas can occur in the sinuses, spinal cord, and soft tissues. The median 5-year survival rate for newly diagnosed patients is 33%.

RISK FACTORS

- Individuals over 70 years
- Blacks have twice the incidence as whites

CLINICAL MANIFESTATIONS AND ASSESSMENT

- Bone pain, usually in the back or ribs, is most common presenting symptom; pain increases with movement and decreases with rest. Patients may report that they have less pain upon awakening, with pain increasing during the day.
- Lytic lesions and osteoporosis may be seen on bone X-rays; bone destruction may cause fractures with vertebral collapse, spinal cord compression, and pain.
- Hypercalcemia may develop secondary to bone destruction. Symptoms include excessive thirst, dehydration, constipation, altered mental status, confusion, and rarely coma.
- Renal failure may also occur secondary circulating immunoglobulins.
- Anemia develops from decreased erythropoietin by the kidney and crowding of the bone marrow by malignant plasma cells; fatigue and weakness may result.
- A reduced number of leukocytes and platelets occur in the later stage.

N u r s i n g   A l e r t
Any elderly patient whose chief complaint is back pain or anemia should be evaluated for possible myeloma.

DIAGNOSTIC FINDINGS

- Elevated levels monoclonal protein or M protein in the serum or urine (light chains or Bence-Jones protein in the urine) are major markers of multiple myeloma; levels are measured by serum or urine protein electrophoresis.
- Elevated serum total protein

M

- Bone marrow biopsy confirms the diagnosis; more than 10% of plasma cells in bone marrow is a hallmark diagnostic criterion.

MEDICAL AND NURSING MANAGEMENT

Initial treatment is often dictated by patient age, with younger patients receiving high-dose chemotherapy and autologous transplant, and older patients being treated with immunomodulatory agents and steroids. There is no cure for multiple myeloma; remission or control of symptoms is the goal.

Pharmacologic Therapy

- Corticosteroids are the mainstay of treatment, particularly dexamethasone (Decadron). Corticosteroids inhibit the expression of cytokines, such as interleukin-6, which are primary growth factors for the development of multiple myeloma. Steroids encourage apoptosis (programmed death) of myeloma cells.
- Steroids are often combined with immunomodulatory agents such as thalidomide, lenalidomide, or bortezomib (used in refractory disease). Medications can cause severe birth defects; use of these agents requires enrollment in a federally regulated safety program.
- Bisphosphonates, such as pamidronate (Aredia) and zoledronic acid (Zometa), strengthen bone by diminishing secretion of osteoclast activating factor, thus controlling bone pain and potentially preventing fracture. These agents are given to patients with lytic lesions or compression fractures.
- Aspirin or aspirin and Plavix may be used to prevent venous thromboembolism (VTE); multiple myeloma and associated pharmacologic therapy increases the risk.

Medical Management

- Radiation therapy is useful in strengthening the bone at a specific lesion, particularly one at risk for fracture or spinal cord compression. It is also useful in relieving bone pain and reducing the size of plasma cell tumors outside the skeletal system.

Because radiation is nonsystemic, it does not decrease the production of malignant plasma cells and is typically used in combination with systemic treatment such as chemotherapy.

- Plasmapheresis is used for signs and symptoms of hyperviscosity, including mental status changes or blurred vision; plasmapheresis may be used to lower the immunoglobulin level.

Surgical Management

- Vertebroplasty, injection of an orthopedic cement, is performed when lytic lesions result in vertebral compression fractures; pain relief is almost immediate for most patients. Concomitant kyphoplasty, the use of a special inflatable balloon to increase the height of the vertebra prior to injecting the cement, may be performed.

Nursing Management

- Nonsteroidal anti-inflammatory drugs (NSAIDs) may be used for mild pain or can be administered in combination with opioid analgesics.
- Educate patients regarding activity restrictions, such as lifting no more than 10 pounds and using proper body mechanics.
- Braces are occasionally needed to support the spinal column.
- Peripheral neuropathy, a common side effect of the immunomodulatory agents, can impact the patient's quality of life and ability to perform activities of daily living (ADLs). Gabapentin, physical therapy, and decreasing doses of immunomodulating medications may be used.
- Observe for bacterial infections (pneumonia); instruct patient in infection prevention measures including hand hygiene, avoiding sick individuals, and contacting the health care provider immediately if fever or other signs and symptoms of infection occur. The patient should receive pneumonia (Pneumovax) and influenza vaccines.
- Prophylactic antibiotics are sometimes used. Intravenous immune globulin (IVIG) can be useful for patients with recurrent infections and low levels of immunoglobulins.
- Monitor for effects of steroids, including hyperglycemia and insomnia (short term), and osteopenia, osteoporosis, cataracts, and diabetes (long term).

M

- Autologous peripheral blood stem cell transplant (PBSCT) is an option that can prolong remission and potentially cure some patients; unavailable to many older people because of age limitations, poor performance status, and comorbidities.

For more information, see Chapter 20 in Pellico, L.H. (2013). *Focus on adult health: Medical-surgical nursing.* Philadelphia: Wolters Kluwer Health | Lippincott Williams & Wilkins.

Multiple Sclerosis

Multiple sclerosis (MS) is an immune-mediated, progressive, demyelinating disease of the CNS.

PATHOPHYSIOLOGY

Demyelination refers to the destruction of myelin, the fatty proteinaceous material that surrounds certain nerve fibers in the brain and spinal cord; demyelination results in impaired transmission of nerve impulses. Plaques appear on demyelinated axons, further interrupting the transmission of impulses. Demyelinated axons are scattered irregularly throughout the CNS. Most frequently affected are the optic nerves, chiasm, and tracts; the cerebrum; the brainstem and cerebellum; and the spinal cord. Eventually, the axons themselves begin to degenerate, resulting in permanent and irreversible damage. Sensitized T cells are implicated in the inflammation and destruction of myelin.

RISK FACTORS

- Typically manifests between the ages of 20 and 40 years; may occur at any age

- Affects women more frequently than men
- Evidence exists for complex interactions between environmental factors and genetically susceptible individuals.
- Increased risk for Caucasians of northern European descent.
- Environmental exposure at a young age may play a role in the development of MS later.

CLINICAL MANIFESTATIONS AND ASSESSMENT

- Signs and symptoms are varied and multiple and reflect the location of the lesion (plaque) or lesions.
- Primary symptoms: Unilateral visual loss, typically preceded or accompanied by orbital pain that increases with eye movement (acute optic neuritis), fatigue, depression, weakness, lower extremity numbness, difficulty in coordination, loss of balance, and pain.
- Visual disturbances: Blurring of vision, diplopia (double vision), nystagmus, patchy blindness (scotoma), and total blindness
- Fatigue, typically worse in the afternoon hours; depression, heat, anemia, deconditioning, and medication may contribute to fatigue.
- Pain and social isolation: Pain may be related to osteoporosis in perimenopausal women secondary to estrogen loss, immobility, and corticosteroid therapy.
- Additional sensory manifestations: Paresthesias (abnormal skin sensations such as tingling, itching, or burning), dysesthesias (unpleasant, abnormal sense of touch), and loss of proprioception (ability to sense the position and location and orientation and movement of the body and its parts) loss. Objective sensory loss of position, vibration, shape, texture may occur.
- Spasticity (muscle hypertonicity) of the extremities, with painful spasms, may interfere with mobility, sleep, and ADLs.
- Gait abnormalities are common and are usually a result of ataxia, weakness, or spasticity; Involvement of the cerebellum or basal ganglia can produce ataxia (impaired coordination of movements) and tremor.

M

- Cognitive impairment may include memory loss and decreased concentration; severe cognitive changes with dementia are rare.
- Emotional lability and euphoria may develop due to loss of the control connections between the cortex and the basal ganglia.
- Bladder dysfunction (urinary urgency, frequency, nocturia, and urge incontinence, and loss of abdominal reflexes) may be noted.

Secondary Manifestations Related to Complications

- Urinary tract infections, constipation
- Pressure ulcers, contracture deformities, dependent pedal edema
- Pneumonia
- Reactive depressions
- Decreased bone density
- Emotional, social, marital, economic, and vocational problems

Exacerbations and Remissions

Exacerbations and remissions are characteristic of MS. During exacerbations, new symptoms appear and existing ones worsen; during remissions, symptoms decrease or disappear.

Relapses may be associated with periods of emotional and physical stress including emotional stress; cold, humid, or hot weather; hot baths or overheating; fever; and fatigue; pregnancy.

DIAGNOSTIC FINDINGS

Magnetic resonance imaging reveals demyelination plaques visualized in the CNS.

MEDICAL AND NURSING MANAGEMENT

There is no cure for MS, therefore the goals of treatment are to treat acute exacerbations, delay the progression of the disease, and manage chronic symptoms. Management strategies target the various motor and sensory symptoms and the effects of immobility that can occur.

Pharmacologic Therapy

Disease-Modifying Therapies

The disease-modifying medications reduce the frequency of relapse, the duration of relapse, and the number and size of plaques observed on MRI.

- Interferon beta-1a (Rebif) and interferon beta-1b (Betaseron) are administered subcutaneously. Another preparation of interferon beta-1a, Avonex, is administered intramuscularly once a week.
- Glatiramer acetate (Copaxone), administered subcutaneously daily, reduces the rate of relapse in the relapsing-remitting course of MS; it may take 6 months for evidence of an immune response to appear.
- Intravenous methylprednisolone shortens the duration of acute relapse in the relapsing-remitting course.
- Mitoxantrone (Novantrone) has immunosuppressive and immunomodulatory properties. It is given by IV infusion every 3 months for patients with secondary-progressive or worsening relapsing-remitting MS. Limited to a lifetime cumulative dose of 140 mg/m^2 due to irreversible cardiotoxicity.

Symptom Management

- Baclofen (Lioresal), orally or intrathecally, is the medication of choice for treating spasticity; benzodiazepines (Valium), tizanidine (Zanaflex), and dantrolene (Dantrium) may also be used.
- Amantadine (Symmetrel), pemoline (Cylert), or fluoxetine (Prozac) are used to treat fatigue.
- Beta-adrenergic blockers (Inderal), antiseizure agents (Neurontin), and benzodiazepines (Klonopin) are used to treat ataxia.

Management of Related Bowel and Bladder Problems

Anticholinergics, alpha-adrenergic blockers, or antispasmodic agents may be used to treat problems related to elimination, and

M

patients may be taught to perform intermittent self-catheterization as well. Additional measures include assessment of urinary tract infections, ascorbic acid to acidify urine, antibiotics when appropriate.

Nursing Interventions

An individualized program of physical therapy, rehabilitation, and education is combined with emotional support. An educational plan of care is developed to enable the person with MS to deal with the physiologic, social, and psychological problems that accompany chronic disease.

Promoting Physical Mobility

- Encourage relaxation and coordination exercises to promote muscle efficiency.
- Encourage progressive resistance exercises to strengthen weak muscles.
- Encourage walking exercises to improve gait.
- Encourage daily exercises for muscle stretching to minimize joint contractures.
- Swimming, stationary bicycling, and progressive weight bearing is used to relieve spasticity in legs.
- Avoid hurrying patient in any activity; rushing increases spasticity.
- Encourage patient to work up to a point just short of fatigue; very strenuous exercise raises body temperature and may aggravate symptoms.
- Advise patient to take frequent short rest periods, preferably lying down; extreme fatigue may exacerbates symptoms.
- Warm packs may be beneficial for muscle spasticity; without treatment, contracture of joints will occur. Avoid hot baths due to risk for burn injury secondary to sensory loss and worsening symptoms that may occur with elevation of the body temperature.
- Prevent complications of immobility by assessing and maintaining of skin integrity and through coughing and deep-breathing exercises.

M

Preventing Injury

- Teach patient to walk with feet wide apart to increase the base of support and improve walking stability.
- Teach patient to watch the feet while walking if there is a loss of position sense.
- Gait training may require assistive devices (walker, cane, braces, crutches) and instruction about their use by a physical therapist.
- Wheelchair or motorized scooter may be needed if gait remains insufficient after gait training.
- Assess skin for pressure ulcers for patients confined to wheelchair.

Enhancing Bladder and Bowel Control

Generally, bladder symptoms fall into the following categories: (1) inability to store urine (hyperreflexic, uninhibited); (2) inability to empty the bladder (hyporeflexic, hypotonic); and (3) a mixture of both types.

- Keep bedpan or urinal readily available for patients with urinary frequency, urgency, or incontinence because the need to void must be heeded immediately.
- Set up a voiding schedule, initially 1.5 to 2 hours, with gradual lengthening of time intervals.
- Instruct patient to drink a measured amount of fluid every 2 hours and to attempt to void 30 minutes after drinking.
- Encourage patient to take prescribed medications for bladder spasticity.
- Teach intermittent self-catheterization, if necessary. For female patients with permanent urinary incontinence, urinary diversion procedures may be considered. The male patient may wear a condom catheter.
- Provide adequate fluids, dietary fiber, and a bowel-training program to prevent or treat constipation, fecal impaction, and incontinence.

Enhancing Communication and Managing Swallowing Difficulties

- Observe for dysarthrias (defects of articulation) marked by slurring, low volume of speech, and difficulties in phonation.

M

- Dysphagia should be evaluated by a speech therapist for strategies to compensate for speech and swallowing problems.
- Reduce the risk for aspiration by careful feeding, proper positioning for eating, having suction apparatus available.

Improving Sensory and Cognitive Function

- Provide an eye patch or covered eyeglass lens to block visual impulses of one eye when diplopia (double vision) occurs. Prism glasses may be helpful for patients who are confined to bed and have difficulty reading in the supine position.
- Advise patient about free talking-book services of the Library of Congress; large-print or audio books are available from local libraries.
- Cognitive impairment, emotional lability, forgetfulness, and easy distractibility may occur, imposing stress on the patient and family. Patients may display denial, depression, withdrawal, and hostility.
- Provide emotional support to assist patients and their families to adapt to the changes, disruptions, and uncertainties associated with MS. Assist the patient to set meaningful and realistic goals, to remain as active as possible, and to keep up social interests, hobbies, and activities.
- Consult with the occupational therapist to assist the family to maintain a structured environment, use lists and other memory aids to maintain a daily routine.

Strengthening Coping Mechanisms

- Alleviate stress, and make referrals for counseling and support to minimize adverse effects of dealing with chronic illness.
- The nurse coordinates a network of services, including social services, speech therapy, physical therapy, and home care services.
- Provide information on the illness to patient and family, including an updated list of available assistive devices, services, and resources.
- Maintain flexibility and a hopeful attitude to assist with psychological and physical adaptation.

M

Improving Home Management

- Suggest modifications that allow independence in self-care activities including assistive eating devices, raised toilet seat, bathing aids, telephone modifications, long-handled comb, tongs, modified clothing.
- Maintain moderate environmental temperature; exposure to heat increases fatigue and muscle weakness. Recommend air conditioning in at least one room; cold may increase spasticity.

Promoting Sexual Functioning

- Inform patients that MS may interfere with sexual activity due to easy fatigability, conflicts arising from dependency and depression, emotional lability, and loss of self-esteem.
- Erectile and ejaculatory disorders in men and orgasmic dysfunction and adductor spasms of the thigh muscles in women, as well as bladder and bowel incontinence and urinary tract infections, may occur.
- Sexual counseling may help identify sexual resources and provide relevant information and supportive therapy.
- Suggest sharing and communicating feelings, planning for sexual activity (to minimize the effects of fatigue), and exploring alternative methods of sexual expression that may open up a wide range of sexual enjoyment and experiences.

> See Chapters 9 and 10 for information related to aspiration; for more information on MS, see Chapter 46 in Pellico, L.H. (2013). *Focus on adult health: Medical-surgical nursing.* Philadelphia: Wolters Kluwer Health | Lippincott Williams & Wilkins.

Musculoskeletal Trauma (Contusions, Strains, Sprains, and Joint Dislocations)

M

A *contusion* is a soft tissue injury produced by blunt force, such as a blow, kick, or fall that results in bleeding into soft tissues (ecchymosis or bruising). A hematoma develops when the bleeding is sufficient to cause an appreciable solid swelling.

A *strain* or "pulled muscle" is an injury to a musculotendinous unit (the tendon connects muscle to bone) and results from overuse, overstretching, or excessive stress.

A *sprain* is an injury to the ligaments and supporting muscle fibers that surround a joint, often caused by a trauma or a wrenching or twisting motion. The injury can range from a mild stretching of the ligament to a complete tear.

A dislocation of a joint is a condition in which the articular surfaces of the bones forming the joint are no longer in anatomic contact. In complete dislocation, the bones are literally "out of joint." A subluxation is a partial dislocation of the articulating surfaces. Traumatic dislocations are orthopedic emergencies because the associated joint structures, blood supply, and nerves are distorted and severely stressed. If dislocation is not treated promptly, avascular necrosis, tissue death due to anoxia and diminished blood supply, and nerve palsy may occur.

RISK FACTORS

- Sports
- Physical fitness activities
- Overuse repetitive injuries or trauma
- Contusions can occur in any soft tissue that suffers blunt trauma.
- Ankles, knees, and wrists are vulnerable to sprains, whereas strains frequently occur in the foot or leg.
- Dislocations may be congenital or present at birth, spontaneous or pathologic, or traumatic.

CLINICAL MANIFESTATIONS AND ASSESSMENT

- Assessment of activity at time of injury:
  - Three "S's": Size, shape, and symmetry of the involved area in comparison to the opposite

- Edema, ecchymosis (bruising), tenderness, abnormal joint motion, and pain
- Contusions, strains, and sprains can present with similar symptoms of pain, edema, and discoloration from the broken blood vessels. The patient may guard or protect the affected area, and he or she may have difficulty moving the affected area; increased warmth may be noted at the injury site.
- Contusion: Local symptoms (pain, swelling, and discoloration), ecchymosis, and edema of the injured area; the patient may complain initially of dull pain at the site that increases as edema develops and subsequent stiffness of the area, usually by the next day. Most contusions resolve in 1 to 2 weeks.
- Strain: Soreness or sudden pain with local tenderness on muscle use and isometric contraction, muscle spasm, ecchymosis, edema, and loss of function. Strains are graded along a continuum based on symptoms and loss of function:
  - A first-degree strain reflects tearing of few muscle fibers and is accompanied by minor edema, tenderness, and mild muscle spasm, without a noticeable loss of function.
  - A second-degree strain involves a tearing of more muscle fibers and is manifested by edema, tenderness, muscle spasm, ecchymosis, and a notable loss of load-bearing strength of the involved extremity.
  - A third-degree strain involves complete disruption of at least one musculotendinous unit that involves separation of muscle from muscle, muscle from tendon, or tendon from bone. An X-ray should be obtained to rule out bone injury with a third-degree strain.
- Sprains are also graded to reflect the degree of injury:
  - A mild sprain or first-degree sprain may cause minor edema, tenderness, and mild muscle spasm without a noticeable loss of function. Patients are able to bear weight with minimal pain.
  - A second-degree sprain is an incomplete tear of the ligament (bone-to-bone). As blood vessels rupture, ecchymosis, edema, and pain in the joint with increasing disability and pain occur. There is restricted motion of the affected limb, and weight bearing is painful.
  - A third-degree sprain involves complete ligament tear with resultant complaints of significant pain, muscle spasm,

M

ecchymosis, edema, and loss of function. Patients are unable to bear weight on the affected limb. Tenderness at the distal tibia (inner ankle) or fibula (outer ankle) associated with an inversion or eversion injury may indicate a fracture.

- Dislocation or subluxation: Acute pain, change in contour of the joint, shortening of the affected limb, loss of mobility, and change in the axis of the dislocated bones

DIAGNOSTIC METHODS

X-ray examination is used to rule out any bone injury or fracture.

MEDICAL AND NURSING MANAGEMENT

Treatment of injury involves providing support for the injured part until healing is complete. Treatment of contusions, strains, and sprains include rest, applying ice, applying a compression bandage, and elevating the affected part (RICE: Rest, ice, compression, elevation).

- Immobilization of the affected extremity until diagnosis is confirmed may be appropriate.
- Monitor "CSM": Circulation by way of pulses, color, temperature, and capillary refill; Sensation by noting awareness of light touch; and Movement by range of motion (ROM) of the most distal digits. The nurse compares the injured limb in relation to the uninjured limb.
- After the acute inflammatory stage (24 to 48 hours after injury), intermittent heat application (for 15 to 30 minutes, four times a day) relieves muscle spasm and promotes vasodilation, absorption, and repair.
- Progressive passive and active exercises may begin in 2 to 5 days, depending on the severity of injury. Excessive exercise early in the course of treatment delays recovery. Splinting may be used to prevent reinjury.
- Severe sprains may require 1 to 3 weeks of immobilization before protected exercises are initiated.

M

- Strains and sprains take weeks or months to heal. Splinting may be used to prevent reinjury.
- A dislocation is promptly reduced (ie, displaced parts are brought into normal position) to preserve joint function. Analgesia, muscle relaxants, and possibly anesthesia are used to facilitate closed reduction (eg, noninvasive or nonsurgical reduction). The joint is immobilized by bandages, splints, casts, or traction, and is maintained in a stable position. Neurovascular status is monitored. After reduction, if the joint is stable, gentle, progressive, active and passive movement is begun to preserve ROM and restore strength. The joint is supported between exercise sessions.

For more information, see Chapter 42 in Pellico, L.H. (2013). *Focus on adult health: Medical-surgical nursing.* Philadelphia: Wolters Kluwer Health | Lippincott Williams & Wilkins.

Myasthenia Gravis

Myasthenia gravis (MG) is an autoimmune disorder affecting the acetylcholine receptors of the myoneural junction.

PATHOPHYSIOLOGY

In myasthenia gravis, antibodies reduce the number of acetylcholine receptor sites, impairing transmission of impulses across the neuromuscular junction. This results in voluntary muscle weakness that escalates with continued activity. Hyperplasia and tumors of the thymus are frequently found in MG patients.

RISK FACTORS

- Three times more common in women before age 40
- Most common age of onset is the second and third decades in females and the seventh and eighth decades in males.

M

CLINICAL MANIFESTATIONS AND ASSESSMENT

Myasthenia gravis is purely a motor disorder with no effect on sensation or coordination.

- Initial manifestation involves ocular muscles, causing diplopia and ptosis.
- Generalized weakness, including weakness of the muscles of the face, results in a bland facial expression; weakness of the throat (bulbar symptoms) may be noted.
- Laryngeal involvement: Dysphonia (voice impairment) and increased risk of choking and aspiration
- Generalized weakness that affects all extremities and the intercostal muscles, resulting in decreasing vital capacity and respiratory failure

DIAGNOSTIC METHODS

- An acetylcholinesterase test using an injection of edrophonium (Tensilon) is used to confirm the diagnosis. Immediate improvement in muscle strength represents a positive test and usually confirms the diagnosis.
- Acetylcholine receptor antibodies are identified in serum.
- Computed tomography (CT) scan of the mediastinum is performed to detect thymoma or hyperplasia of the thymus.
- Repetitive nerve stimulation demonstrates a decrease in successive action potentials.

MEDICAL AND NURSING MANAGEMENT

Management of myasthenia gravis is directed at improving function and reducing and removing circulating antibodies.

Pharmacologic Therapy

- Acetylcholinesterase medications with pyridostigmine bromide (Mestinon) increases concentration of acetylcholine at the neuromuscular junction and is first line of therapy.

- Immunosuppressant agents are used if pyridostigmine bromide does not improve symptoms:
  - Corticosteroids, such as prednisone, suppress immune response and decrease antibody production. As symptoms improve, the medication is tapered. Due to side effects such as diabetes, osteoporosis, and hypertension, steroids are usually reserved for patients with ocular symptoms.
- Cytotoxic medications such as azathioprine (Imuran), an immunosuppressive drug, are used when response to steroids is inadequate. Azathioprine inhibits T lymphocytes and reduces acetylcholine receptor antibody levels; therapeutic effects may not be evident for 3 to 12 months. Leukopenia and hepatotoxicity are serious adverse effects; monthly evaluation of liver enzymes and white blood cell count is necessary.
- Intravenous immune globulin (IVIG) treatment involves the administration of pooled human gamma globulin, which usually produces relatively quick and short-term relief of MG weakness; the response to plasmapheresis is more rapid.

Medical Management

Plasmapheresis or plasma exchange produces a temporary reduction in the titer of circulating antibodies during acute exacerbations; improvement may only last a few weeks.

Surgical Management

Thymectomy can produce antigen-specific immunosuppression and produces improvement in almost all patients; it may take months before benefits are demonstrated.

Nursing Management

Because myasthenia gravis is a chronic disease and most patients are seen on an outpatient basis, much of the nursing care focuses on patient and family teaching.

M

- Teach patients about the actions of medications and need to take them on schedule; teach patients that delaying medications may produce signs and symptoms of myasthenic crisis.

- Teach patients symptoms of cholinergic crisis. A diary can help identify fluctuation and symptoms to determine best times for medication dosing.

☀ NURSING ALERT

Maintenance of stable blood levels of anticholinesterase medications is imperative to stabilize muscle strength; therefore, medications must be administered on time. Any delay in administration of medications may exacerbate muscle weakness and make it impossible for the patient to take medications orally.

- Mealtimes should coincide with peak effects of anticholinesterase medication; rest prior to meals will reduce muscle fatigue.
- Advise patient to sit upright during meals, with the neck slightly flexed to facilitate swallowing.
- Soft foods in gravy or sauces can be swallowed more easily; if choking occurs frequently, suggest puréed food with a pudding-like consistency.
- Ensure suction is available at home and that the patient and family are instructed in its use.
- Supplemental feedings may be necessary in some patients to ensure adequate nutrition.
- Instruct the patient to tape the eyes closed for short intervals and to regularly instill artificial tears to prevent corneal damage. Patients who wear eyeglasses can have "crutches" attached to help lift the eyelids; patching of one eye can help with double vision.
- Remind the patient of the importance of maintaining health promotion practices and of following health care screening recommendations
- Factors that exacerbate symptoms and potentially cause crisis should be noted and avoided: Emotional stress, infections (particularly respiratory infections), vigorous physical activity, some medications, and high environmental temperature.
- Teach the patient strategies to conserve energy; help determine optimal times for rest throughout the day. If living in a two-story home, suggest that frequently used items such as hygiene products, cleaning products, and snacks be kept on each floor to minimize travel between floors.

M

- Encourage the patient to apply for a handicapped license plate to minimize walking and to schedule activities to coincide with peak energy and strength levels.
- Encourage patient to wear a Medic Alert bracelet identifying them as having myasthenia gravis.
- Refer patient to the Myasthenia Gravis Foundation of America, which can provide support groups, services, and educational materials for patients and families.

COMPLICATIONS

- Cholinergic crisis: A problem of overmedication; it results in severe generalized muscle weakness, respiratory impairment, and excessive pulmonary secretions that may cause respiratory failure. Have atropine on hand for treatment.
- Myasthenic crisis: Most commonly precipitated by respiratory infection; it is a sudden, temporary exacerbation of the disease process. Respiratory distress and varying degrees of dysphagia (difficulty swallowing), dysarthria (difficulty speaking), eyelid ptosis, diplopia, and prominent muscle weakness occur:
  - Treatment measures during myasthenic crisis include monitoring lab work, intake and output, and daily weight, along with vigilant pulmonary assessments. Nasogastric feedings may be prescribed for dysphagia. Sedatives and tranquilizers are avoided as they may exacerbate hypoxia and hypercapnia.

For more information, see Chapter 46 in Pellico, L.H. (2013). *Focus on adult health: Medical-surgical nursing*. Philadelphia: Wolters Kluwer Health | Lippincott Williams & Wilkins.

Myocarditis

M

Myocarditis is an inflammation of the heart muscle, commonly resulting from viral infection.

PATHOPHYSIOLOGY

Cardiac muscle inflammation that results in myocyte necrosis (eg, cardiac cell death) is the hallmark of myocarditis. Acute myocarditis is characterized by myocyte damage from viral infection, autoimmunity, or other precipitating event. Myocyte antigens and cytokines are released. In the subacute phase (days 4 to 14), T and B lymphocytes infiltrate the myocardium and the virus is cleared. The immune response continues, and infected myocytes are lysed. During the chronic phase, myocyte injury continues and can lead to dilated cardiomyopathy. Mortality varies with the severity of symptoms. Mild cases with few symptoms may resolve without treatment, whereas more serious cases result in cardiogenic shock and death.

RISK FACTORS

- Viral, bacterial infections
- Immune-mediated mechanisms
- Toxic agents
- Frequently, cause is unknown

CLINICAL MANIFESTATIONS AND ASSESSMENT

The symptoms of myocarditis depend on the type of infection, the degree of myocardial damage, and the capacity of the myocardium to recover.

- Clinical presentation varies widely from mild systemic findings of fever, myalgias, fatigue, and dyspnea to ventricular arrhythmias, cardiogenic shock, and dilated cardiomyopathy.
- Other signs and symptoms include an S_3 gallop, tachycardia, tachypnea, jugular venous distention, edema, ECG abnormalities, orthopnea, and palpitations.
- Fulminant heart failure or sudden cardiac death can quickly develop.

M

DIAGNOSTIC FINDINGS

- Elevated cardiac enzymes and white blood cell count
- Elevated ESR, approximately 60% of the time
- Echocardiography may show impaired heart muscle function or pericardial effusion.
- Myocardial biopsy may be used to confirm diagnosis.

MEDICAL AND NURSING MANAGEMENT

Supportive care is of primary importance, with the goals of care focused on maintaining hemodynamic stability and improvement of symptoms. Treatment of heart failure symptoms with medical therapy and placement of an intra-aortic balloon pump (IABP), ventricular assist device (VAD), total artificial heart (TAH), or heart transplantation are options when no improvement in symptoms or hemodynamic deterioration develops despite maximal medical therapy.

Nursing Management

- Monitor vital signs, heart sounds, lung sounds, and peripheral perfusion.
- Assess hemodynamic, oxygenation, and fluid status.
- Be prepared to use emergency equipment, as the risk of life-threatening ventricular arrhythmias is great.
- Provide emotional support to the patient and family; myocarditis can be particularly stressful due to its variable presentation and course.

For more information, see Chapter 16 in Pellico, L.H. (2013). *Focus on adult health: Medical-surgical nursing.* Philadelphia: Wolters Kluwer Health | Lippincott Williams & Wilkins.

M

N

Nephrotic Syndrome

Nephrotic syndrome is a cluster of clinical findings reflecting underlying organ damage. Nephrotic syndrome can occur with almost any intrinsic renal disease or systemic disease that affects the glomerulus. Although generally considered a disorder of childhood, nephrotic syndrome also occurs in adults, including the elderly.

PATHOPHYSIOLOGY

Nephrotic syndrome is a disorder that causes structural changes in the glomerulus resulting in renal loss of protein (proteinuria), hypoalbuminemia, hyperlipidemia, and edema.

RISK FACTORS

- Diabetic nephropathy
- Chronic glomerulonephritis
- Diabetes mellitus with intercapillary glomerulosclerosis
- Amyloidosis of the kidney
- Systemic lupus erythematosus
- Multiple myeloma
- Renal vein thrombosis.

CLINICAL MANIFESTATIONS AND ASSESSMENT

- Proteinuria, predominately in the form of albuminuria, in which albumin excretion exceeding 3.5 g/day, is the hallmark of the diagnosis of nephrotic syndrome.
- Edema, periorbital edema, or anasarca results from hypoalbuminemia.

⚡ NURSING ALERT

Decreased serum albumin level presents decreased protein binding sites for medications; therefore, the nurse is aware that patients must be observed closely for signs of drug toxicity as the amount of free or unbound drug is increased.

- Hypoimmunoglobulinemia places the patient at risk for infections.
- Hyperlipidemia with increased high-density lipoprotein (HDL) occurs and places the patient at risk for cardiovascular disease.
- Hypertension, irritability, headache, and malaise occur.

DIAGNOSTIC FINDINGS

- Urine may contain increased white blood cells and granular and epithelial casts.
- Needle biopsy of the kidney is used for histologic examination to confirm diagnosis.
- Decreased serum albumin levels are noted.

MEDICAL AND NURSING MANAGEMENT

Patients with nephrotic syndrome need instruction about the importance of following medication and dietary regimens so that their condition can remain stable for as long as possible.

- Low-sodium diet containing liberal amounts of potassium is prescribed if hyperkalemia is absent.
- Reduced dietary cholesterol and saturated fats help with lipidemia.

N

- Moderate protein intake is recommended, avoiding excessive intake that may accelerate renal deterioration and increase urinary protein losses.
- Teach patient to report any signs of acute infection promptly, such as a respiratory tract infection, to prevent further glomerular damage.

Pharmacologic Therapy

- Diuretics may be prescribed for the patient with severe edema; however, caution must be used because of the risk of reducing the plasma volume to the point of impaired circulation.
- Angiotensin-converting enzyme (ACE) inhibitors in combination with loop diuretics often reduces the degree of proteinuria but may take 4 to 6 weeks to be effective.
- Immunosuppressants such as corticosteroids, antineoplastic agents (cyclophosphamide [Cytoxan]), or immunosuppressant medications (azathioprine [Imuran], chlorambucil [Leukeran], or cyclosporine [Neoral]) may be prescribed. It may be necessary to repeat treatment with corticosteroids if relapse occurs.
- Patients should be taught to protect themselves from infection and to report any infections promptly due to immunosuppression.
- Treatment of hyperlipidemia is controversial as typical antilipemics may cause rhabdomyolysis (syndrome associated with rapid destruction of striated muscle fibers), which can damage the kidney.

COMPLICATIONS

- Infection secondary to loss of immunoglobulins
- Accelerated atherosclerosis secondary to hyperlipidemia
- Hypercoagulable state that may result in thromboembolism of the renal vein and pulmonary embolism
- Body image may be altered due to anasarca and edema causing a change in appearance.

For more information, see Chapter 27 in Pellico, L.H. (2013). *Focus on adult health: Medical-surgical nursing.* Philadelphia: Wolters Kluwer Health | Lippincott Williams & Wilkins.

N

O

Obesity, Morbid

Morbid obesity is a term applied to people who are more than two times their ideal body weight or whose body mass index (BMI) exceeds 30 kg/m^2. Another definition of morbid obesity is body weight that is more than 100 pounds over the ideal body weight.

PATHOPHYSIOLOGY

Patients with morbid obesity are at higher risk for health complications, such as diabetes, heart disease, stroke, hypertension, gallbladder disease, osteoarthritis, sleep apnea and other breathing problems, and some forms of cancer (uterine, breast, colorectal, kidney, and gallbladder).

RISK FACTORS

- Low self-esteem
- Impaired body image
- Depression

MEDICAL AND NURSING MANAGEMENT

Conservative management consists of weight loss diet in conjunction with behavioral modification and exercise; however, dietary and behavioral approaches to obesity have had limited success.

Pharmacologic Management

- Orlistat (Xenical, Alli) reduces caloric intake by binding to gastric and pancreatic lipase to prevent digestion of fats. Review side effects; multivitamin supplement is usually recommended.
- Side effects of orlistat: Increased frequency of bowel movements, gas with oily discharge, decreased food absorption, decreased bile flow, and decreased absorption of some vitamins. A multivitamin is usually recommended. Do not use in pregnancy, during lactation, or in transplant recipients.
- Rimonabant (Acomplia) blocks the cannabinoid-1 receptor that is thought to play an important role in metabolism, including obesity.
- Side effects of rimonabant: Depression, anxiety, agitation, sleep disorders; transient effects are nausea, vomiting, diarrhea, headache, and dizziness.
- Depression may contribute to weight gain; use of an antidepressant may be helpful.
- Pharmacologic therapy rarely results in loss of more than 10% of total body weight.

Surgical Management

Bariatric surgery, or surgery for morbid obesity, is performed only after other nonsurgical attempts at weight control have failed.

- Bariatric surgical procedures work by restricting a patient's ability to eat (restrictive procedure), interfering with ingested nutrient absorption (malabsorptive procedures), or both.
- Average weight loss after bariatric surgery is approximately 61% of previous body weight; comorbid conditions such as diabetes mellitus, hypertension, and sleep apnea resolve, and dyslipidemia improves.
- After bariatric surgery, all patients require life-long monitoring of weight, comorbidities, metabolic and nutritional status, diet, and activity due to risk for malnutrition or weight gain.
- Procedures include: Roux-en-Y gastric bypass, gastric banding, vertical-banded gastroplasty, and biliopancreatic diversion with duodenal switch. These procedures may be performed by laparoscopy or by an open surgical technique.

Nursing Management

Nursing management focuses on care of the patient after surgery. General postoperative nursing care is similar to that for a patient recovering from a gastric resection, with attention to the risks associated with morbid obesity.

- Monitor for immediate postoperative complications: Peritonitis, stomal obstruction, stomal ulcers, atelectasis and pneumonia, thromboembolism, and metabolic imbalances resulting from prolonged vomiting and diarrhea or altered gastrointestinal (GI) function.
- Resume oral feeding after bowel sounds have returned, providing six small feedings totaling 600 to 800 calories per day. Encourage fluids to prevent dehydration.
- Instruct the patient to report excessive thirst or concentrated urine, indicative of dehydration.
- Assist the patient to modify eating behaviors and cope with changes in body image.
- Explain that noncompliance by eating too fast, consuming too much food, or eating high-calorie liquids or soft foods results in vomiting and painful esophageal distention.
- Emphasize the importance of follow-up appointments to detect side effects including gallstones, nutritional deficiencies, and potential to regain weight.
- After weight loss, the patient may need lipoplasty to remove fat deposits or a panniculectomy to remove excess abdominal skinfolds.

COMPLICATIONS

- Bleeding
- Blood clots
- Bowel obstruction
- Incisional or ventral hernias
- Infection
- Dumping syndrome
- Long-term complications related to nutritional deficiencies

O

> For more information, see Chapter 23 in Pellico, L.H. (2013).
> *Focus on adult health: Medical-surgical nursing.* Philadelphia:
> Wolters Kluwer Health | Lippincott Williams & Wilkins.

Osteomyelitis

Osteomyelitis is an infection of the bone.

PATHOPHYSIOLOGY

The majority of bone infections are caused by *Staphylococcus aureus*, followed by *Proteus* and *Pseudomonas* species and *Escherichia coli*. The incidence of penicillin-resistant, nosocomial, gram-negative, and anaerobic infections is increasing. Bone infection occurs by:

- Extension of soft tissue infection (eg, infected pressure or vascular ulcer, incisional infection)
- Direct bone contamination from bone surgery, open fracture, or traumatic injury (eg, gunshot wound)
- Hematogenous (bloodborne) spread from other sites of infection (eg, infected tonsils, boils, infected teeth, upper respiratory infections)

RISK FACTORS

- Poorly nourished
- Elderly
- Obese
- Impaired immune system (long-term corticosteroid therapy or immunosuppressive agents)
- Chronic illness (diabetes, rheumatoid arthritis)

- History of previous injury or infection
- Postoperative

CLINICAL MANIFESTATIONS AND ASSESSMENT

- Blood-borne infections cause sudden onset of symptoms of sepsis including chills, high fever, tachycardia, and malaise.
- Infected area becomes painful, swollen, and extremely tender.
- Patient may describe a constant pulsating pain that intensifies with movement due to the pressure of collecting pus.
- When osteomyelitis is caused by adjacent infection or direct contamination, there are no symptoms of sepsis.
- Chronic osteomyelitis: Presents with a nonhealing ulcer that overlies the infected bone, with a connecting sinus that will intermittently drain pus.

DIAGNOSTIC METHODS

- Early X-rays in acute osteomyelitis: Show only soft-tissue swelling, then areas of irregular decalcification, bone necrosis, periosteal elevation, and new bone formation are evident.
- X-ray shows large, irregular cavities, a raised periosteum, sequestra, or dense bone formations in chronic osteomyelitis.
- Radioisotope bone scan, isotope-labeled white blood cell (WBC) scan, and magnetic resonance imaging (MRI) assist with early, definitive diagnosis.
- Blood studies reveal leukocytosis and an elevated erythrocyte sedimentation rate (ESR). Wounds, blood, and abscesses are cultured to identify appropriate antibiotic therapy.
- Magnetic resonance imaging
- Erythrocyte sedimentation rate and the WBC count are usually normal; blood cultures are obtained. Anemia, associated with chronic infection, may be evident.

MEDICAL AND NURSING MANAGEMENT

Initial goal is to control and arrest the infective process.

- General supportive measures including hydration, diet high in vitamins and protein, correction of anemia; affected area is immobilized to prevent pathologic fracture.

Prevention

- Elective orthopedic surgery should be postponed if the patient has a current infection such as urinary tract infection, sore throat, or history of recent infection.
- Prophylactic antibiotics, administered to achieve adequate tissue levels at the time of surgery and for 24 hours after surgery, are administered.

Pharmacology Therapy

- Blood and wound cultures are performed to identify effective antibiotics; antibiotics administered around the clock for 3 to 6 weeks.
- Oral antibiotics are taken for up to 3 months once infection appears to be controlled; take antibiotics on an empty stomach to enhance absorption.

Surgical Management

- Surgical débridement of bone to remove purulent and necrotic material followed by irrigation is performed; IV antibiotics are continued.
- Antibiotic-impregnated beads may be placed directly in the wound.
- Chronic osteomyelitis: Sequestrectomy (removal of necrotic bone) is performed, with sufficient bone removed to convert a deep cavity into a shallow saucer (saucerization). Closed suction irrigation system may be used to remove debris. Wound irrigation using sterile physiologic saline solution may be performed for 7 to 8 days.
- Wounds are closed tightly to obliterate the dead space or packed and closed later by granulation or grafting with muscle flap. Internal fixation or external supportive devices may be needed to stabilize or support the bone to prevent pathologic fracture.

NURSING PROCESS

The Patient With Osteomyelitis

Assessment

- Assess for risk factors (eg, older age, diabetes, long-term steroid therapy) and for previous injury, infection, or orthopedic surgery.
- Assess for acute onset of signs and symptoms (eg, localized pain, edema, erythema, fever) or recurrent drainage of an infected sinus with associated pain, edema, and low-grade fever.
- Observe for guarding or patient avoiding pressure on area.
- Assess for generalized weakness due to systemic reaction to infection.
- Observe for inflammation, edema, tenderness, and purulent drainage.
- Monitor for elevated temperature.
- Patients with chronic osteomyelitis may have minimal temperature elevations, occurring in the afternoon or evening.

Nursing Diagnoses

- Acute pain related to inflammation and edema
- Impaired physical mobility related to pain, immobilization devices, and weight-bearing limitations
- Risk for extension of infection: Bone abscess formation
- Deficient knowledge about treatment regimen

Planning

Goals include relief of pain, improved physical mobility within therapeutic limitations, control and eradication of infection, and knowledge of the treatment regimen.

Nursing Interventions

Relieving Pain

- Splint affected area to decrease pain and muscle spasm.
- Monitor neurovascular status of affected extremity.

(continues on page 500)

- Handle affected part with great care to avoid pain.
- Elevate affected part to reduce swelling and discomfort.
- Administer prescribed analgesics in conjunction with other techniques to reduce pain.

Improving Physical Mobility

- Teach patient to adhere to activity restrictions and reduce stress on the bone, as bone is weakened due to infectious process.
- Encourage activities of daily living within physical limitations.

Controlling Infectious Process

- Monitor response to antibiotic therapy. Observe IV sites for evidence of phlebitis, infection, or infiltration.
- Monitor for signs of superinfection, such as oral or vaginal candidiasis, and loose or foul-smelling stools, secondary to long-term antibiotic therapy.
- If surgery is necessary, maintain wound suction, elevation of area, avoidance of pressure on grafted area; maintain immobility and compliance with weight-bearing restrictions. Change dressings using aseptic technique to promote healing and prevent cross-contamination.
- Monitor general health and nutrition; provide a diet high in protein and vitamin C to promote positive nitrogen balance and healing; encourage adequate hydration.

Teaching Patients Self-Care

- Teach patient and family to adhere strictly to the antibiotic regimen and to prevent falls or other injuries that could result in fracture.
- Teach patient and family how to maintain and manage the IV access site and IV administration equipment.
- Provide education about medication name, dosage, frequency, administration rate, safe storage and handling, adverse reactions, and necessary laboratory monitoring.

- Teach about aseptic dressing and warm compress techniques.
- Monitor for and instruct patient to report elevated temperature, drainage, odor, signs of increased inflammation, adverse reactions, and signs of superinfection.
- Assess need for home care or home infusion.
- Stress importance of follow-up health care appointments and recommend age-appropriate health screening.

Evaluation

Expected Patient Outcomes

- Experiences pain relief
- Increases physical mobility
- Has absence of infection; negative wound cultures, normal WBCs
- Adheres to therapeutic plan

For more information, see Chapter 41 in Pellico, L.H. (2013). *Focus on adult health: Medical-surgical nursing.* Philadelphia: Wolters Kluwer Health | Lippincott Williams & Wilkins.

Osteoporosis

Osteoporosis is characterized by reduction of bone density and a change in bone structure. The bones become progressively porous, brittle, and fragile and fracture easily.

PATHOPHYSIOLOGY

Age-related loss begins in the fourth decade, soon after the peak bone mass is achieved. Calcitonin, which inhibits bone resorption and promotes bone formation, is decreased. Estrogen, which inhibits bone breakdown, decreases with aging. Parathyroid hormone (PTH) increases with aging, increasing bone turnover and resorption. The consequence of these changes is net loss of bone mass over time. Failure to develop optimal peak bone mass during youth or young adulthood contributes to the development of osteoporosis. Secondary osteoporosis is associated with many disease states, nutritional deficiencies, and medications. Multiple compression fractures of the vertebrae result in skeletal deformity (kyphosis) and loss of height.

RISK FACTORS

- Women: Especially postmenopausal, those who have had oophorectomy, and those with small frames, such as Asian and nonobese Caucasian women
- Men may develop osteoporosis at an older age.
- Coexisting medical conditions: Malabsorption syndromes, lactose intolerance, celiac disease, alcohol abuse, renal failure, liver failure, Cushing's syndrome, hypogonadism hyperthyroidism, and hyperparathyroidism
- Medications: Corticosteroids, antiseizure medications, heparin, tetracycline, aluminum-containing antacids, and thyroid supplements; degree of osteoporosis is related to the duration of medication therapy.
- Dietary risks: Inadequate calories and nutrition, inadequate vitamin D and calcium
- Lifestyle: Lack of impact and resistance exercises, immobility, smoking, caffeine intake, and alcohol consumption

Gerontologic Considerations

- The prevalence of osteoporosis in women older than 80 years is 40%.
- The elderly do not absorb dietary calcium efficiently and excrete it more readily through their kidneys; therefore, postmenopausal women and the elderly need to consume liberal amounts of calcium.
- As the population ages, incidence of fractures, pain, and disability associated with osteoporosis is increasing.

CLINICAL MANIFESTATIONS AND ASSESSMENT

- Gradual collapse of vertebrae leads to progressive kyphosis or "dowager's hump" and decreased height.
- Postural changes result in relaxation of the abdominal muscles and a protruding abdomen.
- Pulmonary insufficiency and fatigue may result.

DIAGNOSTIC METHODS

- Osteoporosis is visible on routine X-ray when there has been 25% to 40% demineralization; radiolucency of bones is detected.
- Dual-energy X-ray absorptiometry (DEXA) provides information about spine and hip bone mass and bone mineral density (BMD).
- Bone mineral density studies are useful in identifying osteopenic and osteoporotic bone and in assessing response to therapy.
- Laboratory studies, serum calcium, serum phosphate, serum alkaline phosphatase, urine calcium excretion, urinary hydroxyproline excretion, hematocrit, ESR, and X-ray studies are used to exclude other diagnoses.

MEDICAL AND NURSING MANAGEMENT

All individuals need sufficient calcium, vitamin D, sunshine, and weight-bearing exercise to slow the progression of osteoporosis.

Pharmacologic Therapy

- Selective estrogen receptor modulators (SERMs) such as raloxifene reduce the risk of osteoporosis by preserving BMD without estrogenic effects on the uterus; indicated for both prevention and treatment of osteoporosis.

- Bisphosphonates such as alendronate (Fosamax), risedronate (Actonel), ibandronate (Boniva), and zoledronic acid (Reclast) inhibit osteoclast activity. Side effects include dyspepsia, nausea, flatulence, diarrhea, constipation, esophageal ulcers, gastric ulcers, or osteonecrosis of the jaw.
- Intranasal calcitonin (Miacalcin) for postmenopausal osteoporosis inhibits osteoclasts; alternate nares daily. Side effects include nasal irritation, flushing, GI disturbances, and urinary frequency.
- Teriparatide (Forteo), a subcutaneously administered medication, is given once daily for the treatment of osteoporosis. A recombinant PTH, it stimulates osteoblasts to build bone matrix and facilitates overall calcium absorption.
- Denosumab, a RANK ligand inhibitor, increases BMD by inducing osetoclast formation. This is used for postmenopausal women with osteoporosis who are prone to fractures.

Surgical Management

- Osteoporotic compression fractures of the vertebrae are managed conservatively. Percutaneous vertebroplasty/kyphoplasty with injection of polymethylmethacrylate bone cement into the fractured vertebra, followed by inflation of a pressurized balloon to restore the shape of the affected vertebra, can improve pain and quality of life.
- Fractures of the hip are managed surgically with joint replacement or closed or open reduction with internal fixation (pining). Surgery, early ambulation, intensive physical therapy, and adequate nutrition result in decreased morbidity and improved outcomes.

Nursing Management

- Adequate, balanced diet rich in calcium and vitamin D.
- Instruct patients to consume a high-fiber diet, increase fluids, and use stool softeners to prevent constipation related to immobility and medications.

- Encourage regular weight-bearing and aerobic exercise for 20 to 30 minutes 3 days/week to increase BMD, strengthen muscles, improve balance, and reduce falls and fractures.

For more information, see Chapter 41 in Pellico, L.H. (2013). *Focus on adult health: Medical-surgical nursing.* Philadelphia: Wolters Kluwer Health | Lippincott Williams & Wilkins.

P

Pancreatitis, Acute

Pancreatitis refers to inflammation of the pancreas secondary to autodigestion.

PATHOPHYSIOLOGY

Acute pancreatitis is commonly described as an inflammation and autodigestion of the pancreas. Self-digestion of the pancreas by its own proteolytic enzymes, principally trypsin, causes acute pancreatitis. Activation of the enzymes in the bile duct and subsequent reflux into the pancreatic duct can lead to vasodilation, inflammation, increased vascular permeability, necrosis, erosion, and hemorrhage. This cascade of events may also result in multiorgan failure.

RISK FACTORS

- Alcohol abuse (chronic pancreatitis)
- Biliary tract disease, gallstones
- Drugs including corticosteroids, thiazide diuretics, oral contraceptives
- Abdominal trauma
- Infections, bacterial or viral
- Surgery or instrumentation on or near the pancreas

- Hypercalcemia and hyperlipidemia
- 10% of cases are idiopathic
- Small incidence of hereditary pancreatitis

CLINICAL MANIFESTATIONS AND ASSESSMENT

Severe abdominal pain is the major symptom.

- Acute and severe abdominal pain, typically midepigastric; occurs 24 to 48 hours after a very heavy meal or alcohol ingestion.
- Pain is more severe after meals, unrelieved by antacids or vomiting.
- Pain is accompanied by nausea, abdominal distention, palpable abdominal mass, and decreased peristalsis.
- Patient appears acutely ill.
- Abdominal guarding; rigid or board-like abdomen (generally an ominous sign, usually indicating peritonitis) is noted.
- Ecchymosis in the flank (Grey-Turner sign) or around the umbilicus (Cullen sign), which may indicate severe hemorrhagic pancreatitis.
- Nausea and vomiting, fever, jaundice, mental confusion, agitation are noted.
- Hypotension is related to hypovolemia and shock.
- Patient may develop tachycardia, cyanosis, and cold, clammy skin.
- Acute renal failure is common.
- Respiratory distress is noted.

DIAGNOSTIC FINDINGS

Diagnosis is based on history of abdominal pain, the presence of known risk factor (gallstones, alcohol use, and viral infections), physical examination findings, and diagnostic findings.

- Serum amylase and lipase levels elevated three times the upper limit of normal
- White blood cell (WBC) count is elevated; hematocrit and hemoglobin monitored to assess for hemorrhage.

P

- Hypocalcemia correlates with severity of pancreatitis.
- Transient hyperglycemia; glucosuria and increased serum bilirubin levels may be present in some patients.
- Ultrasound and contrast-enhanced computed tomographic (CT) scans identify an increased pancreatic size, detect pancreatic cysts, abscesses, or pseudocysts. CT imaging is the modality of choice for acute and chronic pancreatitis.
- A history of gallstones, alcohol use, and viral infection are used to diagnose acute pancreatitis.

MEDICAL AND NURSING MANAGEMENT

Acute Phase

During the acute phase, management is symptomatic and directed toward preventing or treating complications.

- Patient is NPO to inhibit pancreatic stimulation and secretion of pancreatic enzymes.
- Provide IV fluid and electrolyte replacement, including calcium and magnesium.
- Monitor skin turgor and moistness of mucous membranes.
- Evaluate intake and output (I & O); assess for ascites.
- Provide jejunal feedings to meet nutritional needs when ordered/prescribed. Monitor lab studies and weights.
- Resume oral feedings when symptoms subside; diet is high carbohydrate, low fat and protein with no alcohol. Instruct patient to avoid heavy meals.
- Nasogastric (NG) suction is used to relieve nausea and vomiting or to decrease painful abdominal distention and paralytic ileus.
- Opioid analgesics are used, such as morphine or hydromorphone. Continued pain is reported to the provider, as hemorrhage may have developed or analgesia is inadequate.
- Bed rest is used to decrease metabolic rate and secretion of pancreatic and gastric enzymes; semi-Fowler's position decreases pressure on the diaphragm and improves respiratory expansion.
- Encourage deep breathing and use of incentive spirometer hourly; intubation and mechanical ventilation may be needed.

- Prevent skin breakdown, especially skin coming in contact with drainage; turn patient every 2 hours and consider use of specialty beds.
- Monitor for hypotension and oliguria indicative of hypovolemia, shock, or renal failure. Hemorrhagic shock may occur with hemorrhagic pancreatitis; blood products may be required.
- Surgery may be performed to assist in the diagnosis of pancreatitis (diagnostic laparotomy), to establish pancreatic drainage, or to resect or débride a necrotic pancreas.
- Monitor for cardiac dysfunction as a result of fluid and electrolyte disturbances, acid–base imbalances, and release of toxic substances into the circulation.
- Provide frequent, repeated, but simple explanations about treatment; patient may have clouded sensorium from pain, fluid imbalances, and hypoxemia.

Promoting Home- and Community-Based Care

The patient who has survived an episode of acute pancreatitis has been acutely ill and is often weak and debilitated for weeks or months.

- Reinforce instructions given in the acute phase using verbal and written materials.
- Reinforce the need to avoid high-fat diet, heavy meals, and alcohol.
- Emphasize signs and symptoms of acute pancreatitis and possible complications that should be reported promptly to the provider.
- Consider referral for home care.
- Provide information about resources and support groups, particularly if alcohol is the cause of acute pancreatitis.

COMPLICATIONS

- Hypotension and shock
- Anoxia
- Fluid and electrolyte imbalances
- Chronic pancreatitis
- Pancreatic necrosis; hemorrhage
- Septic shock and multiple organ failure

For more information, see Chapter 25 in Pellico, L.H. (2013). *Focus on adult health: Medical-surgical nursing.* Philadelphia: Wolters Kluwer Health | Lippincott Williams & Wilkins.

P

Pancreatitis, Chronic

Chronic pancreatitis is an inflammatory disorder characterized by progressive anatomic and functional destruction of the pancreas.

PATHOPHYSIOLOGY

Cells are replaced by fibrous tissue with repeated attacks of pancreatitis. The end result is obstruction of the pancreatic and common bile ducts and duodenum. In addition, there is atrophy of the epithelium of the ducts, inflammation, and destruction of the secreting cells of the pancreas. Long-term alcohol consumption has a direct toxic effect on the cells of the pancreas. Patients with chronic pancreatitis are at increased risk for the development of pancreatic cancer.

RISK FACTORS

- Alcohol consumption and malnutrition
- Smoking, often associated with alcohol abuse
- Dyslipidemia and diet may contribute

CLINICAL MANIFESTATIONS AND ASSESSMENT

- Recurring attacks of severe upper abdominal and back pain, accompanied by vomiting
- Attacks become longer and more severe with disease progression; some patients experience continuous severe pain; others have a dull, nagging constant pain.

- Risk of opioid dependence is high because of the severe pain and recurrent attacks.
- Weight loss is significant, secondary to anorexia or fear that eating will precipitate an attack.
- Malabsorption due to decreased lipase production impairs digestion of proteins and fats; stools become frequent, frothy, and foul-smelling with a high fat content (steatorrhea).
- As disease progresses, calcification of the gland may occur and calcium stones may form within the ducts.
- Diabetes mellitus occurs due to loss of pancreatic beta cells.

DIAGNOSTIC METHODS

- Endoscopic retrograde cholangiopancreatography (ERCP) is the most useful diagnostic study.
- Various imaging procedures, including magnetic resonance imaging (MRI), CT scans, and ultrasound may be performed.
- Steatorrhea is best confirmed by laboratory analysis of fecal fat content and determination of exocrine pancreatic insufficiency via the secretin-cholecystokinin test.

MEDICAL AND NURSING MANAGEMENT

Nonsurgical approaches are primarily focused on complete abstinence of alcohol, pain management, nutritional management, and treatment of diabetes mellitus.

- Pain and discomfort are relieved with nonopioid and opioid analgesics; yoga may be an effective nonpharmacologic method for relief of pain and coexisting symptoms.
- Pancreatic enzyme replacement and fat-soluble vitamin supplements are administered for malabsorption and steatorrhea.
- Proton pump inhibitors (omeprazole [Prilosec], lansoprazole [Prevacid]) are administered with enzyme therapy to reduce gastric acid inactivation of enzymes.

P

- Diabetes mellitus resulting from dysfunction of pancreatic islet cells is treated with diet, insulin, or oral hypoglycemics. Insulin is preferred; however, it should be carefully adjusted to avoid hypoglycemic events
- Patient should avoid alcohol and foods that produce abdominal pain and discomfort. No other treatment will relieve pain if patient continues to consume alcohol.

Surgical Management

The type of surgery performed depends on the anatomic and functional abnormalities of the pancreas, including the location of disease within the pancreas, the presence of diabetes, exocrine insufficiency, biliary stenosis, and pseudocysts of the pancreas.

- Pancreaticojejunostomy (also referred to as Roux-en-Y), with a side-to-side anastomosis or joining of the pancreatic duct to the jejunum, allows drainage of the pancreatic secretions into the jejunum.
- Whipple resection (pancreaticoduodenectomy) can be carried out to relieve the pain of chronic pancreatitis.
- Endoscopy is performed to remove pancreatic duct stones, correct strictures.

Nursing Management

See "Medical and Nursing Management" under "Pancreatitis, Acute" on pages 508–509 for treatment guidelines.

For more information, see Chapter 25 in Pellico, L.H. (2013). *Focus on adult health: Medical-surgical nursing.* Philadelphia: Wolters Kluwer Health | Lippincott Williams & Wilkins.

Parkinson's Disease

Parkinson's disease (PD) is a slowly progressing, degenerative neurologic movement disorder that eventually leads to disability.

PATHOPHYSIOLOGY

Parkinson's disease is associated with decreased levels of dopamine resulting from destruction of pigmented neuronal cells in the substantia nigra in the basal ganglia of the brain. The loss of dopamine stores in this area of the brain results in more excitatory neurotransmitters than inhibitory neurotransmitters, leading to an imbalance that affects voluntary movement. Clinical symptoms do not appear until 60% of the pigmented neurons are lost and the striatal dopamine level is decreased by 80%. Cellular degeneration causes impairment of the extrapyramidal tracts that control semiautomatic functions and coordinated movements; motor cells of the motor cortex and the pyramidal tracts are not affected.

RISK FACTORS

- Men affected more than women; symptoms usually appear in fifth decade of life
- Genetics
- Atherosclerosis
- Excessive accumulation of oxygen free radicals
- Viral infections
- Head trauma
- Chronic use of antipsychotic medications
- Some environmental exposures

CLINICAL MANIFESTATIONS AND ASSESSMENT

Parkinson's disease has a gradual onset, and symptoms progress slowly over a chronic, prolonged course. The cardinal signs are T-R-A-P: Tremor, Rigidity, Akinesia/Bradykinesia (without or decreased body movement), and Postural disturbances.

- Resting tremors that disappear with purposeful movement are a slow, unilateral turning of the forearm and hand (pronation–supination) and a pill-rolling motion of the thumb

P

against the fingers; tremor increases with walking, concentration, and anxiety.

- Rigidity characterized by resistance to passive limb movement; cogwheel rigidity is characterized by ratchet-like rhythmic contractions on passive muscle stretching.
- Involuntary stiffness of passive extremity increases when another extremity is engaged in voluntary active movement.
- *Akinesia,* a lack of movement, and *bradykinesia,* a slowness of initiation and execution of movement occur.
- Loss of postural reflexes: The patient stands with the head bent forward and walks with a propulsive gait. The patient may walk faster and faster, trying to move the feet forward under the body's center of gravity (shuffling gait). Difficulty in pivoting that causes loss of balance (either forward or backward) places the patient at risk for falls.

Other Manifestations

- Autonomic symptoms include excessive and uncontrolled sweating, paroxysmal flushing, orthostatic hypotension, gastric and urinary retention, constipation, and sexual dysfunction
- Cognitive and psychiatric changes are interrelated and include judgment, reasoning, decision making, and memory deficits, although intellect is not usually affected.
- Personality changes, psychosis, depression, dementia, and acute confusion may occur, especially in the elderly.
- Sleep disturbances may occur.
- Auditory and visual hallucinations may be associated with depression, dementia, lack of sleep, or adverse effects of medications.
- Hypokinesia (abnormally diminished movement) is common.
- *Freezing* phenomenon refers to a transient inability to perform active movement and is thought to be an extreme form of bradykinesia.
- As dexterity declines, micrographia (small handwriting) develops.
- Mask-like and expressionless facial expression develops, with decreasing frequency of blinking.
- Dysphonia, soft, low-pitched, and less audible speech, develops.
- Dysphagia, drooling, and risk for choking and aspiration develop.

DIAGNOSTIC METHODS

- Diagnosis based on patient's history and presence of two of the four cardinal manifestations: Tremor, rigidity, akinesia/brady-kinesia, and postural disturbances.
- Medical history, presenting symptoms, neurologic examination, and response to pharmacologic management are carefully evaluated when making the diagnosis.

MEDICAL AND NURSING MANAGEMENT

Treatment is directed at controlling symptoms and maintaining functional independence. Pharmacologic management is the mainstay of treatment.

Pharmacologic Therapy

- Levodopa (Larodopa), which is converted to dopamine in the basal ganglia, is the most effective agent and the mainstay of treatment. Benefits begin to wane and adverse effects become more severe over time. Confusion, hallucinations, depression, and sleep alterations are associated with prolonged use.
- Levodopa, usually administered in combination with carbidopa (Sinemet), an amino acid decarboxylase inhibitor, helps to maximize the beneficial effects of levodopa.
- On–off syndrome in response to the medication causes sudden periods of near-immobility ("off effect"), followed by a sudden return of effectiveness of the medication ("on effect").
- Anticholinergic agents, trihexyphenidyl HCL or benztropine, control tremor.
- Amantadine hydrochloride (Symmetrel), an antiviral agent, reduces akinesia and tremor.
- Dopamine agonists (eg, pergolide [Permax], bromocriptine mesylate [Parlodel]), ropinirole (Requip), and pramipexole (Mirapex) are used to postpone the initiation of carbidopa and levodopa therapy or added when carbidopa/levodopa loses effectiveness.

- Monoamine oxidase inhibitors (MAOIs) selegiline (Eldepryl), rasagiline (Azilect)
- Zydis selegiline HCl (Zelapar) used with a dopamine agonist to delay the use of carbidopa or levodopa therapy.
- Catechol-O-methyltransferase (COMT) inhibitors, entacapone (Comtan) and tolcapone (Tasmar), in combination with carbidopa or levodopa, can increase the duration of action.
- Antidepressant drugs including tricyclics, selective serotonin reuptake inhibitors (SSRIs), and atypical antidepressants.

Surgical Management

Deep brain stimulation is used to deliver high-frequency electrical stimulation to the thalamus; a pulse generator implanted in a subcutaneous subclavicular or abdominal pouch delivers electrical impulses to a lead anchored to the skull. The electrode blocks nerve pathways in the brain that cause tremors.

Additional Strategies

- Progressive exercise program increases muscle strength, improves coordination and dexterity, reduces muscular rigidity, and prevents contractures of unused muscles. Postural exercises are important to counter the tendency of the head and neck to be drawn forward and down. To promote balance, the patient is taught to concentrate on walking erect, to watch the horizon, and to use a wide-based gait (ie, walking with the feet separated).
- To enhance self-care activities, adaptive or assistive devices may be useful. Hospital bed, and a trapeze or rope tied to foot of bed may be helpful. Consider consultation with occupational therapist for recommendations.
- Encourage a regular bowel routine, increasing fluids and fiber as needed, due to weakness of muscles used in defecation, lack of exercise, and medications for PD. A raised toilet seat may be useful as these patients have difficulty rising from a seated position.
- Provide stabilized plate, no-spill cup and utensils with built-up handles, and a warming tray to keep foods warm. Patients eat slowly, suffer from dry mouth and difficulty swallowing, so monitor for aspiration and pneumonia. Tube feedings may be necessary to maintain adequate nutrition.

- Enhance swallowing by keeping the patient upright, provide a semi-solid diet with thick liquids.
- To improve speech, the patient should face the listener, exaggerate the pronunciation of words, speak in short sentences, and take a few deep breaths before speaking. A small electronic amplifier is helpful if the patient has difficulty being heard.
- Support coping by recognizing patients often feel embarrassed, apathetic, inadequate, bored, or lonely; depression and withdrawal can occur. Physiotherapy, psychotherapy, medication therapy, and support group participation may help reduce depression that often occurs.

COMPLICATIONS

- Respiratory and urinary tract infections
- Skin breakdown
- Injury from falls

For more information, see Chapter 46 in Pellico, L.H. (2013). *Focus on adult health: Medical-surgical nursing.* Philadelphia: Wolters Kluwer Health | Lippincott Williams & Wilkins.

Pemphigus

Pemphigus is a group of autoimmune diseases of the skin characterized by the appearance of bullae (blisters) on apparently normal skin and mucous membranes.

PATHOPHYSIOLOGY

Pemphigus is an autoimmune disease involving immunoglobulin G (IgG). It is thought that the pemphigus antibody is directed against a specific cell-surface antigen in epidermal cells. A blister forms from the antigen–antibody reaction. The level of serum antibody is predictive of disease severity.

P

RISK FACTORS

- Genetics, highest among Jewish or Mediterranean descent
- Middle to late adulthood
- Associated with penicillins, captopril, and myasthenia gravis

CLINICAL MANIFESTATIONS AND ASSESSMENT

- Most cases present with oral lesions appearing as irregularly shaped erosions that are painful, bleed easily, and heal slowly.
- Skin bullae enlarge, rupture, and leave large, painful eroded areas with crusting and oozing.
- A characteristic odor emanates from the bullae and the exuding serum.
- Blistering or sloughing of uninvolved skin occurs when minimal pressure is applied (Nikolsky's sign).
- Eroded skin heals slowly, and eventually huge areas of the body are involved. Fluid and electrolyte imbalance and hypoalbuminemia may result from loss of fluid and protein.
- Bacterial superinfection is common.

MEDICAL AND NURSING MANAGEMENT

Goals of therapy are to bring the disease under control as rapidly as possible, prevent loss of serum and development of secondary infection, and promote reepithelialization of the skin.

Pharmacologic Therapy

- High-dose corticosteroids control the disease and keep the skin free of blisters until remission is apparent. (Monitor for serious toxic effects from high-dose corticosteroid therapy.)
- Immunosuppressive agents (eg, azathioprine, cyclophosphamide, gold) may be prescribed to help control the disease and reduce the corticosteroid dose.

- Plasmapheresis decreases serum antibody level; generally reserved for life-threatening cases.

Nursing Management

Infection and Sepsis

- Cleanse skin to remove debris and dead skin and to prevent infection.
- Monitor for secondary infections of the skin and *Candida albicans* of the oral cavity from high-dose corticosteroid therapy; report if noted.
- Monitor for fever and chills; monitor vital signs and for symptoms of local and systemic infection, including culture and sensitivity reports.
- Reduce environmental contamination; use protective isolation when indicated.
- Investigate seemingly "trivial" complaints or minimal changes; corticosteroids mask or alter typical symptoms of infection.
- Administer antimicrobial agents as prescribed, and note response to treatment.

Fluid and Electrolyte Imbalance

- Administer IV saline to replace loss of fluids and sodium chloride through skin.
- Administer blood products to replace plasma proteins, maintain blood volume and hemoglobin.
- Monitor serum albumin, protein, hemoglobin, and hematocrit.
- Encourage oral fluids and small frequent meals or snacks of high-protein, high-calorie foods; parenteral nutrition is considered if nutrition is inadequate.

COMPLICATIONS

- Secondary bacterial infections and sepsis
- Hypoalbuminemia, with extensive blistering
- *Candida albicans* of the mouth secondary to corticosteroid therapy

> For more information, see Chapter 52 in Pellico, L.H. (2013).
> *Focus on adult health: Medical-surgical nursing.* Philadelphia:
> Wolters Kluwer Health | Lippincott Williams & Wilkins.

Peptic Ulcer Disease

A peptic ulcer is an excavation in the mucosal wall of the stomach, pylorus, duodenum, or esophagus. A person with a peptic ulcer has peptic ulcer disease.

PATHOPHYSIOLOGY

Peptic ulcers occur mainly in the gastroduodenal mucosa, as this tissue cannot withstand the digestive action of gastric acid (HCl) and pepsin. The erosion is caused by the increased concentration or activity of acid-pepsin, or by decreased resistance of the mucosa. A damaged mucosa cannot secrete enough mucus to act as a barrier against HCl. Damage to the gastroduodenal mucosa allows for decreased resistance to bacteria, and thus infection from *H. pylori* bacteria may occur.

Esophageal ulcers result from the backward flow of HCl acid from the stomach into the esophagus; this is termed gastroesophageal reflux disease (GERD). Gastrin-secreting tumors and the Zollinger-Ellison syndrome (ZES), which consists of severe peptic ulcers, extreme gastric hyperacidity, and gastrinomas (islet cell tumors of the pancreas), affect the esophagus.

Stress-related mucosal disease (SRMD), also known as stress ulcer, refers to injury to the lining of the stomach and the duodenum during conditions of physiologic stress. The etiology of stress ulcer is multifactorial, beginning with a hypoperfusion state, decreased gastric mucosal blood flow, and gastric ischemia. Catecholamine release furthers vasoconstriction and decreases gastric motility, producing an inability to neutralize hydrogen ions along with increased amount of pepsin. Cushing's ulcers, common in patient's with head injury, and Curling's ulcer, associated with extensive burn injury, are types of gastric ulcers.

RISK FACTORS

- Use of nonsteroidal anti-inflammatory drugs (NSAIDs) or excessive alcohol consumption
- Ingestion of milk, caffeinated beverages, smoking
- Bacterial infection, such as *H. pylori*
- Family history of or predisposition to peptic ulcer
- Ages of 40 and 60 years
- Blood type O
- Stress or stress-related mucosal disease
- Chronic obstructive pulmonary disease (COPD) and chronic renal disease associated with peptic ulcer disease

CLINICAL MANIFESTATIONS AND ASSESSMENT

- Symptoms of an ulcer may last days, weeks, or months and may subside only to reappear without cause. Many patients have asymptomatic ulcers; perforation or hemorrhage may occur in 20% to 30% of patients without symptoms.
- Dull, gnawing pain and a burning sensation in the midepigastrium or in the back are characteristic.
- Pain is relieved by eating or taking alkali; once the stomach has emptied or the alkali wears off, the pain returns.
- Sharply localized tenderness is elicited by gentle pressure to the epigastrium at or slightly right of the midline.
- Other symptoms include pyrosis (heartburn), vomiting, constipation or diarrhea, and bleeding. A burning sensation in the esophagus and stomach, which moves up to the mouth, occasionally with sour eructation (burping) may occur.
- Vomiting may reflect obstruction of pyloric orifice or swelling of inflamed mucous membrane adjacent to the ulcer. Vomiting may occur without nausea; pain and bloating are relieved after emesis.

- Heartburn often accompanied by sour eructation, or burping; common when the patient's stomach is empty.
- Constipation or diarrhea may result from diet and medications.
- Bleeding occurs in 15% of patients, manifested by melena or tarry stools; a small portion of patients with bleeding have mild symptoms or no symptoms.

DIAGNOSTIC METHODS

- Epigastric tenderness, abdominal distention upon physical examination
- Endoscopy allows direct visualization of inflammatory changes, ulcers, and lesions; biopsy may be taken.
- Upper gastrointestinal (GI) barium study may be done.
- Other diagnostic tests include analysis of stool specimens for occult blood, gastric secretory studies, histology of biopsy specimen or, rapid urease test to detect *H. pylori* (serologic testing, stool antigen tests, or a breath test may also detect *H. pylori*).

MEDICAL AND NURSING MANAGEMENT

The goals of treatment are to eradicate *H. pylori* and manage gastric acidity through medications, lifestyle changes, and surgical intervention.

Pharmacologic Therapy

- Antibiotics combined with proton pump inhibitors and bismuth salts suppress *H. pylori* for 10 to 14 days.
- H_2-receptor antagonists or proton pump inhibitors treat NSAID-induced ulcers and others not associated with *H. pylori* infection. Teach the patient to complete the medication regimen even if symptoms disappear.
- Sedatives and tranquilizers may be added as needed for patient comfort.
- High dose H_2 receptor antagonists or octreotide (Sandostatin) for ZES.

- Stress ulcer prophylaxis with IV H_2 receptor antagonists or cytoprotective agents (misoprostol, sucralfate) are used for patients at risk.
- Research is being conducted to develop a vaccine against *H. pylori*.

Surgical Management

Antibiotics therapy for *H. pylori* and of H_2 receptor antagonists has reduced the need for surgical intervention.

- Surgery is usually for intractable ulcers (those that fail to heal after 12 to 16 weeks of medical treatment), life-threatening hemorrhage, perforation, or obstruction and for those with ZES not responding to medications
- Transendoscopic coagulation by laser, heat probe, medication, a sclerosing agent, or a combination of these therapies can halt bleeding and avoid surgical intervention.
- Selective embolization for patients unable to undergo surgery may be used. Autologous blood clots with or without Gelfoam (absorbable gelatin sponge) are introduced through a catheter in the affected artery.
- Surgical procedures include vagotomy, vagotomy with pyloro-plasty, or Billroth I or II.

Nursing Management

Lifestyle Changes

- Stress reduction, smoking cessation, and dietary modifications are included in the plan of care.
- Assist the patient to identify stressful or exhausting situations such as hectic lifestyle and irregular schedules that exacerbate symptoms. Regular rest periods during the acute phase of the disease, biofeedback, hypnosis, behavior modification, mass-age, or acupuncture may also be useful.
- Encourage smoking cessation to decrease duodenal acidity; smoking inhibits ulcer repair. Smoking cessation support groups and other smoking cessation approaches should be discussed.
- Teach patient to avoid extremes of temperature of foods, consumption of meat extracts, alcohol, coffee (including

decaffeinated) and caffeinated beverages, and diets rich in milk and cream, which stimulate acid secretion. Diet is individualized to foods well tolerated; patient avoids foods that produce pain.

- The patient is encouraged to eat three regular meals a day. Small, frequent meals are not necessary if antacids or histamine blockers are part of therapy.

☀ N U R S I N G A L E R T

Teach the patient to report symptoms of hemorrhage (faintness, dizziness or nausea, cool skin, confusion, increased heart rate, labored breathing, and blood in the stool), penetration and perforation (severe abdominal pain, rigid and tender abdomen, vomiting, elevated temperature, and increased heart rate), and pyloric obstruction (nausea, vomiting, distended abdomen, and abdominal pain).

COMPLICATIONS

- Hemorrhage occurs in 28% to 59% of patients; observe for hematemesis, which may be bright red or "coffee ground" appearance; shock may result. Monitor H & H, replace fluids and blood.
- Perforation and penetration: Observe for back and epigastric pain not relieved by medications that were effective in the past. Surgery is required to close the perforation quickly as chemical, then bacterial peritonitis develops within a few hours. Nasogastric suction, antibiotics, and monitoring for peritonitis are performed postoperatively.
- Pyloric obstruction (gastric outlet obstruction): Observe for nausea and vomiting, constipation, epigastric fullness, anorexia, and, later, weight loss. Nasogastric tube with residual of more than 400 mL suggests obstruction and is confirmed with upper GI (UGI) study or endoscopy. Balloon dilation of pylorus via endoscopy, stent placement, or surgery may be done.

For more information, see Chapter 23 in Pellico, L.H. (2013). *Focus on adult health: Medical-surgical nursing.* Philadelphia: Wolters Kluwer Health | Lippincott Williams & Wilkins.

Pericarditis and Cardiac Tamponade

Pericarditis refers to an inflammation of the pericardium, the membranous sac enveloping the heart.

PATHOPHYSIOLOGY

Pericarditis may lead to an accumulation of fluid in the pericardial space, called *pericardial effusion.* This may result in increased pressure on the heart, leading to cardiac tamponade (compression of the heart). Pericarditis may be acute or chronic. Acute pericarditis develops rapidly, causing an inflammatory reaction, whereas chronic pericarditis progresses slowly and can be accompanied by effusion. Constrictive pericarditis results from decreased elasticity of the pericardium and restricts the heart's ability to fill with blood; symptoms of decreased cardiac output and heart failure result.

RISK FACTORS

- Men between ages of 20 and 50
- Viral illness or bacterial infections
- Lupus, scleroderma, rheumatoid arthritis, or other autoimmune disorders
- Post myocardial infarction (MI)
- Post cardiac surgery
- Cause may be unknown.

CLINICAL MANIFESTATIONS AND ASSESSMENT

The diagnosis is most often made on the basis of the history, signs, and symptoms.

- Characteristic symptom is chest pain, which is typically sharp, pleuritic, and felt in mid-chest. Pain may also be located beneath the clavicle and in the neck and left trapezius region. Discomfort is aggravated by deep inspiration, coughing, lying down, or turning, and may be relieved with a forward-leaning or sitting position.

- Pericardial friction rub in the left lower sternal border in the fourth intercostal space may be heard in some patients.

Clinical Manifestations of Cardiac Tamponade

- Pericardial fluid may accumulate slowly without causing noticeable symptoms until a large amount is present.
- The first symptoms of cardiac tamponade are often shortness of breath (SOB), chest tightness, dizziness, or restlessness.
- Patient may report a feeling of fullness within the chest or may have substantial or ill-defined pain.
- Hypotension with narrowing pulse pressure, distended neck veins, and distant (muffled) heart sounds; pulsus paradoxus may be present
- Tachycardia, ECG voltage may be decreased or the QRS complexes may alternate in height (electrical alternans).
- Cough
- Pericardial friction rub is possible.
- Hemodynamic monitoring reveals near equilibration of right and left atrial pressures and left end diastolic pressures.

DIAGNOSTIC METHODS

- Twelve-lead electrocardiogram (ECG) shows diffuse ST elevation that may persist for weeks.
- Atrial dysrhythmia may be present.
- Echocardiography is done to assess for pericardial effusion or tamponade.
- Other signs may include mild fever, increased WBC count, anemia, an elevated erythrocyte sedimentation rate (ESR), or C-reactive protein level.
- Nonproductive cough, or hiccough, dyspnea, and other signs and symptoms of heart failure (HF) may occur.

⚡ *N U R S I N G   A L E R T*

A pericardial friction rub is diagnostic of pericarditis. It has a creaky or scratchy sound and is louder at the end of exhalation. Assess for the presence of a pericardial friction rub by placing the diaphragm of the stethoscope tightly against the thorax at the left lower sternal border in the fourth intercostal space. The rub is best heard when the patient is sitting and leaning forward. The friction rub is caused by the inflamed layers of the pericardium rubbing against each other, and is often intermittent.

Diagnostic Methods for Cardiac Tamponade

- Chest X-ray shows a large pericardial effusion.
- Echocardiogram confirms the diagnosis.
- Diagnostic pericardiocentesis

MEDICAL AND NURSING MANAGEMENT

Surgical Management: Cardiac Tamponade

- Pericardiocentesis: Needle aspiration of pericardial fluid prevents or treats pericardial tamponade; may be performed under guided ultrasound. The patient almost always feels immediate relief. Pericardial fluid is sent to the laboratory for examination for tumor cells, bacterial culture, chemical and serologic analysis, and differential blood cell count.
- Pericardiotomy (pericardial window): A portion of the pericardium is excised, permitting pericardial fluid to drain into the lymphatic system.

Pharmacologic Therapy: Pericarditis

- Nonsteroidal anti-inflammatory drugs
- Corticosteroids if the pericarditis is severe or if the patient does not respond to NSAIDs.

☀️ *N U R S I N G A L E R T*

Nursing assessment skills are key to anticipating and identifying the triad of symptoms of cardiac tamponade: Falling arterial pressure, rising venous pressure, and distant heart sounds. Search diligently for a pericardial friction rub.

NURSING PROCESS

The Patient With Pericarditis

Assessment

- Assess for deep inspiratory pain or pain that intensifies with cough.
- Assess for pericardial friction rub at the fourth intercostal, lower sternal border. Friction rub is continuous and synchronous with heartbeat; it may be intermittent or absent and is best heard with the patient in a seated position.
- Monitor temperature and vital signs frequently; pericarditis causes an abrupt onset of fever in a previously afebrile patient.

Diagnosis

- Decreased cardiac output related to decreased cardiac filling
- Pain related to inflammatory changes

Planning

The nursing plan focuses on two goals: Pain relief and absence of complications.

Nursing Interventions

Relieving Pain

- Assist patients with pericarditis to conserve energy and reduce fatigue.
- Advise chair rest, assuming an upright and forward-leaning position.
- Instruct patient to resume activities of daily living as chest pain and friction rub abate.

- Provide education regarding inflammatory process; offer reassurance that pain is not a heart attack.
- Instruct patient to resume bed rest if chest pain and friction rub recur.
- Teach patient to recognize signs and symptoms of recurrence: Chest pain, malaise, and fever.

Monitoring and Managing Potential Complications

- Observe for pericardial effusion, which can lead to cardiac tamponade.
- Observe for triad of symptoms related to cardiac tamponade.
- Notify health care provider immediately upon observing any of the above symptoms, and prepare for diagnostic echocardiography and pericardiocentesis.

Evaluation

Expected Patient Outcomes

- Free from pain
- Performs activities of daily living without pain, fatigue, or SOB
- Afebrile
- Without pericardial friction rub, normotensive, clearly audible heart sounds
- Without complications

For more information, see Chapters 15 and 16 in Pellico, L.H. (2013). *Focus on adult health: Medical-surgical nursing.* Philadelphia: Wolters Kluwer Health | Lippincott Williams & Wilkins.

Perioperative Nursing Management

SURGERY

Surgery, whether elective or emergent, is a stressful, complex event. Perioperative and perianesthesia nursing addresses the

P

three phases of the surgical experience—preoperative, intraoperative, and postoperative—and is based on the standards of practice (American Society of PeriAnesthesia Nurses, 2008).

Surgical Settings

- Ambulatory surgery: For surgeries, imaging studies and diagnostic tests when anticipated recovery time is limited.
- Inpatient surgery: For trauma patients, acutely ill patients, and/or patients undergoing major surgery.

Surgical Classifications

- Diagnostic: For example, biopsy
- Curative: For example, excision of tumor
- Reconstructive or cosmetic
- Palliative to relieve pain
- May be classed according to degree of urgency (ie, emergency surgery)

Surgical Considerations

Patients Who Are Elderly

Elderly patients account for more than a third of all hospital care days in the United States. In addition, almost one-third of all surgical patients are 65 years of age or older. Important factors that need to be evaluated are (1) disease course versus life expectancy, (2) state of independence, (3) personal motivation, and (4) surgical risk factors versus nonoperative management. Pain assessment and teaching are important in the elderly patient, due to chronic illnesses and health issues.

Patients Who Are Obese

Obesity increases the risk and severity of complications associated with surgery. Fatty tissues are especially susceptible to infection. In addition, obesity increases technical and mechanical problems related to surgery, therefore, wound dehiscence and wound infections are more common. Patient tends to have shallow respirations when supine, which increases the risk of hypoventilation and postoperative pulmonary complications. Increased demands on the heart related to obesity occur.

Patients With Disabilities

Patients with mental or physical disabilities must be identified in the preoperative evaluation and these findings clearly communicated to the appropriate personnel. Include the need for appropriate assistive devices, modifications in preoperative teaching, and additional assistance with and attention to positioning or transferring. Assistive devices include hearing aids, eyeglasses, braces, prostheses, and other devices. People who are hearing-impaired may need a sign interpreter or some alternative communication system perioperatively. If the patient relies on signing or speech (lip) reading and his or her eyeglasses or contact lenses are removed or the health care staff wears surgical masks, an alternative method of communication will be needed.

PREOPERATIVE NURSING

The preoperative phase begins when the decision to proceed with surgical intervention is made and ends with the transfer of the patient onto the OR table.

- Perform baseline physical and emotional assessment, identification of allergies or genetic issues impacting surgery, validate completion of preadmission testing, and provide education regarding anesthesia and postoperative care.
- Ensure informed consent is completed. Consent is voluntary and written in nonemergent situations; obtained by the surgeon. May be signed by patient or their representative.

Preoperative Health Assessment

- Obtain a health history and perform a physical examination to establish vital signs and a database for future comparisons.
- Validate that preoperative blood tests, X-rays, and other diagnostic tests were performed.

Nutritional and Fluid Status

- Identifies factors such as obesity, under-nutrition, weight loss, malnutrition, deficiencies in specific nutrients, metabolic abnormalities, and the effects of medications on nutrition that can affect the patient's surgical course

P

- Correct nutritional deficiencies, dehydration, hypovolemia, and electrolyte imbalances prior to surgery, providing adequate protein for tissue repair.

Drug or Alcohol Use

- Assess for drug or alcohol abuse; for acute intoxication, local, spinal, or regional anesthesia may be used. Nasogastric tube may be needed to prevent aspiration.
- Anticipate and treat withdrawal symptoms related to specific substance use/abuse as it increases postoperative mortality.

Respiratory Status

- Recommend smoking cessation for at least 2 days prior to surgery. Evaluate respiratory infection and neuromuscular diseases, such as Parkinson's disease, which may affect respiratory function.
- Surgery is typically postponed if respiratory infection is present.

Cardiovascular Status

- Ensure hypertension is controlled; uncontrolled hypertension may lead to postponement of surgery.

Hepatic and Renal Function

- Assess renal and hepatic function tests; dysfunction of these organs complicates metabolism and excretion of anesthesia and may increase morbidity and mortality.
- Surgery may need to be postponed for acute renal problems.

Endocrine Function

- Carefully monitor the patient with diabetes who is undergoing surgery due to increased risk for hypoglycemia and hyperglycemia; type 1 diabetics are at risk for diabetic ketoacidosis (DKA).
- Report corticosteroid use during preceding year to anesthesiologist to prevent risk of adrenal insufficiency.
- Assess for control of hypo/hyperthyroidism.

Immune Function

- Identify allergies to medications, blood transfusions, contrast agents, latex, and food products; have patient describe the signs and symptoms produced by these substances.

- Assess immunosuppressed patients, those taking corticosteroids, transplant medications, radiation, chemotherapy, and immune disorder for even slight variations in temperature; use strict aseptic technique.

Medication Use

- Assess medication use, including over-the-counter (OTC) and herbal medications.
- Stop aspirin 7 to 10 days prior to surgery where possible.
- Nurse anesthetists or anesthesiologist evaluates for interaction of medications with anesthesia.

Psychosocial Factors

- Assess for preoperative anxiety, especially fear of the unknown, death, anesthesia, pain, or cancer.
- Recognize a variety of responses and coping, including excessive questions or withdrawal.
- Identify patient's support network.

Spiritual and Cultural Beliefs

- Assist patient to obtain the spiritual support that he or she requests, demonstrating respect for cultural values and beliefs.
- Communicate and document if patient declines blood transfusions for religious reasons (Jehovah's Witnesses).
- Nurses may refer to The Joint Commission standards of cultural competency for health care workers.

Presence of Genetic Disorders

- Assess for risks for malignant hyperthermia, including central core disease, muscular dystrophy, hyperkalemic periodic paralysis, King-Denborough syndrome.

Preoperative Nursing Management

Providing Preoperative Teaching

- Preoperative teaching is initiated as soon as possible; different modalities (verbal, written, electronic, return demonstration) are individualize to the patient.
- Education begins in the surgeon's office or with pre-admission testing (PAT), is continued until the patient arrives in the OR, and extends to discharge.

P

- Include expected sensations, need for ventilator, tubes, drains, or other equipment.
- Teach coughing and deep breathing, incentive spirometry, leg exercises, need for turning, and splinting the incision.

Pain Management

- Assess for acute as well as chronic pain, using a pain intensity scale.
- Teach patients that pain medications will be administered by various routes, IV or patient-controlled analgesia (PCA), epidural or oral based on cardiopulmonary or neurologic status.

Instruction for Patients Undergoing Ambulatory Surgery

- Preoperative education for ambulatory surgery differs in that the teaching environment may include group classes, use of videotape, occur during PAT or by telephone in conjunction with the preoperative interview.
- The patient is reminded not to eat or drink as directed.

Managing Nutrition and Fluids

- The major purpose of withholding food and fluid before surgery is to prevent aspiration.
- Specific recommendations depend on the age of the patient and the type of food eaten; patients may be allowed clear fluids up to 2 to 3 hours prior to surgery, if undergoing minor and very short procedures.

Preparing the Bowel

- Enemas or laxatives may be prescribed the evening prior to and the morning of abdominal or pelvic surgery.
- Antibiotics may be used to reduce intestinal flora.

Preparing the Skin

- If hair must be removed, electric clippers are used for safe hair removal immediately before the operation.
- Patients may be instructed to use a detergent-germicide soap for several days to reduce the number of skin organisms.

Providing Immediate Preoperative Care

- Patient voids and changes into hospital gown, removing hairpins, denture or plates, and jewelry. Valuables are left with family or labeled and stored according to institution policy.
- The chart accompanies the patient to the OR, including the preoperative checklist; Universal Protocol/Safety checklist, anesthesia and surgical consent, and laboratory tests must be completed.
- A standard hand-off procedure is used to communicate critical information to next caregiver.

Administering Preanesthetic Medication

- If a preanesthetic medication is administered, the patient is kept in bed with the side rails raised, to prevent injury due to side effects of lightheadedness or drowsiness.
- Keep immediate surroundings quiet to promote relaxation.

NURSING ALERT

Protecting patients from injury is one of the major roles of the perioperative nurse. Specific nursing interventions to decrease the risk of falling are to elevate the side rails after the premedication is administered and remind the patient not to get out of bed due to potential medication side effects such as dizziness.

Transporting the Patient to the Presurgical Area

- The patient is transferred to the holding area or presurgical suite in a bed or on a stretcher about 30 to 60 minutes before the anesthetic is to be given; prevent chilling.
- A process to verify patient identification, the surgical procedure, and the surgical site is followed to maximize patient safety.

Attending to Family Needs

- A waiting area equipped with comfortable chairs, television, telephones, and facilities for light refreshment is helpful.
- Inform the family and significant others not to judge the seriousness of an operation by the length of time the patient is in the OR.
- The patient is taken to the PACU postoperatively to ensure safe emergence from anesthesia. Many hospitals now adopt the

model of Patient and Family Centered care, allowing visitation in the PACU for short periods.
- The surgeon will relate the outcome of the surgery in the waiting room or PACU to patient and family.

INTRAOPERATIVE NURSING

The intraoperative phase begins when the patient is transferred onto the OR table and ends with admission to the PACU.

- Nursing activities include providing for the patient's safety, maintaining an aseptic environment, ensuring proper functioning of equipment, providing the surgeon with specific instruments and supplies for the surgical field, completing appropriate documentation, providing emotional support during induction of general anesthesia, assisting in positioning the patient on the OR table using appropriate principles of body alignment, or acting as scrub nurse, circulating nurse, or registered nurse first assistant (RNFA).
- Every member of the surgical team verifies the patient's name, procedure, and surgical site as mandated by The Joint Commission. This "time out" or final pause must be performed prior to incision, preferably with the patient involved. If patient's surgical site was marked, it should be visible.

The Surgical Environment

- The OR has special air filtration devices to screen out contaminating particles, dust, and pollutants.
- External precautions include adhering to principles of surgical asepsis; strict control of the OR environment is required, including traffic pattern restrictions.
- Preventing surgical fire is a component of The Joint Commission's 2010 National Patient Safety Goals; sources of ignition include electrocautery units, lasers, and fiberoptic lights, and an environment rich in flammable sources.
- To further improve safety, electrical hazards, emergency exit clearances, and storage of equipment and anesthetic gases are monitored periodically by official agencies, such as the state department of health and The Joint Commission.

- All operating room personnel need to be familiar with and be educated about fire prevention and how to respond in the event of a fire.

Donning Proper Attire

- The surgical area is divided into three zones: The unrestricted zone, where street clothes are allowed; the semi-restricted zone, where attire consists of scrub clothes and caps; and the restricted zone, where scrub clothes, shoe covers, caps, and masks are worn.
- Masks are worn at all times in the restricted zone of the OR to decrease the risk of postoperative wound infection due to microorganisms found in the oropharynx and nasopharynx. Masks should cover mouth and nose tightly, prevent venting from the sides, and should not hang around the neck.
- Headgear should completely cover the hair (head and neckline, including beard) so that single strands of hair, bobby pins, clips, and particles of dandruff or dust do not fall on the sterile field.
- Shoe covers are worn when it is reasonably anticipated that spills or splashes will occur; they are changed if wet, soiled, or torn.
- Short natural fingernails are encouraged; artificial nails can cause nosocomial infections. This is supported by Centers for Disease Control and Prevention (CDC), AORN, and the Association of Professionals in Infection Control.

Using Environmental Controls

- Floors and horizontal surfaces are cleaned frequently with detergent/detergent germicide, soap, and water. Sterilizing equipment is inspected regularly to ensure optimal operation and performance.
- To decrease the amount of bacteria in the air, standard OR ventilation provides 15 air exchanges per hour or laminar airflow is used; high-efficiency particulate air (HEPA) filters may be used.
- Unnecessary personnel are restricted.

Health Hazards Associated With the Surgical Environment

- Safety issues in the OR include exposure to blood and body fluids; and exposure to latex and adhesive substances, radiation, and toxic agents and laser plumes.

- Goggles or a wrap-around face shield are worn to protect against splashing when the surgical wound is irrigated or when bone drilling is performed.
- Early identification of patients with latex allergies, preparation of a latex allergy supply cart, and maintenance of latex allergy precautions throughout the perioperative period is performed.
- While lasers are in use, warning signs must be clearly posted; personnel wear special protective goggles, specific to the type of laser used in the procedure.
- Additional hazard is retention of foreign body; at-risk situations include emergency surgery, unplanned change in procedure, and patient with high body mass index. Patient may require an additional surgery to remove the foreign body.

The Surgical Experience

Anesthesia and Sedation

Anesthesia today is very safe, with anesthesia-related death rate in the United States estimated at less than 1 per 10,000 anesthetics.

- The main types of anesthesia are general anesthesia (inhaled or IV), regional anesthesia, moderate sedation, monitored anesthesia care, and local anesthesia.
- The anesthesiologist or nurse anesthetist monitors vital signs, ECG, blood oxygen saturation level, tidal volume, blood gas levels, blood pH, and alveolar gas concentrations. Electroencephalography (measure of brain waves) is sometimes required.
- Anesthesia is a state of narcosis, analgesia, relaxation, and reflex loss. Patients are not arousable, even to painful stimuli, are unable to maintain ventilatory function, and require assistance in maintaining a patent airway. Cardiovascular function may be impaired as well.

NURSING ALERT

In 2004, The Joint Commission issued an alert regarding the phenomenon of patients being partially awake while under general anesthesia (referred to as anesthesia awareness). Patients at greatest risk of anesthesia awareness are cardiac, obstetric, and major trauma patients. The entire surgical team must be aware of this phenomenon and help prevent or manage it.

- Inhalation anesthetics use a volatile (readily vaporized) anesthetic leading to a state of unconsciousness and amnesia; when combined with additional medications (eg, opioids and benzodiazepines), further sedation/hypnosis, and amnesia is established.
- General anesthesia can be produced by the IV administration of various substances, such as barbiturates, benzodiazepines, nonbarbiturate hypnotics, dissociative agents, and opioid agents.
- Intravenous neuromuscular blockade blocks the transmission of nerve impulses at the neuromuscular junction of skeletal muscles. Neuromuscular blockade is used to relax muscles in abdominal and thoracic surgery, relax eye muscles in certain types of eye surgery, facilitate endotracheal intubation, treat laryngospasm, and assist in mechanical ventilation.
- Local anesthesia is used to block nerves in the peripheral nervous system (PNS) and central nervous system (CNS); they block transmission of pain sensation along nerve fibers. Local anesthesia can be used alone or in conjunction with other type of anesthesia
- Regional anesthesia includes spinal, epidural, and peripheral nerve blocks; the patient is awake and aware of the surroundings. Medications may be given to produce mild sedation or relieve anxiety; the nurse maintains a quiet environment.
  - *Spinal anesthesia* is accomplished when a local anesthetic is introduced into the subarachnoid space at the lumbar level, usually between L4 and L5. If the anesthetic reaches the upper thoracic and cervical spinal cord in high concentrations, a temporary respiratory paralysis results, requiring mechanical ventilation. Headache may be an after-effect; maintaining supine position and hydration are helpful to relieve headache.
  - *Epidural anesthesia,* a commonly used conduction block, is achieved by injecting a local anesthetic into the epidural space that surrounds the dura mater of the spinal cord.
  - *Peripheral nerve block* provides surgical anesthesia and postoperative analgesia for procedures involving the upper and lower extremities. Less physiological stress, avoidance of airway manipulation and the potential complications associated with endotracheal intubation, and potential side effects of general anesthesia are avoided.

- Moderate sedation, administered by nonanesthesiologists, was previously referred to as *conscious sedation.*
- Monitored anesthesia care is a form of anesthesia that involves the IV administration of sedatives and/or analgesic medications to reduce patient anxiety and control pain during diagnostic or therapeutic procedures.
- Moderate sedation and monitored analgesia allow the patient to maintain a patent airway, retain protective airway reflexes, respond to verbal and physical stimuli, and recover more rapidly post procedure. The health care provider or nurse continually monitors vital signs, level of consciousness (LOC), and cardiac function.
- Surgical asepsis through OR personnel scrubbing their hands and arms with antiseptic soap and water, or alternatively using a scrubless process, prevents the contamination of surgical wounds.

Intraoperative Nursing Management

The major goals for care of the patient during surgery are to reduce anxiety, keep patient free of perioperative injury related to positioning, avoid threats to patient safety, maintain patient dignity, and avoid complications.

Reducing Anxiety

- Reduce anxiety by addressing the patient by name, using touch and eye contact, verifying details, providing explanations, and encouraging and answering questions.
- Provide attention to physical comfort (warm blankets, position changes), explain who will be present in the OR, the length of the procedure, and other details to prepare the patient and produce a sense of control.

Preventing Intraoperative Positioning Injury

- Intraoperative position depends on the surgical procedure to be performed and the patient's physical condition.
- Risk for transient discomfort or permanent injury may result from hyperextending joints, compressing arteries, or pressing on nerves and bony prominences.

- Key points with positioning include adequately exposing the operative area, maintaining adequate respirations, and making sure blood vessels and nerves are not impeded by pressure.

Protecting the Patient From Injury

- Verifying information, checking the chart for completeness, and maintaining surgical asepsis and an optimal environment are critical nursing responsibilities.
- The nurse checks that all necessary equipment, nonroutine medications, blood components, instruments, and other equipment are present. Any aspects of the OR environment that may negatively affect the patient are identified and rectified.
- The nurse maintains safety by remaining with sedated patients, using safety straps and side rails, properly positioning grounding pads, decreasing risk for hypothermia and blood loss, and taking steps to avoid retained foreign bodies.

Serving as Patient Advocate

- Advocacy in the OR entails maintaining the patient's physical and emotional comfort, rights, providing physical privacy, and maintaining confidentiality.
- Avoid excessive noise, inappropriate conversation, and derogatory comments.

Monitoring and Managing Potential Complications

- In collaboration with the surgeon and the anesthesiologist or anesthetist, the nurse is alert to and reports changes in vital signs and symptoms of nausea and vomiting, anaphylaxis, hypoxia, hypothermia, malignant hyperthermia, or disseminated intravascular coagulation (DIC).
- Complications include:
  - Nausea, vomiting, gagging, and aspiration
  - Anaphylaxis
  - Hypoxia and respiratory complications
  - Hypothermia
  - Malignant hyperthermia
  - Disseminated intravascular coagulation (DIC)

☀ *N U R S I N G   A L E R T*

Shivering is associated with hypothermia. The nurse is aware that shivering can increase oxygen demand by 300% to 400%, thus supplemental oxygen should be administered and continuous oxygen saturation monitoring used.

POSTOPERATIVE NURSING

The postoperative phase begins with the admission of the patient to the PACU and ends with a follow-up evaluation in the clinical setting or home. The scope of nursing care covers a wide range of activities, including maintaining the patient's airway, monitoring vital signs, assessing the effects of the anesthetic agents, assessing the patient for complications, and providing comfort and pain relief. Nursing activities also focus on promoting the patient's recovery and initiating the teaching, follow-up care, and referrals essential for recovery and rehabilitation after discharge.

Nursing Management During Postanesthesia Care

Postanesthesia care in some hospitals and ambulatory surgical centers is divided into two phases. Phase I, the immediate recovery phase, requires intensive nursing care. In phase II, the patient is prepared for self-care or care in the hospital, extended care setting, or discharge.

- The PACU nurse provides care until the patient has recovered from the effects of anesthesia, is oriented or returns to baseline cognition, has stable vital signs, and shows no evidence of hemorrhage or other complications.
- Transferring the postoperative patient from the OR to the PACU is the responsibility of the anesthesiologist or anesthetist, with attention to airway maintenance. The surgical incision, drains or drainage tubes, and exposure is considered every time the patient is moved.
- The nurse validates that IV fluids and medications are correct and assesses oxygen saturation, airway patency and respiratory function, skin color, LOC, surgical site for hemorrhage, and proper function of drains and equipment. Vital signs are assessed at least every 15 minutes.

- Observe for hypopharyngeal airway obstruction by the tongue; signs include choking, noisy and irregular respirations, decreased oxygen saturation, and cyanosis. Provide supplemental oxygen as needed and elevate head of bed 15 to 30 degrees. If vomiting occurs, turn the patient to the side and suction the airway. Use caution with suction for patients having undergone tonsillectomy or laryngeal surgery due to risk of bleeding.
- Monitor cardiovascular stability by assessing mental status; vital signs; cardiac rhythm; skin temperature, color, and moisture; and urine output to detect shock, hemorrhage, hypertension, and arrhythmias. Provide fluid replacement as needed.

NURSING ALERT

Observe for symptoms of hemorrhage, including restlessness, apprehension, tachycardia, and cool, moist, and pale skin along with rapid deep respirations or "air hunger."

- Administer IV opioid analgesics judiciously; monitor for respiratory depression. Assess for special needs and permit family visitation to decrease anxiety.
- Control nausea before it progresses to vomiting. Metoclopramide (Reglan), prochlorperazine (Compazine), promethazine (Phenergan), dimenhydrinate (Dramamine), hydroxyzine (Vistaril, Atarax), scopolamine (Transderm-Scop), and ondansetron (Zofran) may be used.
- Discharge from the PACU occurs when vital signs are stable, the patient is oriented, pulmonary function is uncompromised, oxygen saturation and urine output are adequate, and pain is minimal. A scoring system such as Aldrete may be used to determine readiness for transfer.
- For same-day or ambulatory surgery, the nurse provides verbal and written instructions for patients and their families, as anesthetics cloud memory. Alternative formats of instruction, including large print, Braille, sign interpreter, or translator may be needed. Instructions should include wound care, activity and dietary recommendations, medications, and follow-up visits to the same-day surgery unit or the surgeon. Activities, such as making important decisions, driving, performing tasks requiring energy or skill, and alcohol consumption are usually limited for 24 to 48 hours.

- For the hospitalized patient, a standardized and comprehensive nurse-to-nurse patient report focused on safety must be given. A standardized mechanism of communicating report should be used across all phases of surgery; SBAR is currently a popular format:
  - The nurse prepares to receive the patient on the clinical unit by ensuring necessary equipment and supplies: IV pole, drainage receptacle holders, suction equipment, oxygen, emesis basin, tissues, disposable pads, blankets, and postoperative documentation forms are available.
  - The PACU nurse communicates demographic data, medical diagnosis, procedure performed, comorbid conditions, allergies, unexpected intraoperative events, estimated blood loss, types and amounts of fluids received, medications administered for pain, types of IV fluids or medications infused, whether the patient has voided, and information that the patient and family have received about the patient's condition.
  - The receiving nurse reviews the postoperative orders, admits the patient to the unit, performs an initial assessment, and attends to the patient's immediate needs.
- In the first 24 hours after surgery, the nurse assists the patient to recover from anesthesia, and frequently assesses physiologic status focusing on vital signs, adequate ventilation, hemodynamic stability, incisional pain, surgical site integrity, nausea and vomiting, neurologic status, and spontaneous voiding.
  - Patients usually begin to return to their usual state of health several hours after surgery or the next day. They may have pain, but many feel more alert and less anxious. Breathing, leg exercises, leg dangling at the side of the bed, ambulating, getting out of bed to a chair, and eating may begin. The focus of care shifts from physiologic management to regaining independence with self-care and preparing for discharge.

NURSING PROCESS

The Hospitalized Patient Recovering From Surgery

Assessment

Postoperative assessment includes monitoring vital signs and completing a review of the systems, and observing for postoperative complications upon arrival of the patient to the clinical unit and at regular intervals thereafter.

- The nurse recognizes pulmonary complications are among the most frequent and serious problems:
  - Monitor for airway patency, including quality of respirations. Respirations may be slow due to anesthesia. Rapid shallow respirations may be caused by pain, constricting dressings, gastric dilation, abdominal distention, or obesity. Noisy breathing may be due to obstruction by secretions or the tongue.
  - Assess pain level using a verbal or visual analogue scale; include characteristics of pain.
  - Monitor cardiovascular function, including vital signs, skin temperature, and if skin is cool and clammy or warm and dry.
  - Observe for bleeding and function of all tubes and drains.
  - Assess mental status and LOC; recognize that changes in mental status or postoperative restlessness may be related to anxiety, pain, urinary retention, or medications, as well as hypoxemia hypoglycemia or hemorrhage.

Diagnosis

- Risk for ineffective airway clearance related to depressed respiratory function, pain, and bed rest
- Acute pain related to surgical incision
- Decreased cardiac output related to shock or hemorrhage
- Risk for activity intolerance related to generalized weakness secondary to surgery
- Impaired skin integrity related to surgical incision and drains
- Ineffective thermoregulation related to surgical environment and anesthetic agents
- Risk for imbalanced nutrition, less than body requirements related to decreased intake and increased need for nutrients secondary to surgery
- Risk for constipation related to effects of medications, surgery, dietary change, and immobility
- Impaired urinary elimination related to urinary retention
- Risk for injury related to surgical procedure/positioning or anesthetic agents
- Anxiety related to surgical procedure

(continues on page 546)

P

- Risk for ineffective self-health management of therapeutic regimen related to wound care, dietary restrictions, activity recommendations, medications, follow-up care, or signs and symptoms of complications

Planning

The major goals for the patient include optimal respiratory function, relief of pain, optimal cardiovascular function, increased activity tolerance, successful wound healing, maintenance of body temperature, and maintenance of nutritional balance.

- Further goals include resumption of usual pattern of bowel and bladder elimination, identification of any perioperative positioning injury, acquisition of sufficient knowledge to manage self-care after discharge, and absence of complications.

✴ N U R S I N G   A L E R T

Unless indicated more frequently, record the pulse, blood pressure, and respirations every 15 minutes for the first hour and every 30 minutes for the next 2 hours. Thereafter, they are measured less frequently if they remain stable. Monitor patient's temperature every 4 hours for the first 24 hours.

Gerontologic Considerations

- Elderly patients recover more slowly, have longer hospital stays, and are at greater risk for development of postoperative complications including pneumonia, decline in functional ability, exacerbation of comorbid conditions, pressure ulcers, decreased oral intake, GI disturbance, and falls:
  - Plan for progressive ambulation and avoid prolonged sitting.
  - Place the call bell within reach and prompt the patient to void to prevent incontinence.
  - Plan high-protein meals with sufficient fiber, calories, and vitamins to promote wound healing and return of bowel function. Consider liquid nutritional supplements, multivitamins, iron, and vitamin C for wound healing and hematopoiesis.
  - Provide extensive discharge teaching and repetition if sensory deficits are present; coordinate discharge planning

with professional and family care providers, social worker, or nurse care manager to ensure continuity of care.
- Postoperative delirium, characterized by confusion, perceptual and cognitive deficits, altered attention levels, disturbed sleep patterns, and impaired psychomotor skills, is a significant problem for older adults:
  - Interventions for delirium include keeping the patient in a well-lit room, close to the nurses' station, minimizing distracting and unfamiliar noises, and ensuring adequate pain control. Reorient the patient as necessary, engage the patient in conversation, provide clock and calendar nearby, and continue with physical activity. Avoid restraints, have a family member or staff member stay with the patient; consider brief use of antianxiety medications.

Nursing Interventions

Promoting Respiratory Function

- Identify patients at risk for postoperative pulmonary complication: Increased age, smoking, COPD, long duration of surgery, incision site (chest and upper abdomen), as well as comorbidities such as HF, arrhythmias, diabetes mellitus, and patients with swallowing disorders.
- Assist patients to improve respiratory function affected by opiates, pain, and surgical positioning by encouraging deep-breathing, coughing, sitting in the upright position, turning frequently, promoting early mobility, and using incentive spirometer to prevent atelectasis and pneumonia:
  - Observe for hypoxemia particularly in those having undergone major surgery of thorax or abdomen, patients who are obese, or those with pre-existing pulmonary problems.

⚡ N U R S I N G   A L E R T
Coughing is contraindicated in patients who have head injuries or who have undergone intracranial surgery due to increased intracranial pressure (ICP); and in patients following eye surgery or plastic surgery due to increase in intraocular pressure (IOP) or stress on delicate tissues

(continues on page 548)

P

Relieving Pain

The degree and severity of postoperative pain and the patient's tolerance for pain depend on the incision site, the nature of the surgical procedure, the extent of surgical trauma, the type of anesthetic agent, and how the agent was administered.

- Conduct a thorough preoperative pain evaluation and develop pain goals for the surgical patient.
- Providing information on what to expect, how the pain will be managed, and reassurance can contribute to reducing anxiety and possibly the postoperative pain experienced.
- Intrapleural anesthesia provides sensory anesthesia without affecting motor function to the intercostal muscles when pain in the thoracic region would interfere with breathing; useful after cholecystectomy, renal surgery, and rib fractures. It has fewer adverse effects than systemic opioids and is associated with a lowered incidence of nausea, vomiting, and pruritus.
- A subcutaneous pain management system with a silicone catheter inserted into the affected area may be used. The catheter is attached to a pump that delivers a slow, continuous amount of local anesthetic.
- Teach the patient that poor pain control contributes to postoperative complications and increased length of stay. Taking analgesic agents before the pain becomes intense is more effective; provide around-the-clock dosing rather than waiting for the patient to request it.
- Nonpharmacologic measures including imagery, music, relaxation, massage, application of heat or cold (if prescribed), and distraction.

Promoting Cardiac Output

If signs and symptoms of shock or hemorrhage occur, treatment and nursing care are implemented as described in the discussion of care in the PACU.

- Intravenous fluid replacement is standard for up to 24 hours after surgery or until the patient is stable and tolerating oral fluids.
- Monitor patients at risk for fluid volume excess secondary to existing cardiovascular or renal disease, advanced age, or

the release of adrenocorticotropic hormone and antidiuretic hormone as a result of the stress of surgery.

- Maintain accurate I & O including output from wounds and drains, emesis, urine output. Report urine output of less than 30 mL/hr.
- Monitor H & H; hemodilution secondary to fluids administered during surgery; may contribute to decreasing H & H.
- Encourage patient to perform leg exercises and frequent position changes and early ambulation. Apply sequential compression devices (SCDs).

Encouraging Activity

- Encourage early ambulation to reduce the incidence of postoperative complications, such as atelectasis, hypostatic pneumonia, GI discomfort and distention, and circulatory problems such as deep vein thrombosis (DVT).
- Monitor for orthostatic hypotension due to changes in circulating blood volume or bedrest. Tachycardia with a 15 mm Hg drop in systolic pressure indicates orthostasis.
- Assist the patient to perform as much routine hygiene as possible by setting up the patient to bathe with a bedside wash basin or assisting the patient to sit in a chair at the sink.
- To be safely discharged to home, patients need to be able to ambulate a functional distance, get in and out of bed unassisted, and be independent with toileting. Collaborate with the patient on a progressive schedule of activity. Involve physical therapist for patients having orthopedic surgery or needing mobility aids such as a walker or crutches.

Promoting Wound Healing

Ongoing assessment of the surgical site involves inspection for approximation of wound edges, integrity of sutures or staples, redness, discoloration, warmth, swelling, unusual tenderness, or drainage. The area around the wound should also be inspected for a reaction to tape or trauma from tight bandages.

- Inform patients that surgical wound healing occurs in three phases: Inflammatory, proliferative, and maturation phases. The nurse recognizes wounds heal by first-intention,

(continues on page 550)

P

second-intention, and third-intention. Wounds closed with cyanoacrylate tissue adhesive should not receive a dressing. Postoperative wounds healing by secondary or tertiary intention are usually packed with saline-moistened sterile dressings.

- Wound drains such as Penrose, Hemovac, and Jackson-Pratt drains allow escape of blood and serous fluid that can serve as a culture medium for bacteria. Output of drains is monitored and recorded in the I & O; multiple drains are numbered or labeled for consistent record keeping. Report increasing amounts of bloody drainage to the surgeon.

Changing the Dressing

- Change the dressing using aseptic or clean technique based on institutional policy; more evidence is needed regarding influence of sterile versus clean gloves.
- Provide for patient privacy, and avoid dressing changes at mealtime or when visitors are present. Teach the patient about incision care and dressing changes at this time, assessing readiness to learn, such as looking at the incision, expressing interest, or assisting in the dressing change.
- Avoid referring to the incision as a scar, which may carry negative connotation.

Maintaining Normal Body Temperature

- Recognize that the patient is still at risk for malignant hyperthermia and hypothermia in the postoperative period.
- Monitor for hypothermia; provide blankets, maintain a comfortable room temperature. Prolonged surgery in the elderly increases the risk of hypothermia. Report symptoms of hypothermia to the surgical team; anticipate administering oxygen, hydration, and nutrition.

Managing Gastrointestinal Function and Resuming Nutrition

- Anticipate post anesthesia nausea and vomiting; this is more common in women, obese individuals, those prone to motion sickness, and those undergoing lengthy procedures.
- An NG tube may be inserted preoperatively, or for postoperative vomiting or distention, and when emergency surgery is required.

- Hiccups may occur secondary to intermittent spasms of the diaphragm related to irritation of the phrenic nerve. GI discomfort, nausea, and vomiting may occur after anesthesia. If persistent vomiting occurs, an antiemetic is used.
- Encouraging oral intake will promote normal GI function and is begun when the patient is fully awake and alert, and bowel sounds are present. Liquids are begun first.
- Encourage frequent position changes and turning to prevent abdominal distention caused by swallowed air and accumulation of gas and GI secretions. Observe for symptoms of paralytic ileus and intestinal obstruction, most common after intestinal or abdominal surgery.

Promoting Bowel Function

- Constipation is common after surgery secondary to decreased mobility, decreased oral intake, and opioid analgesics. Notify the surgeon if the patient does not have a bowel movement by the second or third postoperative day so that a laxative can be ordered.

Managing Voiding

- Postoperative urinary retention can occur due to anesthesia, anticholinergic agents, and opioids. Abdominal, pelvic, and hip surgery may increase the likelihood of retention secondary to pain.
- Assess for bladder distention and the urge to void upon arrival to the unit and frequently thereafter. If the patient does not void within 8 hours after surgery, a portable ultrasound bladder scan should be performed and all methods tried to encourage the patient to void; after voiding, rescan the bladder for residual. Consider a commode; suggest that a male patient stand. Intermittent catheterization is preferred over indwelling catheterization due to risk of infection; it may be performed every 4 to 6 hours until the postvoid residual is less than 100 mL. If bladder scanning is unavailable, palpate the suprapubic area for distention or tenderness after voiding.

(continues on page 552)

P

Maintaining a Safe Environment

- Immediately postoperatively, maintain three side rails up and the bed in low position.
- Assess LOC and provide eyeglasses, hearing aid, or call bell to reduce risk for injury.
- Instruct patient to ask for assistance with activity.
- Avoid restraints; if needed, follow institutional policy.

Providing Emotional Support to the Patient and Family

- Provide information, reassurance, and active listening to address anxiety, pain, the unfamiliar environment, inability to control one's circumstances or care for oneself, fear of the long-term effects of surgery, fear of complications, fatigue, spiritual distress, altered role responsibilities, ineffective coping, and altered body image.
- Keep patients informed about hospital routines, assessment and interventions, when they will be able to drink or eat, when they will be getting out of bed, and when tubes and drains will be removed. This helps them to gain a sense of control, to participate in recovery, and engages them in the plan of care.
- Modify the environment to enhance rest and relaxation by providing privacy, reducing noise, adjusting lighting, providing enough seating for family members, and encouraging a supportive atmosphere.

Managing Potential Complications

- Monitor for symptoms of MI, which may be silent or present with dyspnea, hypotension, or atypical pain. Alert the surgical team; obtain vital signs and oxygen saturation; and perform a cardiac, peripheral vascular, and pulmonary assessment and ECG.
- Observe for congestive heart failure (CHF) around postoperative day 2 or 3 related to fluid shifts. Monitor for crackles, dyspnea, wheezing, cough, fatigue, weight gain, and jugular vein distention (JVD).
- Monitor for DVT, heralded by pain or cramp in the calf followed by swelling of the leg, fever, chills, and diaphoresis. Maintain elastic compression stockings, administer low-dose heparin as ordered, and encourage early ambulation, hydration, and leg exercises.

- Observe for symptoms of pulmonary embolism (PE) including sudden onset of SOB, tachypnea, tachycardia, chest pain, and apprehension.
- Observe the wound for hematoma, which can delay healing; prepare the patient for evacuation of clot if necessary.
- Follow current guidelines to prevent surgical site infections. Administer prophylactic antibiotic within 1 hour before surgical incision and continue for a maximum of 24 hours (48 hours for cardiothoracic surgery, if vancomycin and fluoroquinolones are administered within 2 hours of incision):
  - Emphasize proper wound care and signs and symptoms of infection, which may not develop until at least postoperative day 5; most patients are discharged by that time. Teach the patient to observe for increased pulse rate and temperature; an elevated WBC count; wound swelling, warmth, tenderness, or discharge; and incisional pain.
  - Risk factors for wound infection include wound contamination, foreign body, faulty suturing technique, devitalized tissue, hematoma, debilitation, dehydration, malnutrition, anemia, advanced age, extreme obesity, shock, length of preoperative hospitalization, duration of surgical procedure, and associated disorders (eg, diabetes mellitus, immunosuppression).
  - Treatment may require incision and drainage, wound care, and antimicrobial therapy.
- Observe for wound dehiscence (disruption of surgical incision or wound) and evisceration (protrusion of wound contents) manifested by a gush of serosanguineous fluid from the wound or bowel loops protruding from the wound. Cover an evisceration with moist saline dressings, notify the surgeon, and assess vital signs and pulse oximetry. Maintain an IV and NPO status, and bed rest with knees bent to reduce abdominal muscle tension. Postoperatively, have the patient splint the abdomen and consider use of an abdominal binder.

Providing Discharge Teaching

Dramatically reduced hospital lengths of stay have greatly increased the amount of information needed while reducing the amount of time in which to provide it.

(continues on page 554)

Evaluation

Expected patient outcomes may include the following:

- Maintains optimal respiratory function
- Indicates that pain is decreased in intensity
- Increases activity as prescribed
- Wound heals without complication
- Maintains body temperature within normal limits
- Resumes oral intake, free from nausea and vomiting
- Reports resumption of usual bowel elimination pattern
- Resumes usual voiding pattern
- Is free of injury
- Exhibits decreased anxiety
- Acquires knowledge and skills necessary to manage therapeutic regimen
- Experiences no complications

For more information, see Chapter 5 in Pellico, L.H. (2013). *Focus on adult health: Medical-surgical nursing.* Philadelphia: Wolters Kluwer Health | Lippincott Williams & Wilkins.

Peripheral Arterial Disease

Peripheral artery disease (PAD) refers to any disease process that affects the arteries. Various peripheral arterial diseases result in ischemia.

PATHOPHYSIOLOGY

Peripheral artery disease is one manifestation of atherosclerosis, which narrows the vessel lumen. Obstructive lesions may extend from the aorta below the renal arteries to the popliteal artery. Atherosclerosis involves changes of the intima consisting of accumulation of lipids, calcium, blood components, complex carbohydrates, and fibrous tissue, referred to as atheromas or plaques. Atherosclerosis causes arterial stenosis, obstruction by thrombosis, aneurysm, ulceration, and vessel rupture.

RISK FACTORS

Similar to those of coronary atherosclerosis

- Nonmodifiable: Age, race, sex (male)
- Modifiable: Tobacco use, hypertension (HTN), diabetes
- Obesity, stress, and sedentary lifestyle
- Hyperhomocysteinemia
- Acute arterial occlusion may be caused by aneurysm, arterial dissection, emboli, trauma, tumor compression, drug abuse, low cardiac output, massive iliofemoral venous thrombosis, or compartment syndrome.

CLINICAL MANIFESTATIONS AND ASSESSMENT

Most patients with PAD are asymptomatic. Clinical signs and symptoms are manifested in the end organ supplied.

- Intermittent claudication: Pain, aching, or cramping in a muscle of the feet or hands during exercise and relieved by rest. Pain is reproducible with similar activities.
- In lower extremity PAD, monitor progression of disease by documenting ambulatory distance before pain is perceived.
- Rest pain indicates severe disease and limb threatening ischemia. Pain is persistent, often worse at night, and may interfere with sleep; it improves by placing the leg in the dependent position.
- Upper extremity arterial occlusion may cause arm fatigue and pain with exercise (forearm claudication) and inability to hold or grasp objects (eg, painting, combing hair, placing objects on shelves above the head).

- Coldness or pallor of extremity
- Extremities may develop rubor, a reddish-blue color, when lowered to a dependent position.
- Cyanosis, a bluish tint to the skin, may be present and is more subtle in dark-skinned patients.
- Sluggish capillary refill time may be present; recent evidence questions reliability of intraobserver reliability.
- Skin and nail changes, ulcers, gangrene, and muscle atrophy may be evident in chronic disease.
- Unequal pulses between extremities or absence of a normally palpable pulse; a good pulse does not exclude PAD in the presence of leg pain.
- Bruits may be auscultated just distal to arterial stenosis.

DIAGNOSTIC METHODS

- Hand-held continuous wave (CW) Doppler
- Doppler with ankle-brachial index (ABI) tests
- Exercise testing for ankle systolic blood pressure in response to walking on treadmill
- Duplex ultrasonography, computed tomography angiography (CTA), magnetic resonance angiography (MRA), angiography, vascular endoscopy (angioscopy).

MEDICAL AND NURSING MANAGEMENT

Medical management includes exercise, pharmacologic treatment, and invasive options.

- Exercise program: Patient walks to point of pain, pauses until pain subsides, and continues walking.
- Smoking cessation and weight loss

Pharmacologic Therapy

- Cilostazol (Pletal), a phosphodiesterase III inhibitor, is a vasodilator that interferes with platelet aggregation.

- Antiplatelet agents such as aspirin or clopidogrel (Plavix) prevent the formation of thromboemboli, which can lead to MI and stroke secondary to atherosclerosis.
- Thrombolytics for stenosis or occlusion are injected via catheter into affected vessel.

Surgical Management

- Revascularization or arterial bypass to reroute blood flow around the occlusion is first-line intervention. Native/autologous veins (from the patient) are preferred, although synthetic materials or cryopreserved saphenous veins or umbilical veins are available.
- Angioplasty, also called percutaneous transluminal balloon angioplasty (PTA), may be performed. Balloons are inserted into the vessels via a catheter and expanded to open the vessel lumen; a stent may be placed for support and patency.
- Complications from PTA include hematoma, embolization, dissection of the vessel, bleeding, intimal damage (dissection), and stent migration.

Nursing Management

The primary objective in the postprocedure period is to maintain adequate circulation.

- Perform neurovascular checks of limb; use Doppler for pulses if needed. Report cool, dusky skin; weakened pulses; delayed capillary refill; and decreased sensory/motor function to surgeon immediately.
- Assess for hemorrhage, metabolic abnormalities, renal failure, and compartment syndrome.
- Monitor vital signs, I & O; perform assessment of pulmonary, cardiac, pulmonary, GI, mental status, and laboratory data.
- Encourage patient to move extremity and be active as ordered by surgeon.
- Administer pain medication, usually narcotic analgesic, to manage rest pain; following intervention, patient may need higher than usual doses of analgesic due to tolerance.
- Teach patient to avoid tissue damage; infection may develop and amputation may be needed due to poor blood flow. Patients are

taught to wear sturdy, well-fitting shoes or slippers, and to use neutral soaps and body lotions. Provide detailed instructions for wound care and foot care (same as for diabetic patients). Avoid extremes of temperature, nicotine and second-hand smoke, emotional upset, and constrictive clothing or accessories.

☀ NURSING ALERT

Elevation of the lower extremities is associated with decreased flow, which lessens perfusion and increases pain. A dependent position improves flow and decreases pain.

For more information, see Chapter 18 in Pellico, L.H. (2013). *Focus on adult health: Medical-surgical nursing.* Philadelphia: Wolters Kluwer Health | Lippincott Williams & Wilkins.

Peritonitis

Peritonitis is inflammation of the peritoneum, the serous membrane lining the abdominal cavity and covering the viscera. Peritonitis is typically a life-threatening emergency that requires prompt surgical intervention and typically requires critical care postoperatively.

PATHOPHYSIOLOGY

Peritonitis is caused by leakage of contents from abdominal organs into the abdominal cavity, usually as a result of inflammation, infection, ischemia, trauma, or tumor perforation. Bacterial proliferation occurs. Edema of the tissues ensues, and exudation of fluid into the peritoneal cavity develops in a short time. Peritoneal fluid becomes turbid, with increasing amounts of protein, WBCs, cellular debris, and blood. The immediate response of the intestinal tract is hypermotility, soon followed by paralytic ileus, with an accumulation of air and fluid in the bowel.

RISK FACTORS

- Abdominal surgery
- Organisms from GI tract or internal reproductive organs in women
- External injury or trauma
- Inflammation extending from kidney or peritoneal dialysis
- Appendicitis, perforated ulcer, diverticulitis, and perforated bowel.

CLINICAL MANIFESTATIONS AND ASSESSMENT

Symptoms depend on the location and extent of inflammation. Early clinical manifestations, frequently the symptoms of the underlying disorder, are aptly called an "acute abdomen."

- Diffuse pain that becomes constant, localized, and more intense near site of the inflammation
- Pain aggravated by movement
- Affected area of the abdomen becomes extremely tender and distended, and muscles become rigid; patients with diabetes, ascites, those taking corticosteroids or analgesics may have decreased perception of pain.
- Rebound tenderness and paralytic ileus may be present.
- Anorexia, nausea, and vomiting occur, and peristalsis is diminished.
- Temperature and pulse increase; hypotension may develop.

DIAGNOSTIC METHODS

- Leukocytosis and altered serum electrolytes (potassium, sodium, and chloride)
- H & H decreased if blood loss occurs
- Abdominal X-ray may show air and fluid levels, as well as distended bowel loops.
- Computed tomography scan of the abdomen may show abscess formation, acute inflammation or infection of one of the major abdominal organs, or a perforation of the small or large bowel.

- Peritoneal aspiration with culture and sensitivity studies may reveal causative organisms.

MEDICAL AND NURSING MANAGEMENT

Fluid, colloid, and electrolyte replacement is the major focus of medical management.

- Plan to administer several liters of isotonic fluid; decreased vascular volume develops due to massive fluid shifts from intestinal lumen into peritoneal cavity.
- Analgesics are administered for pain; antiemetics are administered for nausea and vomiting.
- Insert NG tube for suction to relieve abdominal distention.
- Oxygen therapy by nasal cannula or mask is instituted to improve ventilatory function. Observe need for intubation and ventilatory assistance.
- Administer high-dose, broad-spectrum antibiotics and antifungicides IV until the specific organism causing the infection is identified.
- Surgical objectives include removal of infected material and correcting the cause. Surgeries may include appendectomy, resection with or without anastomosis of intestine, repair of perforation, or drainage of abscess. Fecal diversion may be created if sepsis is present.

Nursing Management

Intensive care is often needed.

- Prepare the patient for emergency surgery.
- Monitor the patient's blood pressure by arterial line if shock is present.
- Monitor I & O and central venous or pulmonary artery pressures to calculate fluid replacement.
- Provide ongoing assessment of pain, GI function, and fluid and electrolyte balance.
- Bladder pressure is also routinely measured to identify abdominal compartment syndrome.

- Assess nature of pain, location in the abdomen, and shifts of pain and location.
- Administer analgesic medication and position for comfort; side lying with knees flexed decreases tension on abdominal organs.
- Administer and monitor IV fluids closely; NG intubation may be necessary.
- Signs indicating peritonitis is subsiding include a decrease in temperature and pulse rate, softening of the abdomen, return of peristaltic sounds, passing of flatus, and bowel movements.
- Increase food and oral fluids gradually, decreasing parenteral fluid as prescribed.
- Observe and record character of drainage from surgical drains; move and turn the patient carefully to avoid dislodging drains. Consider pinning drains to patient gown.
- Postoperatively, prepare patient and family for discharge; teach care of incision and drains if still in place at discharge.
- Refer for home care or rehabilitation as necessary.

COMPLICATIONS

- Sepsis
- Hypovolemic or septic shock
- Intestinal obstruction secondary to adhesions
- Pulmonary embolism

For more information, see Chapter 24 in Pellico, L.H. (2013). *Focus on adult health: Medical-surgical nursing*. Philadelphia: Wolters Kluwer Health | Lippincott Williams & Wilkins.

Pharyngitis, Acute

Acute pharyngitis is a sudden inflammation of the pharynx involving the back portion of the tongue, soft palate, and tonsils.

P

PATHOPHYSIOLOGY

Most cases of acute pharyngitis are caused by viral infection. Responsible viruses include the adenovirus, influenza virus, Epstein-Barr virus, and herpes simplex virus. Bacterial organisms account for the remainder of the cases. Ten percent of adults with pharyngitis have group A beta-hemolytic streptococcus (GABHS), which is commonly referred to as group A streptococcus (GAS) or streptococcal pharyngitis. Other bacterial organisms found in acute pharyngitis include *Mycoplasma pneumoniae, Neisseria gonorrhoeae,* and *Haemophilus influenzae* type B.

RISK FACTORS

- Patients under 25 years
- Exposure to ill individuals

CLINICAL MANIFESTATIONS AND ASSESSMENT

- Fiery-red pharyngeal membrane and tonsils; creamy exudates in tonsillar pillars
- Lymphoid follicles swollen and freckled with white-purple exudate
- Cervical lymph nodes enlarged and tender
- Fever, malaise, and sore throat
- Patients with group A streptococcus pharyngitis may exhibit vomiting, anorexia, and a scarlatina-form rash with urticaria known as scarlet fever.

DIAGNOSTIC METHODS

Accurate diagnosis of pharyngitis is essential to determine the causative organism and to initiate treatment early.

- Rapid streptococcal antigen test (RSAT, sometimes called STCX) used with professional clinical evaluation.

MEDICAL AND NURSING MANAGEMENT

- Viral pharyngitis is treated with supportive measures.
- Antibiotics, usually penicillins, are used to treat bacterial pharyngitis.
- Nasal congestion may be relieved by nasal sprays or medications containing ephedrine sulfate or phenylephrine HCL. Antihistamine decongestants may be used along with ASA or acetaminophen.

COMPLICATIONS

- Rhinosinusitis
- Otitis media
- Peritonsillar abscess, mastoiditis, and cervical adenitis.
- Rarely bacteremia, pneumonia, meningitis, rheumatic fever
- Acute poststreptococcal glomerulonephritis (APSGN) with resulting temporary kidney failure may develop; manifested by gross hematuria, edema, HTN, respiratory distress, and pulmonary edema.

For more information, see Chapter 9 in Pellico, L.H. (2013). *Focus on adult health: Medical-surgical nursing.* Philadelphia: Wolters Kluwer Health | Lippincott Williams & Wilkins.

Pharyngitis, Chronic

Chronic pharyngitis is a persistent inflammation of the pharynx.

RISK FACTORS

Chronic pharyngitis is common in adults who work or live in dusty surroundings, use their voice to excess, suffer from chronic cough, or habitually use alcohol and tobacco.

P

CLINICAL MANIFESTATIONS AND ASSESSMENT

- Constant sense of irritation or fullness in the throat
- Mucus that collects in the throat and is expelled by coughing
- Difficulty in swallowing

MEDICAL AND NURSING MANAGEMENT

- Treatment of chronic pharyngitis is based on relieving symptoms, avoiding exposure to irritants, and correcting any upper respiratory, pulmonary, or cardiac condition that might cause a chronic cough.
- For adults with chronic pharyngitis, tonsillectomy is an effective option.

For more information, see Chapter 9 in Pellico, L.H. (2013). *Focus on adult health: Medical-surgical nursing.* Philadelphia: Wolters Kluwer Health | Lippincott Williams & Wilkins.

Pheochromocytoma

A pheochromocytoma is a benign catecholamine-secreting tumor of the adrenal gland causing HTN and severe hypertensive crisis.

PATHOPHYSIOLOGY

Pheochromocytoma begins with benign growth of a catecholamine-secreting tumor inside the adrenal gland. Most tumors arise from the adrenal medulla, but can arise in the extra-adrenal chromaffin tissue located in or near the aorta, ovaries, spleen, or other organs. Massive release of catecholamines causes severe HTN. The annual incidence of pheochromocytoma is 2 to 8 cases per million. In most cases, 10% of the tumors are bilateral, and 10% are malignant.

RISK FACTORS

- Multiple endocrine neoplasia type 2 (MEN-2), a rare inherited disease that leads to overactivity and enlargement of endocrine glands, may predispose to pheochromocytoma.
- Family members of affected patients
- Symptoms usually develop in the fifth decade

CLINICAL MANIFESTATIONS AND ASSESSMENT

The nature and severity of symptoms depend on epinephrine and norepinephrine secretion.

- Typical symptoms include five H's: Hypertension (severe), headache, hyperhidrosis (excessive sweating), hypermetabolism, and hyperglycemia.
- Blood pressures may exceed 250/150.
- About 8% of patients are asymptomatic.
- Characterized by acute, unpredictable attacks with headache, vertigo, blurring of vision, tinnitus, air hunger, and dyspnea. Other symptoms include polyuria, nausea, vomiting, diarrhea, abdominal pain, and a feeling of impending doom.
- Palpitations and tachycardia are common; postural hypotension may occur.

DIAGNOSTIC METHODS

- Twenty-four hour urine for plasma levels of catecholamines and metanephrine (MN), a catecholamine metabolite, and vanillylmandelic acid (VMA) are conclusive tests for adrenal

P

overactivity. Teach the patient to avoid coffee and tea (including decaffeinated varieties), bananas, chocolate, vanilla, and aspirin to ensure accuracy of tests.

- Total plasma catecholamine is collected with the patient at rest and supine for 30 minutes. The patient must avoid the dietary items listed above and tobacco, emotional and physical stress, and use of many prescription and OTC medications (eg, amphetamines, nose drops or sprays, decongestant agents, bronchodilators) prior to the test.

MEDICAL AND NURSING MANAGEMENT

Once diagnosed, surgery is indicated after appropriate preparation. Laparoscopic removal is often treatment of choice.

Pharmacologic Therapy

- Careful administration of alpha-adrenergic blocking agents (eg, phentolamine [Regitine]) or smooth muscle relaxants (eg, sodium nitroprusside [Nipride]) lower the blood pressure quickly.
- Phenoxybenzamine (Dibenzyline), a long-acting alpha blocker, may be used once stabilized. Nifedipine (Procardia) is associated with low morbidity and mortality. Beta-adrenergic blockers are used with caution due to increased sensitivity.
- Catecholamine synthesis inhibitors, such as alpha-methyl-p-tyrosine (metyrosine) also may be used preoperatively if adrenergic blocking agents do not reduce the effects of catecholamines.
- Insulin may be required to maintain normal serum glucose levels.

Nursing Management

- The patient will be admitted to the ICU for close monitoring of ECG and vital signs; watch for precipitous hypotension that may reduce perfusion to vital organs (brain and kidneys).
- Monitor mental status, acute ECG changes, arterial pressures, fluid and electrolyte balance, and blood glucose levels.

- Give encouragement and support, because patient may be fearful of repeated attacks.

COMPLICATIONS

- Cardiac dysrhythmias
- Dissecting aneurysm
- Stroke
- Acute renal failure

For more information, see Chapter 31 in Pellico, L.H. (2013). *Focus on adult health: Medical-surgical nursing*. Philadelphia: Wolters Kluwer Health | Lippincott Williams & Wilkins.

Pleural Effusion

Pleural effusion, a collection of fluid in the pleural space, is usually secondary to other disease processes.

PATHOPHYSIOLOGY

In certain disorders, fluid may accumulate in the pleural space to a point at which it becomes clinically evident. This almost always has pathologic significance. A pleural effusion can be composed of a relatively clear fluid, or it can be bloody or purulent. An effusion of clear fluid may be a transudate or an exudate. A transudate, filtrate of plasma that moves across intact capillary walls, occurs with imbalances in hydrostatic or oncotic pressures, common in HF. An exudate, extravasation of fluid into tissues or a cavity, usually results from inflammation by bacterial products or tumors involving the pleural surfaces.

Empyema is a purulent, exudative effusion, occurring frequently as complications of bacterial pneumonia, lung abscess, or penetrating chest trauma. At first, the pleural fluid is thin, with a low leukocyte count, but it frequently progresses to a fibropurulent stage and, finally, to a stage at which it encloses the lung within a thick exudative membrane (loculated empyema).

RISK FACTORS

- Heart failure
- Tuberculosis (TB)
- Pneumonia
- Pulmonary infections
- Nephrotic syndrome
- Connective tissue diseases
- Pulmonary embolus
- Neoplastic tumors, especially bronchogenic carcinoma and breast cancer

CLINICAL MANIFESTATIONS AND ASSESSMENT

Usually, the clinical manifestations are caused by the underlying disease.

- Pneumonia causes fever, chills, and pleuritic chest pain, whereas a malignant effusion may result in dyspnea when lying flat and coughing.
- The size of the effusion, the speed of its formation, and the underlying lung disease determine the severity of symptoms.
- Large effusions cause SOB; a small to moderate effusion causes minimal or no dyspnea.
- Decreased or absent breath sounds over the area, decreased fremitus, dullness or flatness to percussion, tracheal deviation away from the affected side, hypoxemia, hypotension, and tachycardia may be noted.

DIAGNOSTIC METHODS

- Physical examination
- Chest X-ray, lateral decubitus chest X-ray with patient lying on unaffected side, chest CT
- Thoracentesis
- Pleural fluid analysis including Gram stain, acid-fast bacillus (AFB), red and white blood cell counts, chemistry studies, cytology for malignant cells
- Pleural biopsy may be performed

MEDICAL AND NURSING MANAGEMENT

Objectives of treatment are to discover the underlying cause; to prevent reaccumulation of fluid; and to relieve discomfort, dyspnea, and respiratory compromise. Treatment is directed at the underlying cause.

- Thoracentesis with or without guided ultrasound is performed to remove fluid, collect specimen for analysis, and relieve dyspnea and respiratory.
- Chest tube with water-seal drainage and suction may be used for drainage and lung reexpansion.
- Chemical pleurodesis uses a chemically irritating agent (eg, talc, bleomycin, doxycycline) instilled into the pleural space to obliterate the space and prevent further fluid accumulation.
- Other treatment modalities include surgical pleuracotomy, with a small tube attached to a drainage bottle for outpatient management (Pleurx catheter, Denver Biomedical).
- An implanted pleuroperitoneal shunt that carries fluid from the pleural space to the peritoneal cavity via a manual pump may be used.
- Decortication is the surgical removal of fibrous tissue in the pleural space; also called a *pleural peel.*

Nursing Management

See "Nursing Management" under the disorder describing the underlying condition.

- Prepare and position patient for thoracentesis and offer support; record amount of fluid removed and ensure it is sent for appropriate diagnostic testing.
- Monitor chest tube drainage and water-seal system; monitor proper function of system and record amount of drainage at prescribed intervals.
- Provide nursing care specific to the underlying cause of the pleural effusion.
- Assist patient in pain relief and to assume positions that are least painful.
- Prepare patient for pleurodesis by premedicating with narcotic analgesic; consider antianxiety agent as well. Turn patient frequently to ensure pleurodesic agent contacts the pleural surface.
- Teach the patient to use hands or pillow to splint the rib cage while coughing.
- Administration and assessment of the effects of narcotics or NSAIDs is necessary.

For more information, see Chapter 10 in Pellico, L.H. (2013). *Focus on adult health: Medical-surgical nursing.* Philadelphia: Wolters Kluwer Health | Lippincott Williams & Wilkins.

Pleurisy

Pleurisy refers to inflammation of the visceral and parietal pleurae.

PATHOPHYSIOLOGY

When the inflamed pleural membranes rub together during respiration, the result is severe, sharp, knife-like pain, which is worse on inspiration.

RISK FACTORS

- Pneumonia or an upper respiratory tract infection
- Tuberculosis or collagen disease
- Chest trauma and after thoracotomy
- Pulmonary infarction or PE
- Patients with primary or metastatic cancer

CLINICAL MANIFESTATIONS AND ASSESSMENT

- Pain related to respiration; deep breaths, coughing, or sneezing worsens the pain.
- Pain is minimal or absent when the breath is held. Pain is unilateral, localized, and may radiate to the shoulder or abdomen.
- As pleural fluid accumulates, pain lessens.

DIAGNOSTIC METHODS

Assess for underlying condition.

MEDICAL AND NURSING MANAGEMENT

Objectives of management are to discover the underlying condition causing the pleurisy and to relieve the pain.

- Patient is monitored for signs and symptoms of pleural effusion: SOB, pain, assumption of a position that decreases pain, and decreased chest wall excursion.
- Prescribed analgesics, such as NSAIDs, occasionally narcotic analgesic, application of heat or cold, are used to promote coughing and deep breathing and provide pain relief.
- An intercostal nerve block is done for severe pain.

Nursing Management

- Enhance comfort by turning patient frequently on affected side to splint chest wall.
- Teach patient to use hands or pillow to splint rib cage while coughing.

See "Medical and Nursing Management" under "Pneumonia" on pages 575–579 for additional information.

> For more information, see Chapter 10 in Pellico, L.H. (2013). *Focus on adult health: Medical-surgical nursing.* Philadelphia: Wolters Kluwer Health | Lippincott Williams & Wilkins.

Pneumonia

Pneumonia is the infection of the lower respiratory tract caused by a variety of microorganisms including bacteria, viruses, fungi, protozoa, and parasites. Pneumonia is common and is associated with considerable mortality and morbidity. It is the most common infectious cause of death and the eighth leading cause of death in the United States.

A wide variety of ways exist to classify pneumonia, including by its microbiologic cause, host condition, and host setting. Overlap occurs in how specific pneumonias are classified because they may occur in differing settings. Currently, the most common classifications for pneumonia are:

- Community-acquired pneumonia (CAP): Occurs in the community-dwelling person or within the first 48 hours after hospitalization or institutionalization. Higher incidence in winter and early spring, in men and African Americans.
- Hospital-acquired (nosocomial) pneumonia (HAP): Onset of pneumonia symptoms more than 48 hours after admission in patients with no evidence of infection at the time of hospitalization.

- Ventilator-associated pneumonia (VAP): Type of HAP associated with endotracheal intubation and mechanical ventilation of at least 48 hours duration.
- Health care-associated pneumonia (HCAP): Occurs in patients who have had extensive health care contact, such as residents of nursing homes or long-term care facilities, acute care hospitalization for 2 or more days within in the last 90 days, IV antibiotic therapy, wound care, or chemotherapy or attended a hospital or hemodialysis clinic within the last 30 days.
- Pneumonia in the immunocompromised host: Occurs with use of corticosteroids or immunosuppressive agents, chemotherapy, nutritional depletion, use of broad-spectrum antimicrobial agents, AIDS, genetic immune disorders, and long-term mechanical ventilation.

PATHOPHYSIOLOGY

Pneumonia can be caused by normal flora present in patients with altered resistance; aspiration of flora from the nasopharynx or oropharynx; inhalation of airborne microorganisms from sneezing, coughing, or talking; from contaminated water sources or respiratory equipment, or from blood borne organisms trapped in the pulmonary capillary beds.

Once the microorganisms reach the lower airways and alveoli, their presence activates an inflammatory response causing migration of WBCs (mainly neutrophils), plasma fluid, and immune complexes into the alveoli, filling them with exudative liquids and cellular debris. This causes alveolar edema and lung tissue consolidation. Additional damage can occur when some microorganisms release toxins that further damage respiratory cells. Alveolar and bronchial tissues become swollen and infiltrated with WBCs, causing consolidation of lung tissue that can be seen on X-ray. The damage caused by toxins and inflammatory mediators and immune complexes interferes with the diffusion or oxygen and carbon dioxide, leading to clinical manifestations of pneumonia.

P

RISK FACTORS

- Smoking
- Alcohol abuse and malnutrition
- Chronic underlying disorders such as renal failure
- Chronic obstructive pulmonary disease
- Severe acute illness, such as pulmonary edema
- Suppressed immune system
- Immobility, acute-care hospitalization, resident of long-term care facility
- Family members with drug-resistant organism
- Age older than 65 years

CLINICAL MANIFESTATIONS AND ASSESSMENT

Clinical features vary depending on the causative organism and the patient's disease.

- Classic clinical manifestations of pneumonia are fever, cough (productive or nonproductive), dyspnea, and leukocytosis.
- Rigors (shaking chills), pleuritic chest pain, tachypnea, use of accessory muscles, tachycardia, fatigue, and anorexia may be noted.
- Some patients initially exhibit an upper respiratory tract infection (nasal congestion, sore throat), with gradual and nonspecific onset of symptoms. The predominant symptoms may then be headache, low-grade fever, pleuritic pain, myalgia, rash, and pharyngitis.

DIAGNOSTIC METHODS

- History, particularly recent respiratory infection, physical examination
- Chest X-rays, blood and sputum cultures, Gram stain
- Rapid bacterial antigen testing of urine or oropharyngeal swabs
- Arterial blood gas (ABG) analysis, pulse oximetry

MEDICAL AND NURSING MANAGEMENT

Pharmacologic Therapy

The treatment of pneumonia includes prompt administration of the appropriate antibiotic based on Gram stain results and antibiotic guidelines (resistance patterns, risk factors, etiology must be considered).

- Emerging data demonstrate that shorter durations of antibiotics produce good clinical responses and fewer emergences of multidrug-resistant (MDR) pathogens.
- Nebulized bronchodilators or mucolytics

Nursing Interventions

- Provide oxygen therapy to prevent or treat hypoxemia and tissue hypoxia.
- Observe for manifestations of hypoxemia: Agitation, anxiety, confusion and disorientation, lethargy, tachycardia, arrhythmia, and changes in blood pressure. Cyanosis is a late sign of hypoxemia.
- Supportive treatment includes hydration, antipyretics, nutritional assessment and support, DVT prophylaxis.
- Respiratory support may include high inspiratory oxygen concentrations, endotracheal intubation, and mechanical ventilation.

Gerontologic Considerations

Pneumonia in elderly patients may occur as a primary diagnosis or as a complication of a chronic disease. Pulmonary infections in older people frequently are difficult to treat and result in a higher mortality rate than in younger people. General deterioration, weakness, abdominal symptoms, anorexia, confusion, tachycardia, and tachypnea may signal the onset of pneumonia. The diagnosis of pneumonia may be missed because the classic symptoms of cough, chest pain, sputum production, and fever may be absent or masked in elderly patients. Abnormal breath sounds may be caused by decreased mobility, decreased lung volumes, or other respiratory function changes. Chest X-rays may be needed to differentiate chronic HF from pneumonia.

Supportive treatment includes hydration and observing for fluid overload in the elderly. Supplemental oxygen therapy and vaccination against pneumococcal and influenza infections is recommended.

Prevention

Pneumococcal vaccination has been demonstrated to prevent pneumonia in otherwise healthy populations by 50%. Vaccination is advised for persons 2 to 64 years of age with chronic illnesses and in people 65 year or older.

NURSING PROCESS

The Patient With Pneumonia

Assessment

- Assess for fever, chills, dyspnea, and cough.
- Perform respiratory assessment for pleuritic-type pain, fatigue, tachypnea, use of accessory muscles for breathing, tachycardia, coughing, and purulent sputum.
- Monitor the patient for changes in temperature and pulse; amount, odor, and color of secretions; frequency and severity of cough; degree of tachypnea or SOB; changes in physical assessment findings (primarily assessed by inspecting and auscultating the chest); and changes in the chest X-ray findings.
- Assess the elderly patient for change in mental status, dehydration, excessive fatigue, and concomitant HF.

Nursing Diagnoses

- Ineffective airway clearance related to copious tracheobronchial secretions
- Impaired gas exchange
- Activity intolerance related to impaired respiratory function

- Risk for deficient fluid volume related to fever, rapid respiratory rate, and sepsis
- Imbalanced nutrition, less than body requirements
- Deficient knowledge about treatment regimen and preventive health measures

Planning

The major goals of the patient may include improved airway patency, rest to conserve energy, maintenance of fluid volume, maintenance of adequate nutrition, an understanding of the treatment protocol and preventive measures, and absence of complications.

Nursing Interventions

Improving Airway Patency

- Encourage hydration: 2 to 3 L of fluid/day to thin and loosen secretions.
- Provide humidified air or oxygen using high-humidity face mask.
- Encourage patient to cough effectively, and provide correct positioning, chest physiotherapy, and incentive spirometry. Provide nasotracheal suctioning for weak or ineffective cough.
- Monitor effectiveness of oxygen therapy.

✴ *N u r s i n g   A l e r t*

In general, the dependent lung or "good lung down" is associated with improved perfusion. However, any position for a prolonged period of time is associated with stagnation of secretions and pressure on the dependent lung, increasing the risk of atelectasis in the dependent lung. Therefore, the nurse turns the patient at regular intervals.

Promoting Rest and Conserving Energy

- Encourage the debilitated patient to rest and avoid overexertion and exacerbation of symptoms. Engage in moderate activity early in treatment.

(continues on page 578)

P

- Assist patient into a comfortable position, such as semi-Fowler's, to promote rest and breathing; change positions frequently to enhance secretion clearance and pulmonary ventilation and perfusion.

Promoting Fluid Intake and Maintaining Nutrition

- Encourage fluids intake of 2 L/day unless contraindicated.
- Nutritional supplement drinks with fluids, electrolytes, and protein may be prescribed for anorexia secondary to SOB and fatigue.
- Administer IV fluids and nutrients, if necessary.

Promoting Patients' Knowledge

- Instruct on cause of pneumonia, management of symptoms, signs and symptoms that should be reported to the health care provider or nurse, and the need for follow-up.
- The patient also needs information about factors that may have contributed to development of pneumonia and strategies to promote recovery and prevent recurrence.
- Provide written instructions using alternative formats for patients with hearing or vision loss, if necessary. The patient may require instructions and explanations to be repeated several times.

Monitoring Symptoms After Initiation of Therapy

- Patients usually begin to respond to treatment within 24 to 48 hours after antibiotic therapy.
- Assess for deterioration of condition, persistent or recurrent fever, medication allergy (rash, medication resistance, pleural effusion).
- Failure of pneumonia to resolve or persistent symptoms raises suspicion of other disorders, such as lung cancer.
- Monitor for respiratory failure, shock, multisystem failure.
- Monitor for pleural effusion, atelectasis.
- Monitor for superinfection related to overgrowth of normal flora (ie, white coating of tongue or oral mucosa, vaginal discharge, and diarrhea).

Promoting Health

- Encourage the patient to stop smoking, to avoid stress, fatigue, sudden changes in temperature, and excessive alcohol intake, all of which lower resistance to pneumonia.
- Review principles of adequate nutrition and rest; an episode of pneumonia may make a patient susceptible to recurring respiratory tract infections.
- Recommend influenza vaccine (Pneumovax) to all patients at risk.

Evaluation

- Demonstrates improved airway patency, as evidenced by adequate oxygenation by pulse oximetry or ABG analysis, normal temperature, normal breath sounds, and effective coughing
- Rests and conserves energy by limiting activities and remaining in bed while symptomatic and then slowly increasing activities
- Maintains adequate hydration, as evidenced by an adequate fluid intake and urine output and normal skin turgor
- Consumes adequate dietary intake, as evidenced by maintenance or increase in body weight without excess fluid gain
- States explanation for management strategies
- Complies with management strategies
- Exhibits no complications:
  - Reports productive cough diminishing over time
  - Has absence of signs or symptoms of shock, respiratory failure, or pleural effusion
  - Remains oriented and aware of surroundings
  - Maintains or increases weight

For more information, see Chapter 10 in Pellico, L.H. (2013). *Focus on adult health: Medical-surgical nursing.* Philadelphia: Wolters Kluwer Health | Lippincott Williams & Wilkins.

Pneumothorax and Hemothorax

Pneumothorax occurs when the parietal or visceral pleura is punctured and the pleural space is exposed to positive atmospheric pressure. Hemothorax refers to collection of blood in the pleural space resulting from torn intercostal vessels, lacerations of the great vessels, or lacerations of the lungs.

TYPES OF PNEUMOTHORAX

Types of pneumothorax include simple, traumatic, and tension pneumothorax.

Simple Pneumothorax

A simple, or spontaneous, pneumothorax occurs when air enters the pleural space through a ruptured bleb (blister) or a bronchopleural fistula. This may occur in an apparently healthy person (generally in young men), in the absence of trauma. It may be associated with bullous lung disease such as emphysema or pulmonary fibrosis.

Traumatic Pneumothorax

A traumatic pneumothorax occurs when air enters the pleural space from a wound in the chest wall or laceration in the lung. It may result from blunt trauma, penetrating chest or abdominal trauma, or diaphragmatic tears. Traumatic pneumothorax may occur during thoracentesis, transbronchial lung biopsy, insertion of a subclavian line, or from barotrauma from mechanical ventilation. A traumatic pneumothorax resulting from major injury to the chest is often accompanied by hemothorax. Open pneumothorax, a form of traumatic pneumothorax, occurs when a wound in the chest wall is large enough to allow air to be "sucked" freely in and out of the thoracic cavity with each breath.

⚡ N U R S I N G A L E R T

Traumatic open pneumothorax calls for emergency interventions. Stopping the flow of air through the opening in the chest wall is a life-saving measure.

Tension Pneumothorax

A tension pneumothorax occurs when air is drawn into the pleural space from a lacerated lung or through a small opening or wound in the chest wall and is trapped. With each breath, positive pressure or tension builds up in the pleural space, collapsing the affected lung. The heart, great vessels, and the trachea shift toward the unaffected side (mediastinal shift), causing a life-threatening situation. Poor cardiac output, impairment of peripheral circulation, and cardiac arrest may ensue.

CLINICAL MANIFESTATIONS AND ASSESSMENT

Signs and symptoms associated with pneumothorax depend on its size and cause:

- Pain that develops suddenly and may be pleuritic
- Respiratory distress and chest discomfort varies from minimal with small pneumothorax; acute respiratory distress if large.
- Anxiety, dyspnea, air hunger, use of accessory muscles with severe hypoxemia
- In a simple pneumothorax, the trachea is midline, expansion of the chest is decreased, breath sounds may be diminished, and percussion of the chest may reveal normal sounds or hyperresonance depending on the size of the pneumothorax.
- In a tension pneumothorax, the trachea shifts away from the affected side, chest expansion may be decreased or fixed in a hyperexpansion state, breath sounds are diminished or absent, and percussion to the affected side is hyperresonant. Air hunger, agitation, increasing hypoxemia, central cyanosis, hypotension, and tachycardia are present.

MEDICAL AND NURSING MANAGEMENT

The goal is evacuation of air or blood from the pleural space.

Surgical Intervention

- A thoracostomy tube (chest tube) is used to evacuate any accumulated air or fluid.
- A small chest tube or pigtail catheter may be inserted near the second intercostal space for simple pneumothorax.
- Larger pneumothoraces, especially if there is fluid or blood present, are managed with larger sized tubes (32 to 36 French), placed in the fourth or fifth intercostal space, midaxillary line.
- In an emergency, a tension pneumothorax can be decompressed quickly by inserting a large-bore needle (14-gauge) at the second intercostal space, midclavicular line on the affected side to relieve the pressure and vent the positive pressure to the external environment.
- If more than 1,500 mL of blood is aspirated initially by thoracentesis (or is the initial chest tube output), or if chest tube output continues at greater than 200 mL/hr, thoracotomy is performed.
- Observe for subcutaneous emphysema, indicating air entering tissue spaces and passing under the skin. A crackling sensation is palpated, and the face, neck, body, and scrotum become misshapen. A tracheostomy is indicated if the airway is threatened.
- Assist in chest tube insertion; maintain chest drainage or water-seal.

For more information, see Chapter 10 in Pellico, L.H. (2013). *Focus on adult health: Medical-surgical nursing.* Philadelphia: Wolters Kluwer Health | Lippincott Williams & Wilkins.

Polycythemia

Polycythemia, literally meaning "too many cells in the blood," refers to an increased volume of erythrocytes. The term refers to a hematocrit level of more than 55% in men or more than 50% in women. Polycythemia is classified as either primary or secondary.

POLYCYTHEMIA VERA (PRIMARY)

Polycythemia vera, or primary polycythemia, is a myeloproliferative disorder in which the myeloid stem cells have escaped normal control mechanisms. The bone marrow is hypercellular, and the erythrocyte, leukocyte, and platelet counts in the peripheral blood are elevated. Eventually, the bone marrow may become fibrotic and unable to produce as many cells ("burnt out" or spent phase). The disease evolves into myeloid metaplasia with myelofibrosis (MDS) or refractory acute myeloid leukemia (AML).

CLINICAL MANIFESTATIONS AND ASSESSMENT

- Patients typically have a ruddy complexion and splenomegaly.
- Symptoms are due to the increased blood volume (headache, dizziness, tinnitus, fatigue, paresthesias, and blurred vision) or to increased blood viscosity (angina, claudication, dyspnea, and thrombophlebitis), particularly in the presence of atherosclerosis.
- Blood pressure and uric acid are often elevated.
- Pruritus, possibly secondary to histamine release, may occur; exposure to water triggers pruritus (aquagenic pruritus).
- Erythromelalgia (a burning sensation in the fingers and toes) may be reported and is partially relieved by cooling.

DIAGNOSTIC METHODS

- Blood counts
- *JAK 2* mutation is present in more than 95% of patients.

MEDICAL AND NURSING MANAGEMENT

The objective of management is to reduce the high red blood cell mass.

- Phlebotomy, to maintain a hematocrit level of less than 45% in men and less than 42% in women and to deplete the iron stores, improves survival.

Pharmacologic Therapy

- Chemotherapeutic agents such as hydroxyurea, to suppress marrow function, may be administered (may increase risk for leukemia).
- Interferon alfa-2b (Intron-A) is given to manage pruritus; may be difficult for patients to tolerate because of its frequent side effects of flu-like syndrome and depression.
- Antiplatelet therapy such as ASA should be used with caution secondary to the underlying risk of bleeding in these patients. Aspirin or ASA may reduce the pain of erythromelalgia (redness, warmth, and burning pain of the extremities).
- Allopurinol is used to prevent gout when the uric acid level is elevated.

Nursing Management

The nurse's role is primarily that of educator.

- Assess for risk factors for thrombotic complications: Smoking, obesity, and poorly controlled HTN. Teach patient to recognize signs and symptoms of thrombosis.
- Prevent DVT by encouraging activity and walking frequently on long airplane flights. Avoid crossing the legs and wearing tight or restrictive clothing.
- Advise patient to avoid aspirin and medications containing aspirin if history of bleeding is present.
- Advise patient to minimize alcohol intake.
- Advise patient to avoid iron and vitamins containing iron.
- Suggest a cool or tepid bath for pruritus, along with cocoa butter–based lotions and bath products, add colloidal oatmeal to bath water, or take ASA to relieve itching.

COMPLICATIONS

- Cerebrovascular accident (CVA; stroke)
- Myocardial infarction
- Thrombotic complications
- Bleeding: Nosebleeds, ulcers/ GI bleeding, hematuria, and intracranial hemorrhage

SECONDARY POLYCYTHEMIA

Secondary polycythemia is caused by excessive production of erythropoietin. This may occur in response to a reduction of oxygen such as in cigarette smoking, COPD, cyanotic heart disease, or living at high altitude. It can result from certain hemoglobinopathies in which the hemoglobin has an abnormally high affinity for oxygen, or from a neoplasm, such as renal cell carcinoma.

MEDICAL AND NURSING MANAGEMENT

- Management of secondary polycythemia may not be necessary.
- When management is necessary, the goal is to treat the primary conditions.
- If the cause cannot be corrected, therapeutic phlebotomy may be performed in symptomatic patients.

For more information, see Chapter 20 in Pellico, L.H. (2013). *Focus on adult health: Medical-surgical nursing.* Philadelphia: Wolters Kluwer Health | Lippincott Williams & Wilkins.

Prostatitis

Prostatitis is an inflammation of the prostate gland that is caused by infectious agents or other conditions (eg, urethral stricture, prostatic hyperplasia).

P

PATHOPHYSIOLOGY

Escherichia coli is the most commonly isolated organism. Microorganisms are usually carried to the prostate from the urethra. Prostatitis syndromes are classified as:

- Acute bacterial (type I), chronic bacterial (type II)
- Chronic prostatitis/chronic pelvic pain syndrome (CP/CPPS) (type IIIa)
- Inflammatory, chronic prostatitis/chronic pelvic pain syndrome (CP/CPPS) (type IIIb)
- Noninflammatory and asymptomatic inflammatory prostatitis (type IV)

CLINICAL MANIFESTATIONS AND ASSESSMENT

- Symptoms of prostatitis may include perineal discomfort, dysuria, urgency, frequency, and pain with or after ejaculation.
- Prostatodynia (pain in the prostate) is manifested by pain on voiding or perineal pain without evidence of inflammation or bacterial growth in the prostate fluid.
- Acute bacterial prostatitis may produce sudden fever, chills, perineal, rectal or low back pain, dysuria, frequency, urgency, and nocturia.
- Chronic bacterial prostatitis produces mild symptoms of frequency, dysuria, and occasionally, urethral discharge.

DIAGNOSTIC FINDINGS

- Digital rectal examination (DRE) after collection of a urine sample commonly reveals many WBCs.
- Avoid DRE if acute prostatitis is suspected due to risk of causing bacteremia and septicemia.

MEDICAL AND NURSING MANAGEMENT

The goal of therapy for acute bacterial prostatitis is to avoid the complications of abscess formation and septicemia.

- Complete blood count (CBC), blood and urine culture
- A prostate-specific antigen (PSA) test may not be obtained since in many patients the acute inflammatory process causes elevation. However, it can also provide a means to track the success of treatment, as it should lessen with the use of antibiotics.

Pharmacologic Therapy

- Antibiotics, such as trimethoprim-sulfamethoxazole or a fluoroquinolone, are administered.
- Analgesic agents, antispasmodic medications, bladder sedatives, and stool softeners
- Alpha-adrenergic blockers such as tamsulosin (Flomax) promote relaxation of the bladder and prostate.

Nursing Management

- Supportive, nonpharmacologic therapies may be prescribed (eg, biofeedback, pelvic floor training, physical therapy, sitz baths, stool softeners).
- Administer antibiotics as prescribed; instruct patient to complete course of antibiotics.
- Promote comfort with analgesics and sitz baths for 10 to 20 minutes several times daily.
- Caution patient to avoid activities that results in repetitive perineal trauma, such as mountain biking.
- Teach patient to recognize recurrent signs and symptoms of prostatitis.
- Encourage fluids to satisfy thirst but do not "force" them, because effective drug levels must be maintained.
- Instruct patient to avoid foods and drinks that have diuretic action or increase prostatic secretions, including alcohol, coffee, tea, chocolate, cola, and spices.

- Advise patient to avoid sitting for long periods to minimize discomfort.

COMPLICATIONS

- Prostatic swelling
- Urinary retention
- Epididymitis
- Bacteremia
- Pyelonephritis

> For more information, see Chapter 34 in Pellico, L.H. (2013).
> *Focus on adult health: Medical-surgical nursing.* Philadelphia:
> Wolters Kluwer Health | Lippincott Williams & Wilkins.

Psoriasis

Psoriasis is a chronic, noninfectious, inflammatory disease of the skin that stems from a hereditary defect that causes overproduction of keratin. Psoriasis has a tendency to improve and then recur periodically throughout life.

PATHOPHYSIOLOGY

Epidermal cells are produced at a rate that is about six to nine times faster than normal. The basal layer of the skin cells divides too quickly, and the newly formed cells move so rapidly to the skin surface that they become evident as profuse scales or plaques of epidermal tissue. The psoriatic epidermal cell may travel from the basal cell layer of the epidermis to the stratum corneum and be cast off in 3 to 4 days, which is in sharp contrast to the normal 26 to 28 days. Current evidence supports an immunologic basis for the disease, although genetic makeup and environmental stimuli may trigger the onset. Periods of emotional stress and anxiety aggravate the condition, and trauma, infections, and seasonal and hormonal changes also are trigger factors.

RISK FACTORS

- Hereditary component
- European ancestry
- Aged 15 to 35

CLINICAL MANIFESTATIONS AND ASSESSMENT

Symptoms range from a cosmetic annoyance to a physically disabling and disfiguring disorder.

- Lesions appear as red, raised patches of skin covered with silvery scales.
- If scales are scraped away, the dark red base of lesion is exposed, with multiple bleeding points.
- Patches are dry and may itch.
- A variation of this condition, guttate (drop shaped) psoriasis, consists of 1 cm lesions, scattered like raindrops over the body. Believed to be associated with a recent streptococcal throat infection.
- Most common areas affected include the scalp, extensor surface of the elbows and knees, the lower part of the back, and the genitalia. Bilateral symmetry is a feature of psoriasis.
- The condition may involve nail pitting, discoloration, crumbling beneath the free edges, and separation of the nail plate.
- When psoriasis occurs on the palms and soles, it can cause pustular lesions called *palmar pustular psoriasis.*

DIAGNOSTIC METHODS

- Presence of classic plaque-type lesions confirms the diagnosis.
- Skin biopsy is of little value as lesions change rapidly.
- Signs of nail and scalp involvement and positive family history

P

MEDICAL AND NURSING MANAGEMENT

Goals of management are to slow the rapid turnover of epidermis, promote resolution of the psoriatic lesions, and control the natural cycles of the disease. There is no known cure. The therapeutic approach should be understandable, cosmetically acceptable, and not too disruptive of lifestyle. First, any precipitating or aggravating factors are addressed. An assessment is made of lifestyle, because psoriasis is significantly affected by stress.

Removal of Scales

- The most important principle of psoriasis treatment is gentle removal of scales.
- Oils such as olive, mineral, Aveeno Oilated Oatmeal bath, or coal tar preparations can be added to the bath water, and a soft brush used to gently scrub the plaques.
- After bathing, the application of emollient creams containing alpha-hydroxy acids (Lac-Hydrin, Penederm) or salicylic acid will continue to soften thick scales.

Pharmacologic Therapy

Four types of therapy are now commonly used: Topical, intra-lesional, oral, and injectable.

Topical Therapy

- Topical treatment is used to slow the overactive epidermis without affecting other tissue. Medications may be in the form of lotions, ointments, pastes, creams, and shampoos.
- Topical corticosteroids of varying strengths are used to reduce inflammation; occlusive dressings may be applied for up to 8 hours.
- Nonsteroidal treatments include calcipotriene (Dovonex), a form of vitamin D_2; not recommended for use by elderly patients because of their more fragile skin.
- Tazarotene (Tazorac), a retinoid, decreases cell division. This is a Category X drug in pregnancy, indicating evidence of fetal risk; a negative pregnancy test should be obtained prior to use in childbearing women.

- Intralesional injections of triamcinolone acetonide (Aristocort, Kenalog-10, Trymex) can be administered into highly visible or isolated patches of psoriasis resistant to other forms of therapy.
- Methotrexate, a cytotoxic preparation, may be used for extensive psoriasis not responding to other forms of therapy. The patient should avoid alcohol and have hepatic, renal, and hematopoietic functions assessed. It should not be used during pregnancy.
- Hydroxyurea (Hydrea) inhibits cell replication by affecting DNA synthesis.
- Cyclosporine A, a cyclic peptide used to prevent rejection of transplanted organs, has shown some success in treating severe, therapy-resistant cases of psoriasis. Its use is limited due to development of HTN and nephrotoxicity.
- Oral retinoids, such as Etretinate, are synthetic derivatives of vitamin A and its metabolite, vitamin A acid. Etretinate modulates the growth and differentiation of epithelial tissue and is useful for severe pustular or erythrodermic psoriasis. This drug has a long half-life and should not be used by women with childbearing potential.

Photochemotherapy

- A psoralen (phototoxic) medication (eg, methoxsalen) combined with ultraviolet-A (PUVA) light therapy may be used for severely debilitating psoriasis. This has been associated with long-term risks of skin cancer, cataracts, and premature aging of the skin.
- Ultraviolet B (UVB) light therapy may be used to treat generalized plaques.
- Patient may expose themselves to sunlight, if access to above treatments are not feasible.

NURSING ALERT

Biologic agents act by inhibiting activation and migration of T cells, slowing postsecretory cytokines, or inducing immune deviation. These agents include infliximab (Remicade), etanercept (Enbrel), efalizumab (Raptiva), alefacept (Amevive), and adalimumab (Humira), may be used. Biological agents have significant side effects, making close monitoring essential.

COMPLICATIONS

- Asymmetric rheumatoid factor–negative arthritis of multiple joints
- Erythrodermic psoriasis, an exfoliative psoriatic state, involves the total body surface

For more information, see Chapter 52 in Pellico, L.H. (2013). *Focus on adult health: Medical-surgical nursing.* Philadelphia: Wolters Kluwer Health | Lippincott Williams & Wilkins.

Pulmonary Edema, Acute

Pulmonary edema is the abnormal accumulation of fluid in the interstitial spaces and alveoli of the lungs. Pulmonary edema can be categorized into two subsets depending on the etiology: cardiogenic and noncardiogenic.

PATHOPHYSIOLOGY

Cardiogenic pulmonary edema is an acute event that results from HF. It can occur acutely, as with MI, or it can occur as an exacerbation of chronic HF. With increased resistance to left ventricular filling, blood backs up into the pulmonary circulation. The patient quickly develops pulmonary edema, sometimes called *flash pulmonary edema,* from the blood volume overload in the lungs. Pulmonary edema can also be caused by noncardiac disorders, such as renal failure and other conditions that cause the body to retain fluid. The pathophysiology is similar to that seen in HF, in that the left ventricle cannot handle the volume overload, and blood volume and pressure builds up in the left atrium. The rapid increase in atrial pressure results in an acute increase in pulmonary venous pressure, causing increased hydrostatic pressure that forces fluid out of the pulmonary capillaries and into the interstitial spaces and alveoli. Impaired lymphatic drainage contributes to the accumulation of fluid in the lung tissues.

The classic symptom of pulmonary edema is frothy pink (blood-tinged) sputum. Because of the fluid within the alveoli, gas exchange is impaired, causing hypoxemia.

CLINICAL MANIFESTATIONS AND ASSESSMENT

- As a result of decreased cerebral oxygenation, the patient becomes increasingly restless and anxious.
- Sudden onset of breathlessness; sense of suffocation; cough that produces a large amount of pink, frothy sputum; cold and moist skin, cyanotic nail beds; a weak and rapid pulse; pulmonary rales; expiratory wheezing; and distended neck veins is noted.
- The patient, nearly suffocated by the blood-tinged, frothy fluid filling the alveoli, is literally drowning in secretions. The situation demands emergent action.

For noncardiogenic pulmonary edema, see "Acute Respiratory Distress Syndrome" on pages 24–27.

MEDICAL AND NURSING MANAGEMENT

- Management of symptoms follows the similar clinical management plan for treating acute decompensated HF: Oxygen, diuretics, pharmacologic preload and afterload reduction, and possibly hemodynamic monitoring.
- Additional therapies may include early rescue with noninvasive mask ventilation and bronchodilator therapy with select beta$_2$ agonist medications like albuterol.

For more information, see Chapter 15 in Pellico, L.H. (2013). *Focus on adult health: Medical-surgical nursing.* Philadelphia: Wolters Kluwer Health | Lippincott Williams & Wilkins.

Pulmonary Embolism

P

Pulmonary embolism refers to the obstruction of the pulmonary artery or one of its branches by a thrombus (or thrombi) that originates somewhere in the venous system or in the right side of the heart. Hospitalized patients are at a high risk for PE.

PATHOPHYSIOLOGY

Most commonly, PE is due to a blood clot or thrombus. Other types of emboli include air, fat, amniotic fluid, tumor cells, intravenously injected particulates, and sepsis (from bacterial invasion of the thrombus). Venous thrombosis can result from slowing of blood flow (stasis) secondary to damage to the blood vessel wall or changes in the blood coagulation mechanism. In atrial fibrillation, blood stagnates in the fibrillating atria, forming clots that may travel into the pulmonary circulation.

When a thrombus completely or partially obstructs a pulmonary artery or its branches, the area is ventilated but receives little or no blood flow, which impairs gas exchange. Vasoactive substances are released from the clot causing vasoconstriction, bronchoconstriction, and the loss of alveolar surfactant. Increased workload of the right ventricle, atelectasis, and hypoxemia result. Right ventricular failure occurs, leading to a decrease in cardiac output, and shock develop.

RISK FACTORS

- Trauma
- Arrhythmia
- Surgery
- Pregnancy
- Heart failure
- Malignancy and hypercoagulable states
- Age older than 50 years
- Prolonged immobility

CLINICAL MANIFESTATIONS AND ASSESSMENT

- Symptoms depend on the size of the thrombus and the area of the pulmonary artery occlusion.
- Dyspnea is the most common symptom. Tachypnea is the most frequent sign.
- Chest pain, cough, leg pain, hemoptysis, and palpitations occur.
- Tachypnea, crackles, tachycardia, and presence of an S_4 heart sound, split S_2, and cyanosis (hypoxemia) are common signs.
- Typically, patients report sudden onset of pain and/or swelling and warmth of the proximal or distal extremity, skin discoloration, and superficial vein distention.
- Shock can develop with massive PEs ("saddle" embolisms) or in patients with preexisting HF.
- Clinical picture may mimic that of bronchopneumonia or HF.
- In atypical instances, PE causes few signs and symptoms, whereas in other instances it mimics various other cardiopulmonary disorders.

DIAGNOSTIC METHODS

- Because the symptoms of PE can vary, a diagnostic workup is performed to rule out other diseases.
- The initial diagnostic workup may include chest X-ray, ECG, peripheral vascular studies (ultrasound, venogram), ABG analysis, D-dimer assay, and ventilation–perfusion (VQ) scan. A ventilation and perfusion scan was once the second choice for diagnosis of a PE (with pulmonary angiogram [discussed below] considered the best diagnostic procedure). It is still used, especially in facilities that do not have access to a spiral CT scanner.
- Spiral CT scan of the lung with contrast or pulmonary arteriogram may be performed.
- Pulmonary angiography was considered the best method to diagnose PE; however, it may not be feasible, cost-effective, or easily performed, especially with critically ill patients.

PREVENTION

- Early ambulation or active leg exercises in patients on bed rest
- Application of sequential compression devices or elastic compression stockings
- Prophylactic anticoagulant therapy for patients over 40 who are undergoing major elective abdominal or thoracic surgery where hemostasis is adequate

MEDICAL AND NURSING MANAGEMENT

Immediate objective is to stabilize the cardiopulmonary system.

- Oxygen is administered immediately to relieve hypoxemia, respiratory distress, and central cyanosis.
- Intravenous infusion lines are established for medications or fluids that will be needed.
- A perfusion scan, hemodynamic measurements, and ABG determinations are performed. Spiral (helical) CT or pulmonary angiography may be performed.
- Hypotension is treated with IV fluid resuscitation, vasopressors (dopamine, norepinephrine), or inotropic support (dobutamine).
- The ECG is monitored continuously for arrhythmias and right ventricular failure, which may occur suddenly.
- Blood is drawn for serum electrolytes, complete blood cell count, and coagulation studies (PT, INR, PTT, D-dimer).
- Intubation and mechanical ventilation is initiated if clinical assessment and ABGs indicate the need.
- An indwelling urinary catheter is inserted to monitor urinary output when hypotension results from a massive embolism.

Pharmacologic Therapy

- Digitalis glycosides, IV diuretics, and antiarrhythmic agents are administered when appropriate.
- Small doses of IV morphine or sedatives are administered to relieve patient anxiety, alleviate chest discomfort, improve tolerance of the endotracheal tube, and to ease adaptation to the mechanical ventilator.

- Intravenous thrombolytic agents (tissue plasminogen activase: Alteplase or Reteplase) maybe used in patients who are hemodynamically unstable (hypotension, ECG strain patterns), to lyse the clot.
- Initiation of low-molecular-weight heparins (SC route) or IV heparin should be considered.

Anticoagulation Therapy

- Anticoagulant therapy, using unfractionated or low-molecular-weight heparins, is the primary method for managing acute DVT and PE. Heparins prevent recurrence of emboli, but do not effect emboli already present.
- Enoxaparin has the advantage over heparin as its levels do not need to be monitored daily and IV access is not an issue.
- Therapy may be changed to an oral regimen, such as warfarin, as soon as the patient is able to take oral medications. Heparin is continued until the international normalized ratio (INR) is therapeutic (2.0 to 3.0)
- Lepirudin (Refludan) and argatroban, direct thrombin inhibitors, are alternatives for patients in whom heparin or heparinoids are contraindicated (eg, patients with heparin-induced thrombocytopenia [HIT]).
- Patients must continue to take some form of anticoagulation for at least 3 to 6 months after the embolic event.
- Major side effects include bleeding anywhere in the body and anaphylactic reaction resulting in shock or death. Other side effects include fever, abnormal liver function, and allergic skin reaction.

Thrombolytic Therapy

- Thrombolytic therapy may include urokinase, streptokinase, alteplase, anistreplase, and reteplase for patient with severe hemodynamic instability. Indications include hypotension, RV dysfunction, patent foramen ovale, large or saddle embolism, or significant hypoxemia despite oxygen supplementation.
- Bleeding is a significant side effect; nonessential invasive procedures are avoided.
- After the thrombolytic infusion is completed, anticoagulant therapy is initiated.

P

Surgical Management

- A surgical embolectomy is rarely performed but may be indicated if the patient has a massive PE or hemodynamic instability, or if there are contraindications to thrombolytic therapy.
- Venous catheter embolectomy via rheolytic (injection of pressured saline) or rotating blades can be used to break up clots in the pulmonary vasculature. An inferior vena cava filter is usually inserted at the time of surgery to prevent recurrence.

Nursing Management

Minimizing the Risk of Pulmonary Embolism

The nurse must have a high degree of suspicion for PE in all patients, but particularly in those with conditions predisposing to a slowing of venous return.

Preventing Thrombus Formation

- Encourage early ambulation and active and passive leg exercises.
- Instruct patient to move legs in a "pumping" exercise to increase venous flow.
- Advise patient to avoid prolonged sitting, immobility, crossing the legs, and constrictive clothing.
- Do not permit dangling of legs and feet in a dependent position; instead, rest the feet on the floor or chair.
- Do not leave peripheral catheters for parenteral therapy or central venous catheters in place for prolonged periods.
- Assess potential for PE through health history, family history, medication record, and pain or discomfort in extremities for unilateral leg warmth, redness, and inflammation.

Monitoring Anticoagulant and Thrombolytic Therapy

- During thrombolytic infusion, the patient remains on bed rest, vital signs are assessed every 15 minutes for 2 hours, then every 2 hours for 4hours. Limit invasive procedures.
- Partial thromboplastin time (PTT) testing is performed every 6 hours after thrombolytics or heparins are started.

☀ *N U R S I N G   A L E R T*

The activated partial thromboplastin time (aPTT) is a more sensitive test than the PTT for monitoring of heparin therapy. A normal aPTT is 21 to 35 seconds. The goal of heparin therapy is to extend the aPTT to 2 or 2.5 the normal level. When the aPTT is over 70 seconds, the risk for spontaneously bleeding increases. The nurse follows hospital protocol but antici-pates that if the aPTT is over 90 seconds, the anticoagulant is stopped for 1 hour and restarted per protocol, typically at a lower rate. If no protocols are available, the nurse contacts the provider immediately.

- Measure INR for patients receiving Coumadin. The goal of therapy is to extend the INR to 2 to 3. Teach patient the impor-tance of monitoring anticoagulant therapy.

☀ *N U R S I N G   A L E R T*

Any INR of over 3.6 is a critical value that necessitates notification of the patient's provider.

Managing Pain

- Pain is usually pleuritic; place patient in semi-Fowler's posi-tion, turn and reposition frequently.
- Administer opioid analgesics as prescribed for severe pain.

Managing Oxygen Therapy

- Assess the patient frequently for signs of hypoxemia, and moni-tor the pulse oximetry to evaluate effectiveness of therapy.
- Assist patient with deep breathing and incentive spirometry to prevent atelectasis and improve ventilation.
- Nebulizer therapy or percussion and postural drainage may be necessary for management of secretions.

Relieving Anxiety

- Encourage patient to express feelings and concerns.
- Answer questions concisely and accurately.
- Explain therapy, and describe how to recognize untoward effects early.

Monitoring for Complications

Be alert for the potential complication of cardiogenic shock or right ventricular failure.

Providing Postoperative Care

- Measure pulmonary arterial pressure and urinary output.
- Assess insertion site of arterial catheter for hematoma formation and infection.
- Maintain blood pressure to ensure perfusion of vital organs.
- Encourage isometric exercises, antiembolism stockings, and walking when permitted out of bed; elevate foot of bed when patient is resting.
- Discourage sitting; hip flexion compresses large veins in the legs.

For more information, see Chapter 10 in Pellico, L.H. (2013). *Focus on adult health: Medical-surgical nursing.* Philadelphia: Wolters Kluwer Health | Lippincott Williams & Wilkins.

Pulmonary Arterial Hypertension

Pulmonary arterial HTN (PAH) exists when the mean pulmonary artery pressure exceeds 25 mm Hg at rest or 30 mm Hg with activities. Pulmonary arterial HTN is a condition that is not clinically evident until late in its progression.

PATHOPHYSIOLOGY

There are two types of PAH: idiopathic PAH (formerly known as primary) and PAH due to a known cause. As the pulmonary arterial pressure increases, the pulmonary vascular resistance also increases. This increased workload affects right ventricular function. The myocardium ultimately cannot meet the increasing demands imposed on it, leading to right ventricular hypertrophy (enlargement and dilation) and failure.

RISK FACTORS

- Women 20 to 40 years of age (idiopathic)
- Left ventricular failure, mitral stenosis
- Pulmonary diseases
- Collagen vascular diseases

CLINICAL MANIFESTATIONS AND ASSESSMENT

- Dyspnea, the main symptom, occurs first with exertion and then at rest.
- Other signs and symptoms include chest pain, weakness, fatigue, syncope, occasional hemoptysis, and signs of right-sided HF (peripheral edema, ascites, distended neck veins, hepatomegaly, crackles, heart murmur, splitting of second heart sound).

DIAGNOSTIC METHODS

Diagnosis of idiopathic PAH is made by exclusion of secondary causes such as COPD, pulmonary embolism, HIV, and cardiac disease.

- Complete diagnostic evaluation includes a history, physical examination, chest X-ray, pulmonary function studies, ECG, echocardiogram, ventilation–perfusion scan, CT or MRA, sleep studies, autoantibody tests (to identify diseases of collagen vascular origin), HIV tests, liver function testing, hypercoagulation studies, and cardiac catheterization.
- Pulmonary function studies may be normal or show a slight decrease in vital capacity and lung compliance, with a mild decrease in the diffusing capacity.
- The PaO_2 also is decreased (hypoxemia).

P

- The ECG demonstrates right atrial enlargement, tall peaked P waves in inferior leads, right axis deviation, right ventricular hypertrophy, and ST-segment depression or T-wave inversion in V 1 through 4.
- An echocardiogram can assess the progression of the disease and rule out other conditions with similar signs and symptoms.
- A ventilation–perfusion scan or pulmonary CT or MRA detects defects in pulmonary vasculature, such as pulmonary emboli.
- Acute vasodilator testing can be performed to determine if there is a reduction in mean pulmonary artery pressure when a short-acting vasodilator (adenosine, epoprostenol, or inhaled nitric oxide) is administered.

MEDICAL AND NURSING MANAGEMENT

The goal of treatment is to manage the underlying condition related to PAH of known cause.

- Provide supplemental oxygen for hypoxemia at rest or with exercise to reverse vasoconstriction and pulmonary HTN.

Pharmacologic Therapy

- Pharmacologic agents such as diuretics, digoxin, anticoagulant therapy, and calcium-channel blockers (nifedipine, diltiazem) may be prescribed.
- Vasodilating agents include epoprostenol, treprostinil, bosentan, sildenafil, and iloprost may be used. Current therapies are not curative, have considerable side effects, and are often quite expensive.
- Because calcium-channel blockers are effective in only a small percentage of patients, other treatment options, including prostacyclin, are often necessary.

Surgical Management

Lung or heart-lung transplantation is reserved for patients who have advanced disease despite maximal medical therapy.

Nursing Management

- Identify patients at high risk for developing PAH, such as those with COPD, pulmonary emboli, congenital heart disease, and mitral valve disease.
- Be alert for signs and symptoms of deterioration such as worsening dyspnea, hypoxemia, and right ventricular failure.
- Administer oxygen as ordered; teach patient and family about use of home oxygen.
- Inform patients treated with prostacyclin (ie, epoprostenol or treprostinil) about the need for central venous access (epoprostenol) or subcutaneous infusion (treprostinil).
- Emotional and psychosocial aspects of this disease must be addressed.

For more information, see Chapter 10 in Pellico, L.H. (2013). *Focus on adult health: Medical-surgical nursing*. Philadelphia: Wolters Kluwer Health | Lippincott Williams & Wilkins.

Pyelonephritis, Acute

Pyelonephritis, an upper urinary tract infection (UTI), is a bacterial infection of the renal pelvis, tubules, and interstitial tissue of one or both kidneys. Pyelonephritis may be acute or chronic.

PATHOPHYSIOLOGY

Causes involve either the upward spread of bacteria from the bladder or spread from systemic sources reaching the kidney via the bloodstream. An incompetent ureterovesical valve or obstruction occurring in the urinary tract increases the susceptibility of the kidneys to infection. Acute pyelonephritis is usually manifested by enlarged kidneys with interstitial infiltrations of inflammatory cells. Abscesses may be noted on the renal capsule and at the corticomedullary junction. Atrophy and destruction of tubules and the glomeruli may result.

RISK FACTORS

- Bladder tumors
- Strictures
- Benign prostatic hyperplasia
- Urinary stones

CLINICAL MANIFESTATIONS AND ASSESSMENT

- The patient with acute pyelonephritis is acutely ill with chills, fever, leukocytosis (elevated WBCs), bacteriuria, and pyuria.
- Low back pain, flank pain, nausea and vomiting, headache, malaise, and painful urination are common findings.
- Physical examination reveals pain and tenderness in the area of the costovertebral angle.
- Symptoms of lower urinary tract involvement, such as dysuria and frequency, are common.

DIAGNOSTIC METHODS

- Ultrasound or CT scan.
- Urine culture and sensitivity test

MEDICAL AND NURSING MANAGEMENT

- Uncomplicated cases are treated on an outpatient basis with a 2-week course of antibiotics; commonly prescribed agents include TMP-SMZ, ciprofloxacin, gentamicin with or without ampicillin, or a third-generation cephalosporin.

- Pregnant women may be hospitalized for 2 or 3 days of parenteral antibiotic therapy.
- Oral antibiotic agents may be prescribed once the patient is afebrile and showing clinical improvement.
- For chronic or recurring symptoms, the patient may need antibiotic therapy for up to 6 weeks if a relapse occurs. A follow-up urine culture is obtained 2 weeks after completion of antibiotic therapy to document clearing of the infection.
- Hydration is essential when there is adequate kidney function, to facilitate "flushing" of the urinary tract, and it reduces pain and discomfort.

Nursing Management

The plan of care is the same as that for upper UTIs.

For more information, see Chapter 28 in Pellico, L.H. (2013). *Focus on adult health: Medical-surgical nursing.* Philadelphia: Wolters Kluwer Health | Lippincott Williams & Wilkins.

Pyelonephritis, Chronic

Repeated bouts of acute pyelonephritis may lead to chronic pyelonephritis.

PATHOPHYSIOLOGY

When pyelonephritis becomes chronic, the kidneys become scarred, contracted, nonfunctional, and cause chronic kidney disease that can result in the need for therapies such as transplantation or dialysis.

CLINICAL MANIFESTATIONS AND ASSESSMENT

- Patient usually has no symptoms of infection unless an acute exacerbation occurs.
- Fatigue, headache, and poor appetite may occur.
- Polyuria, excessive thirst, and weight loss may result.
- Persistent and recurring infection may produce progressive scarring resulting in renal failure.

DIAGNOSTIC METHODS

- Intravenous urogram
- Measurement of blood urea nitrogen (BUN), creatinine levels, and creatinine clearance

MEDICAL AND NURSING MANAGEMENT

Long-term use of prophylactic antimicrobial therapy may help limit recurrence of infections and renal scarring. Impaired renal function alters the excretion of antimicrobial agents and necessitates careful monitoring of renal function, especially with use of nephrotoxic agents.

Nursing Management

The plan of care is the same as that for upper UTIs.

- If patient is hospitalized, encourage fluids (3 to 4 L/day) unless contraindicated.
- Monitor and record I & O.
- Assess temperature every 4 hours and administer antipyretic and antibiotic agents as prescribed.
- Patient teaching focuses on prevention of further infection by consuming adequate fluids, emptying the bladder regularly, and performing recommended perineal hygiene.

- Stress the importance of taking antimicrobial medications exactly as prescribed, along with the need for keeping follow-up appointments.

For more information, see Chapter 28 in Pellico, L.H. (2013). *Focus on adult health: Medical-surgical nursing.* Philadelphia: Wolters Kluwer Health | Lippincott Williams & Wilkins.

R

Raynaud's Disease and Raynaud's Phenomenon

Primary *Raynaud's disease* refers to vasospasm that occurs with cold or stress. Patients with scleroderma or systemic lupus erythematosus may have the same signs and symptoms. This is called *Raynaud's phenomenon*.

PATHOPHYSIOLOGY

Raynaud's disease is of unknown etiology. Although its exact cause is unknown, it may be associated with immunologic disorders. It may cause skin and muscle atrophy.

Prognosis varies; patients may slowly improve, become progressively worse, or show no change.

RISK FACTORS

- Women between 16 and 40 years of age
- More frequent in cold climates and winter

CLINICAL MANIFESTATIONS AND ASSESSMENT

- The patient's skin becomes cyanotic due to vasospasm, then vasodilation causes redness (rubor).
- Numbness, tingling, and burning pain occur.

MEDICAL AND NURSING MANAGEMENT

With appropriate patient teaching and lifestyle modifications, the disorder is generally benign and self-limiting.

- Instruct patient to avoid stimuli (eg, cold, tobacco) that provoke vasoconstriction.
- Calcium channel blockers may relieve symptoms.
- Sympathectomy, interrupting the sympathetic nerves, may help some patients.

R

> For more information, see Chapter 18 in Pellico, L.H. (2013). *Focus on adult health: Medical-surgical nursing.* Philadelphia: Wolters Kluwer Health | Lippincott Williams & Wilkins.

Regional Enteritis (Crohn's Disease)

Regional enteritis is a subacute and chronic inflammation of the gastrointestinal (GI) tract wall that extends through all layers (ie, transmural lesion).

PATHOPHYSIOLOGY

Although it can occur anywhere in the GI tract, regional enteritis most commonly occurs in the distal ileum but can be seen in the ascending colon. It is characterized by periods of remission and exacerbation. The disease process begins with edema and thickening of the mucosa, then ulceration. The ulcerations are separated by normal tissue and have a classic "cobblestone" appearance on colonoscopy. Fistulas, fissures, and abscesses form as the inflammation extends down into the peritoneum. As the disease advances, the bowel wall thickens and becomes fibrotic, and the intestinal lumen narrows; adhesions may develop.

RISK FACTORS

- Adolescent or young adult, but may appear at any age
- Family history
- Possibly environmental agents such as pesticides, food additives, tobacco, and radiation
- Allergies and immune disorders

R

CLINICAL MANIFESTATIONS AND ASSESSMENT

- Onset of symptoms is usually insidious, with prominent right lower quadrant abdominal pain and diarrhea unrelieved by defecation.
- Abdominal tenderness and spasm is present.
- Crampy abdominal pains occur after meals; the patient tends to limit intake, causing weight loss, malnutrition, and secondary anemia.
- Chronic diarrhea; patient is thin and emaciated in appearance.
- The weeping, edematous intestine continually empties a colonic and skin-irritating discharge, secondary to ulceration and inflammation.
- The inflamed intestine may perforate and form intra-abdominal and anal abscesses.
- Fever and leukocytosis occur.
- Steatorrhea may occur.
- Abscesses, fistulas, and fissures are common.
- Symptoms extend beyond the GI tract to include joint disorders (eg, arthritis), skin lesions (eg, erythema nodosum), ocular disorders (eg, conjunctivitis), and oral ulcers.

DIAGNOSTIC METHODS

- Proctosigmoidoscopy is usually performed initially to determine whether the rectosigmoid area is inflamed.

- Stool is examined for occult blood and steatorrhea.
- Barium study of the upper GI tract is the most conclusive diagnostic aid; shows the classic "string sign" of the terminal ileum indicating constriction of a segment of intestine.
- Barium enema may show ulcerations as cobblestone appearance, fistulas, and fissures.
- Endoscopy, colonoscopy, and intestinal biopsies may be used to confirm the diagnosis.
- Computed tomography (CT) scan may show bowel wall thickening and fistula formation.
- Complete blood cell count (CBC) shows decreased hemoglobin (Hbg) and hematocrit (Hct) levels and leukocytosis.
- Erythrocyte sedimentation rate (ESR) is elevated; albumin and protein levels are usually decreased due to malnutrition.

MEDICAL AND NURSING MANAGEMENT

See "Medical and Nursing Management" under "Ulcerative Colitis" on pages 670–671 for additional information.

COMPLICATIONS

- Intestinal obstruction or stricture
- Perianal disease
- Fluid and electrolyte imbalance
- Malnutrition
- Fistula and abscess formation
- Increased risk of colon cancer

For more information, see Chapter 24 in Pellico, L.H. (2013). *Focus on adult health: Medical-surgical nursing.* Philadelphia: Wolters Kluwer Health | Lippincott Williams & Wilkins.

Renal Failure, Acute

Acute renal failure (ARF) is a typically reversible clinical syndrome in which there is an abrupt loss of kidney function over a period of hours to days.

PATHOPHYSIOLOGY

Acute renal failure is classified by its three major etiologies, which helps to focus the treatment.

- Prerenal ARF is caused by reduced blood flow to the kidney. Volume-depletion states, which include dehydration, hemorrhage, or GI losses; decreased cardiac output such as occurs with myocardial infarction, heart failure, or cardiogenic shock; and vasodilated states such as sepsis or anaphylaxis are prerenal causes.
- Intrarenal ARF is the result of actual parenchymal damage to the glomeruli or kidney tubules. Acute tubular necrosis (ATN), nephrotoxic agents, ischemia due to decreased renal perfusion, burns, crush injuries, infections, and severe blood transfusion reactions are intrarenal causes.
- Postrenal ARF is the result of an obstruction that develops anywhere from the collecting ducts of the kidney to the urethra. Blockage such as from bilateral renal calculi or benign prostatic hypertrophy (BPH) are postrenal causes.

Phases of Acute Renal Failure

- Initiation period is a period of initial insult to cellular injury and oliguria
- Oliguric period is accompanied by an increase in the serum concentration of wastes such as urea, creatinine, organic acids, and the electrolytes potassium, phosphorous, and magnesium (urine volume <400 mL/day); average time is 7 to 14 days.
- Diuretic phase is marked by gradual increase in urine output signaling beginning of glomerular filtration's recovery. Laboratory values plateau and begin to decrease.

- Recovery period shows improving renal function and energy level (may take 6 to 12 months).
- If residual damage to the glomerular basement membrane occurs, residual renal impairment may result.

CLINICAL MANIFESTATIONS AND ASSESSMENT

Almost every system of the body is affected when the renal regulatory mechanisms fail.

- Patient may appear critically ill and lethargic with oliguria.
- Nausea, vomiting, lethargy, headache, muscle twitching, and seizures may occur secondary to increasing blood urea nitrogen (BUN).

DIAGNOSTIC METHODS

- Blood urea nitrogen (BUN) level increases steadily, along with creatinine, a more sensitive indicator of renal function.
- I & O reveals oliguria or anuria.
- Hyperkalemia occurs with decreased urine output; electrocardiogram (ECG) may show tall, tented, or peaked T waves, absent P wave, widened QRS, or bradyarrhythmia.
- Metabolic acidosis demonstrated on arterial blood gases (ABG), with low CO_2 indicating rapid and deep breathing to "blow off" CO_2 and compensate for acidosis.
- Serum phosphate levels increase. Calcium levels may decrease.
- Hematuria may be present, and the urine has a low specific gravity due to inability to concentrate the urine
- Decreased urine sodium levels and urinary casts and other cellular debris may be present.
- Anemia from reduced erythropoietin production, blood loss due to uremic GI lesions, reduced red blood cell life-span is noted.

PREVENTION

- Assess for use of potentially nephrotoxic agents and exposure to environmental toxins, including amphotericin B, vancomycin, cyclosporine; aminoglycosides (gentamicin, tobramycin, neo-mycin); certain antineoplastics or anesthetics; heavy metals such as cisplatin or bismuth; and radiological contrast agents.

- Chronic use of analgesics, particularly nonsteroidal anti-inflammatory agents (NSAIDs), may cause interstitial nephritis (inflammation within the renal tissue) and papillary necrosis. Patients with heart failure or cirrhosis with ascites are at par-ticular risk for NSAID-induced renal failure.
- Increased age, preexisting renal disease, and the co-administra-tion of nephrotoxic agents increase the risk for kidney damage.
- Identify patients at risk for radiocontrast-induced nephropathy; patients with creatinine levels greater than 2 mg/dL are at risk and should receive preprocedure hydration and acetylcysteine (Mucomyst) the day prior to tests requiring contrast media.

MEDICAL AND NURSING MANAGEMENT

Management includes maintaining fluid and electrolyte balance, avoiding fluid excesses, and supporting the patient until repair of renal tissue and restoration of function occur. Dialysis may be used on a temporary basis to restore homeostasis.

- Treatment of prerenal azotemia consists of optimizing renal perfusion with fluids or treating decreased cardiac output.
- Intrarenal problems are treated with supportive therapy, removal of causative agents, and aggressive management of shock and infection.
- Treatment of postrenal failure is to relieve the obstruction. Sur-gery such as prostatectomy, nephrostomy tubes, or indwelling catheters may be used.
- Observe for fluid excess manifested by dyspnea, crackles, tachy-cardia, hypertension, distended neck veins, and generalized edema in the presacral and pretibial areas. The central venous pressure (CVP), where measured, will be elevated.
- Fluid restriction becomes important to prevent fluid overload and pulmonary edema. Diuretics such as furosemide (Lasix) may be prescribed to initiate diuresis and maintain renal perfusion.

- Dialysis or continuous renal replacement therapy may be used to maintain homeostasis when hyperkalemia, metabolic acidosis, pericarditis, fluid volume excess, and pulmonary edema occur.

Pharmacologic Therapy

- Hyperkalemia may be reduced by administering sodium polystyrene sulfonate (Kayexalate) orally, via nasogastric (NG) tube or by retention enema. Kayexalate, a cation-exchange resin, works by exchanging sodium ions for potassium ions in the intestinal tract.
- Symptomatic hyperkalemia requires rapid treatment: IV dextrose, insulin, and calcium replacement may be administered to shift potassium back into the cells. Albuterol sulfate (Ventolin HFA) by nebulizer can lower plasma potassium concentration
- Acidosis may require sodium bicarbonate therapy, if the serum bicarbonate concentration is below 15 mmol/L or arterial pH is less than 7.2.
- Phosphate-binding agents such as calcium acetate (PhosLo) or aluminum hydroxide gel (short-term only) are given to decrease the absorption of phosphate from the intestinal tract.
- Dosage adjustments are needed with antibiotics, especially aminoglycosides, digoxin, angiotensin-converting enzyme (ACE) inhibitors, and magnesium-containing agents.

Nursing Management

Nutritional Therapy

- Restrict dietary protein; caloric requirements are met with high-carbohydrate meals, due to their protein-sparing effect.
- Avoid dietary potassium including bananas, citrus, tomatoes, melons. Phosphorus, found in dairy, beans, nuts legumes, and carbonated beverages, is restricted.
- Caffeine is restricted.
- The patient may require enteral or parenteral nutrition.
- Fluid is restricted; administering fluids (PO or IV) may require replacing both sensible and insensible loss.

Reducing Metabolic Rate

- Bed rest may be indicated to reduce exertion and the metabolic rate.
- Fever and infection increase the metabolic rate and may lead to catabolism; these are prevented or treated promptly.

Preventing Infection

- Asepsis is essential with invasive lines and catheters.
- Avoid indwelling urinary catheter.

Providing Skin Care

- The skin may be dry or susceptible to breakdown as a result of edema; therefore, meticulous skin care is important.
- Excoriation and itching of the skin may result from the deposit of uremic toxins in the patient's tissues.
- Turn the patient frequently, bathing him or her with cool water, and keep the skin clean and well moisturized, and the fingernails trimmed to avoid injury.

Providing Support

- Provide frequent explanations of the purpose and rationale of the treatments as rising BUN leads to confusion and lethargy.
- Explain length of illness and that duration of treatment varies.

Gerontologic Considerations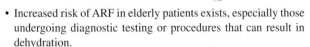

- Increased risk of ARF in elderly patients exists, especially those undergoing diagnostic testing or procedures that can result in dehydration.
- Suppression of thirst, decreased mobility with lack of access to drinking water, and confusion contribute to the older patient's failure to consume adequate fluids, causing dehydration and further compromise of already decreased renal function.
- Muscle mass and glomerular filtration rate (GFR) can decrease with age; therefore, even small elevations or changes in creatinine may indicate significant renal impairment in the elderly and should be investigated.

For more information, see Chapter 27 in Pellico, L.H. (2013). *Focus on adult health: Medical-surgical nursing.* Philadelphia: Wolters Kluwer Health | Lippincott Williams & Wilkins.

R

Renal Failure, Chronic and End-Stage Renal Disease

Chronic renal failure is a progressive and irreversible deterioration in renal function taking place over months to years. When a patient has sustained enough kidney damage to require renal replacement therapy on a permanent basis, the patient has moved into the final stage of chronic kidney disease or end-stage renal disease (ESRD).

PATHOPHYSIOLOGY

Chronic renal failure results in the body's inability to maintain metabolic and fluid and electrolyte balance, resulting in azotemia and subsequent uremia. In ESRD, renal replacement therapy with dialysis or renal transplant is needed to sustain life.

As renal function declines, the end products of protein metabolism, normally excreted in urine, accumulate in the blood. Uremia develops and adversely affects every system in the body. The greater the buildup of waste products, the more severe the symptoms. The disease tends to progress more rapidly in patients who excrete significant amounts of protein or have elevated blood pressure than in those without these conditions.

RISK FACTORS

- Diabetes
- Hypertension

- Proteinuria
- Family history
- Increasing age
- Chronic glomerulonephritis, or chronic pyelonephritis
- Obstruction of the urinary tract
- Polycystic kidney disease
- Vascular and autoimmune disorders (such as systemic lupus erythematosus)
- Infections, medications, or toxic agents
- Environmental and occupational agents: Lead, cadmium, mercury, and chromium.
- African Americans, Hispanics and Native Americans

CLINICAL MANIFESTATIONS AND ASSESSMENT

Severity of signs and symptoms depends on the degree of uremia and renal impairment, other underlying conditions, and the patient's age.

- Neurologic manifestations: Weakness, fatigue, confusion or behavioral changes, inability to concentrate, muscle twitching, agitation, confusion, seizure, restless leg syndrome, or peripheral neuropathy
- Cardiovascular manifestations: Hypertension, pitting/periorbital edema pericarditis, pericardial effusion or tamponade, distended neck veins, heart failure or pulmonary edema, fluid volume excess. Major cause of death in ESRD is cardiovascular disease.
- Pulmonary manifestations: Crackles, thick, tenacious sputum, depressed cough reflex, pleuritic pain, shortness of breath, tachypnea, Kussmaul respirations, uremic pneumonitis
- Gastrointestinal manifestations: Anorexia, nausea, vomiting, hiccups, ammonia or urine odor to breath (uremic fetor), metallic taste in the mouth, constipation or diarrhea, GI bleeding
- Immunologic/hematologic manifestations: Defective granulocyte, B-cell, and T-cell function, anemia, thrombocytopenia
- Genitourinary manifestations: Erectile dysfunction, decreased libido, pain during intercourse (women), amenorrhea, testicular atrophy, infertility

- Dermatologic manifestations: Pruritus, gray-bronze or waxy yellow skin, dry flaky skin
- Musculoskeletal manifestations: Muscle cramps, loss of muscle strength, renal osteodystrophy, bone pain, fractures, foot drop

DIAGNOSTIC FINDINGS

- Elevated BUN and creatinine
- Oliguria or anuria
- Hyponatremia often dilutional, occasional sodium excess
- Hyperkalemia, hypermagnesemia
- Hypocalcemia/hyperphosphatemia
- Metabolic acidosis
- Hypoproteinemia
- Symptoms of fluid volume excess, heart failure, or pulmonary edema
- Evidence of related diseases

MEDICAL AND NURSING MANAGEMENT

Goals of management are to retain kidney function and homeostasis for as long as possible, while continuing to treat the underlying disorder(s). Management is accomplished primarily with medications and diet therapy. Renal replacement therapy is planned for in stage 4 kidney disease.

Pharmacologic Management

- Hyperphosphatemia and hypocalcemia are treated with medications that bind dietary phosphorus in the GI tract (eg, calcium carbonate, calcium acetate, sevelamer hydrochloride); administer with food.
- Hypertension is managed by sodium and fluid restriction. Antihypertensive medication, diuretics, inotropics (digoxin or dobutamine) may be used.
- Metabolic acidosis is treated with Bicitra (Shohl's solution/sodium citrate and citric acid) or sodium bicarbonate

supplements (rarely used) to correct acidosis. Dialysis may be needed.

- IV diazepam (Valium), lorazepam (Ativan), or phenytoin (Dilantin) is usually administered to control seizures, which may develop as azotemia worsens.
- Recombinant human erythropoietin (e-poietin, Epogen/Procrit) is used to treat anemia to a target hemoglobin level of 11 to 12 g/dL. Iron, in the form of iron sucrose (Venofer) and ferric gluconate (Ferrlecit), may be prescribed as an adjunct.

Nutritional Therapy

- Limit protein to 0.7 to 1.0 g/kg of ideal body weight; plan diet low sodium, potassium, and phosphorus.
- Daily fluid allowance of approximately 500 to 800 mL plus the previous day's 24-hour urine output.
- Teach the patient strategies to control intake and thirst, such as sucking on hard candies or mints, chewing gum, rinsing the mouth with cold water, sucking on a lemon wedge, using small glasses instead of large ones, and moisturizing the lips.

Renal Replacement Therapy

- Renal replacement therapy is a term used to encompass life-supporting treatments for renal failure including hemodialysis, peritoneal dialysis, hemofiltration, and renal transplantation.
- The patient with increasing symptoms of chronic renal failure is referred to a dialysis and transplantation center early in the course of progressive renal disease.
- Dialysis is used to remove fluid and uremic waste products from the body when the kidneys are unable to do so. Methods of therapy include hemodialysis, peritoneal dialysis, and continuous renal replacement therapy (CRRT). Temporary or permanent vascular access is needed.
- Kidney transplantation has become the treatment of choice for most patients with ESRD. Waiting times across the country continue to increase, with the median time to transplant projected to be nearly 4 years for candidates added to the list in 2008. Patients must take immunosuppressive drugs for the life of the kidney to prevent rejection.

Nursing Management

The patient with chronic renal failure requires astute nursing care to avoid the complications of reduced renal function and the stresses and anxieties of dealing with a life-threatening illness.

- Provide frequent, clear explanations and information to the patient and family concerning ESRD, treatment options, and potential complications.
- Reinforce the renal diet and explain the correlation between symptoms and nonadherence; encourage home blood pressure monitoring to illustrate effect of fluid retention, increasing blood pressure, and shortness of breath.
- The patient and family should report the following symptoms of worsening renal function to the health care provider:
  - Worsening signs and symptoms of renal failure including nausea, vomiting, change in usual urine output, or ammonia/urine odor to the breath
  - Signs and symptoms of hyperkalemia including muscle weakness, diarrhea, abdominal cramps
  - If receiving dialysis, observe for signs and symptoms of access problems, such as clotted fistula or graft or signs of infection at the site.
- Continuing care includes importance of follow-up to prevent or detect progression, assessment of coping strategies, adherence to diet, reinforcement of the renal diet, and participation in health promotion and health screenings.

Gerontologic Considerations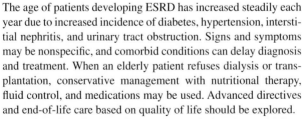

The age of patients developing ESRD has increased steadily each year due to increased incidence of diabetes, hypertension, interstitial nephritis, and urinary tract obstruction. Signs and symptoms may be nonspecific, and comorbid conditions can delay diagnosis and treatment. When an elderly patient refuses dialysis or transplantation, conservative management with nutritional therapy, fluid control, and medications may be used. Advanced directives and end-of-life care based on quality of life should be explored.

A plan of nursing care for a patient with chronic renal failure is available online at http://thePoint.lww.com/Pellico1e.

COMPLICATIONS

- Atherosclerotic cardiovascular disease, angina, stroke, and peripheral vascular disease
- Gastric ulcers
- Renal osteodystrophy, bone pain, fractures
- Malnutrition
- Infection
- Neuropathy
- Heart failure

For more information, see Chapter 27 in Pellico, L.H. (2013). *Focus on adult health: Medical-surgical nursing.* Philadelphia: Wolters Kluwer Health | Lippincott Williams & Wilkins.

S

Seborrheic Dermatitis

Seborrheic dermatitis is a chronic inflammatory disease of the skin occurring in areas that are well supplied with sebaceous glands or that lie between skin folds, where the bacteria count is high.

PATHOPHYSIOLOGY

Seborrhea is an excessive production of sebum (secretion of sebaceous glands) in areas where sebaceous glands are normally found in large numbers. The face, scalp, eyebrows, eyelids, sides of the nose and upper lip, malar regions (cheeks), ears, axillae, under the breasts, the groin, and the gluteal crease of the buttocks are common areas affected There are remissions and exacerbations of this condition.

RISK FACTORS

- Genetic predisposition
- Hormones
- Nutritional status
- Infection
- Emotional stress

CLINICAL MANIFESTATIONS AND ASSESSMENT

Two forms can occur: An oily form and a dry form. Either form may start in childhood and continue throughout life.

Oily Form

Moist or greasy patches of yellowish-red or gray-white, greasy skin, with or without scaling, and slight erythema; small pustules or papulopustules appear on the trunk, resembling acne.

Dry Form

Flaky desquamation of the scalp (dandruff); asymptomatic mild forms or scaling often are accompanied by pruritus, leading to scratching and secondary infections and excoriation.

MEDICAL AND NURSING MANAGEMENT

Because there is no known cure for seborrhea, the objectives of therapy are to control the disorder and allow the skin to repair itself.

Pharmacologic Therapy

- Topical corticosteroid cream to body and face (use with caution near eyes, may produce glaucoma)
- Topical antifungal (eg, ciclopirox or ketoconazole) may be needed for secondary yeast infection in body creases.
- Medicated shampoos containing selenium sulfide suspension, zinc pyrithione, salicylic acid, or sulfur compounds, or tar shampoo that contains sulfur or salicylic acid. Shampoos are left on 5 to 10 minutes; two or three different types are used in rotation to prevent resistance.

Nursing Management

- Advise patient to avoid external irritants, excess heat, and perspiration; rubbing and scratching prolong the disorder.

- Aerating skin and carefully cleanse creases or folds to prevent candidal yeast infection (evaluate patients with persistent candidiasis for diabetes).
- Reinforce instructions for using medicated shampoos; frequent shampooing is contrary to some cultural practices—be sensitive to these differences when providing teaching.
- Caution patient that seborrheic dermatitis is a chronic problem that tends to reappear. The goal is to keep it under control through adherence to treatment program.
- Treat patients with sensitivity and an awareness of their need to express their feelings when they become discouraged by the disorder's effect on body image.

For more information, see Chapter 52 in Pellico, L.H. (2013). *Focus on adult health: Medical-surgical nursing.* Philadelphia: Wolters Kluwer Health | Lippincott Williams & Wilkins.

Shock, Cardiogenic

Cardiogenic shock occurs when the heart's ability to contract and to pump blood is impaired and the supply of oxygen is inadequate for cardiac and tissue perfusion.

PATHOPHYSIOLOGY

In cardiogenic shock, cardiac output, a function of stroke volume and heart rate, is compromised. When stroke volume and heart rate decrease or become erratic, blood pressure falls, and systemic tissue perfusion is compromised, causing decreasing urine output, cold, clammy skin, mental status changes, anxiety, and delayed capillary refill. Blood supply for the heart muscle itself is inadequate, resulting in further decreases in cardiac output. This can occur rapidly or over a period of days. Patients in cardiogenic shock may experience angina pain and develop arrhythmias and hemodynamic instability.

RISK FACTORS

- Myocardial infarction
- Stress to the myocardium, severe hypoxemia, acidosis, hypoglycemia, and hypocalcemia
- Cardiomyopathies
- Valvular disease
- Arrhythmias

CLINICAL MANIFESTATIONS AND ASSESSMENT

- Classic signs include hypotension, rapid and weak pulse.
- Arrhythmias are common.
- Anginal pain may be experienced.
- Hemodynamic instability
- Complaints of fatigue
- Jugular vein distention (JVD), crackles, shortness of breath (SOB), and S_3
- Oliguria

DIAGNOSTIC METHODS

- Cardiac enzyme levels (ie, CK-MB and troponin-I)
- Serial laboratory markers for ventricular dysfunction (eg, brain-derived natriuretic peptide [BNP])
- Serial 12-lead electrocardiogram (ECG)
- Echocardiogram to assess the degree of myocardial damage or dysfunction

MEDICAL AND NURSING MANAGEMENT

Goals of management include limiting further myocardial damage, preserving the healthy myocardium, and improving cardiac contractility, preload, afterload, or both. These goals are achieved by increasing oxygen supply to the heart muscle while reducing oxygen demands.

- Correct the underlying cause of cardiogenic shock.
- Provide supplemental oxygen, control chest pain, control heart rate with medication or pacemaker.
- Administer vasoactive medications and fluids if warranted.
- Hemodynamic monitoring and laboratory marker monitoring are performed.
- Mechanical cardiac support may be necessary.
- Coronary cardiogenic shock may be treated with thrombolytic therapy, angioplasty, coronary artery bypass graft surgery, and/or intra-aortic balloon pump therapy.
- Noncoronary cardiogenic shock may be treated with cardiac valve replacement, correction of arrhythmia, correction of acidosis and electrolyte disturbances, or treatment of the tension pneumothorax.

Pharmacologic Therapy

- Analgesia
- Antiplatelets
- Beta blockers
- Vasoactive medications
- Diuretics
- Antiarrhythmic medications

Nursing Management

Prevention

- Early on, identify patients at risk for cardiogenic shock.
- Promote adequate tissue perfusion of the heart muscle and decreased cardiac workload (eg, conserve energy, relieve pain, administer oxygen, ASA, and beta blockers).

Monitoring Hemodynamic Status

- Monitor hemodynamic and cardiac status: Maintain arterial lines and ECG equipment.
- Anticipate need for medications, IV fluids, and additional equipment.

- Document and promptly report changes in hemodynamic, cardiac, pulmonary status, renal status, and laboratory values.

Administering Fluids and Medications

- Administer IV fluids accurately, observing for fluid overload and pulmonary edema.
- Monitor for desired effects and side effects (eg, hypotension after administering morphine or nitroglycerin, bleeding at arterial and venipuncture sites after receiving thrombolytics).
- Monitor urine output, blood urea nitrogen (BUN), and serum creatinine levels to detect any decrease in renal function.

Enhancing Safety and Comfort

- Take an active role in ensuring patient's safety and comfort and in reducing anxiety.
- Offer explanations regarding treatments to patient and families; provide opportunities for family to see and talk to patient.

For more information, see Chapter 54 in Pellico, L.H. (2013). *Focus on adult health: Medical-surgical nursing.* Philadelphia: Wolters Kluwer Health | Lippincott Williams & Wilkins.

Shock, Hypovolemic

Hypovolemic shock, the most common type of shock, is characterized by decreased intravascular volume.

PATHOPHYSIOLOGY

Hypovolemic shock can be caused by sudden fluid losses, as in traumatic blood loss, or by internal fluid shifts, as in severe dehydration, severe edema, or ascites. Decreased blood volume results in decreased venous return and subsequent decreased ventricular filling, decreased stroke volume and cardiac output, and decreased tissue perfusion.

RISK FACTORS

- Trauma
- Surgery
- Vomiting
- Diarrhea
- Diuresis
- Diabetes insipidus
- NPO status
- Hemorrhage
- Burns
- Ascites
- Peritonitis
- Dehydration

CLINICAL MANIFESTATIONS AND ASSESSMENT

- Signs of poor tissue perfusion and decreased cardiac output
- Tissue hypoxia with increased lactic acid levels
- Tachycardia, peripheral vasoconstriction, and anxiety are common.
- Cool and clammy skin, pallor, thirst, diaphoresis
- Altered sensorium, oliguria, metabolic acidosis, tachypnea
- Blood pressure readings alone are not reliable indicators of tissue perfusion.

MEDICAL AND NURSING MANAGEMENT

Goals of treatment are to restore intravascular volume, support the respiratory system, correct the underlying cause and, when necessary, involve patient and family in end-of-life decisions.

- Hemorrhage is treated by applying pressure; invasive procedure or surgery is used to stop internal bleeding.
- Diarrhea and vomiting are treated with medications.
- Insulin is used for osmotic diuresis, desmopressin (DDAVP) is administered for diabetes insipidus.

Nursing Management

Fluid Replacement

- Prevent hypovolemic shock by closely monitoring patients who are at risk for fluid deficits and to assist with fluid replacement before intravascular volume is depleted.
- Insert two large-bore IV catheters to administer fluid, medications, and/or blood.
- Obtain a baseline complete blood count (CBC) and type and cross-match in anticipation of blood transfusions.
- Crystalloids (Lactated Ringer's solution or 0.9% sodium chloride solution [normal saline]) or colloids (albumin or blood) are administered to restore intravascular volume.
- Position the patient in modified Trendelenburg position to promote venous return, unless evidence of head injury exists.

Vasoactive Medication Therapy

- Vasoactive medications are titrated to improve the patient's hemodynamic stability when fluid therapy alone cannot maintain adequate mean arterial pressure (MAP).
- Administer medications via infusion pump, through a central venous line. Infiltration and extravasation of some medications can cause tissue necrosis and sloughing.
- Monitor blood pressure by arterial line when possible.

Nutritional Support

- Increased metabolic rates during shock increase energy requirements and therefore caloric requirements.
- Administer enteral nutrition to maintain integrity of the GI tract; parenteral nutrition may be used.
- Administer antacids, H_2 blockers, or proton pump inhibitors to prevent ulcer formation.

Respiratory Support

- Administer oxygen; provide explanations about the need for oxygen mask if patient is apprehensive.
- Observe for need for ventilator support.
- Monitor oxygen saturation continuously.

Nursing Interventions

- Monitor for cardiovascular overload including difficulty breathing, JVD, changes in lung sounds, and pulmonary edema, especially in the elderly or those with cardiovascular diseases.
- Monitor and trend hemodynamic pressure, vital signs, arterial blood gases (ABGs), serum lactate levels, hemoglobin and hematocrit levels, and fluid intake and output (I & O).

For more information, see Chapter 54 in Pellico, L.H. (2013). *Focus on adult health: Medical-surgical nursing.* Philadelphia: Wolters Kluwer Health | Lippincott Williams & Wilkins.

Shock, Septic

Septic shock, the most common type of distributive (or circulatory) shock, is caused by widespread infection. Mortality rates for severe sepsis are 25% to 30% and 40% to 70% for septic shock.

PATHOPHYSIOLOGY

Microorganism invasion causes an inflammatory immune response caused by biochemical cytokines and mediators. The cascade of events begins with increased capillary permeability, fluid loss from the capillaries, and vasodilation, and results in inadequate perfusion of oxygen and nutrients to the tissues and cells. Proinflammatory and anti-inflammatory cytokines released during this process activate the coagulation system, causing clots to form in areas where they may not be needed. This further compromises tissue perfusion. Systemic inflammatory response syndrome (SIRS) presents clinically like sepsis but without an identifiable source of infection. Despite an absence of infection, antibiotic agents may still be administered because of the possibility of unrecognized infection.

RISK FACTORS

- Invasive procedures and indwelling medical devices
- Antibiotic-resistant microorganisms, gram-negative organisms, fungi, and viruses
- Elderly population
- Malnutrition or immunosuppression
- Chronic illness (eg, diabetes mellitus, hepatitis)

CLINICAL MANIFESTATIONS AND ASSESSMENT

- In the early stage of septic shock:
  - Blood pressure may remain within normal limits or be hypotensive but responsive to fluids.
  - Tachycardia and tachypnea
  - High cardiac output with vasodilation
  - Hyperthermia (febrile) with warm, flushed skin, bounding pulses
  - Urinary output normal or decreased
  - Gastrointestinal status is compromised (eg, nausea, vomiting, diarrhea, or decreased bowel sounds).
  - Subtle changes in mental status; confusion or agitation
  - Hypermetabolism with increased serum glucose and insulin resistance
- As sepsis progresses:
  - Low cardiac output with vasoconstriction
  - Hypotension unresponsive to fluids
  - Skin cool and pale
  - Temperature normal or below normal

- Heart and respiratory rates rapid
- Acidosis
- Signs of end-organ damage (eg, renal failure/anuria, respiratory failure, hepatic failure

Gerontologic Considerations

Septic shock may be manifested by atypical or confusing clinical signs. Suspect septic shock in any elderly person who develops an unexplained acute confused state, tachypnea, or hypotension.

MEDICAL AND NURSING MANAGEMENT

Current treatment of septic shock involves identification and elimination of the cause of infection and aggressive cardiopulmonary support.

- Blood, sputum, urine, and wound drainage specimens are collected to identify and eliminate the cause of infection.
- Tips of central lines may be cultured; however, recently that practice has been called into question.
- Potential routes of infection are eliminated, IVs removed and reinserted, urinary catheters replaced, abscesses are drained, and necrotic areas débrided.
- Fluid replacement is instituted using crystalloids, colloids, and blood products.
- Early goal-directed therapy is associated with decreased mortality and is used to guide fluid resuscitation: Central venous pressure (CVP) 8 to 12, MAP greater than 65, urinary output more than 0.5 mL/kg, and SVO_2 greater than 70%.

Pharmacologic Therapy

- Broad-spectrum antibiotics are started after cultures have been obtained. When culture and sensitivity reports become available, antibiotics are changed to those more specific to the infecting organism.

- Glucocorticoids alleviate physiologic stress and possibly mortality. Drawbacks include increased infection rate, worsening glycemic control, and impaired wound healing.

> ☀ **N U R S I N G   A L E R T**
> SVO_2 measures venous oxygen saturation, which reflects the amount of oxygen that has been extracted or used from the body. Tissue hypoxia can be determined by the mixed venous oxygen level, obtained from a special pulmonary artery, or a venous blood gas obtained from a central venous catheter. When the SVO_2 drops below the normal 60% to 80%, it reflects the increased consumption of oxygen and the need for intervention.

Nutritional Therapy and Glycemic Control

- Aggressive nutritional supplementation should be initiated within 24 to 48 hours of admission; malnutrition further impairs the patient's compensatory mechanisms.
- Enteral feeding, rather than parental nutrition, is associated with improved outcomes although reasons for this remain unclear.
- Glycemic control to a target blood glucose of 140 to 180 mg/dL has been shown to reduce mortality.

Nursing Management

- Identify patients at risk for sepsis, severe sepsis, and septic shock, including elderly and immunosuppressed patients and those with extensive trauma, burns, or diabetes.
- Carry out all invasive procedures with correct aseptic technique after careful hand hygiene.
- Collaborate with the health care team to identify the site and source of sepsis and organisms involved; obtain specimens for culture and sensitivity.
- Monitor IV lines, arterial and venous puncture sites, surgical incisions, trauma wounds, urinary catheters, and pressure ulcers for signs of infection.

- Reduce patient's temperature to reduce oxygen demand for fevers over 40°C (104°F) or if the patient is uncomfortable. Administer acetaminophen or apply hypothermia blanket; monitor for shivering, which increases oxygen demand.
- Administer prescribed IV fluids and antibiotics.
- Monitor and report blood levels (antibiotic, BUN, and creatinine levels; white blood cell count; hemoglobin and hematocrit levels; platelet count; coagulation studies).
- Provide aggressive nutrition, monitor daily weights and serum albumin to determine protein requirements.

S

For more information, see Chapter 54 in Pellico, L.H. (2013). *Focus on adult health: Medical-surgical nursing*. Philadelphia: Wolters Kluwer Health | Lippincott Williams & Wilkins.

Spinal Cord Injury

Spinal cord injuries (SCIs) are a major health problem, with an estimated 259,000 people in the United States living with this disability. An estimated 12,000 new injuries occur each year.

PATHOPHYSIOLOGY

Damage to the spinal cord ranges from transient concussion (from which the patient fully recovers) to contusion, laceration, compression, or complete transection (severing) of the cord. The latter renders the patient paralyzed below the level of the injury.

The vertebrae most frequently involved in SCIs are C5 to C7, the 12th thoracic vertebra (T12), and the first lumbar vertebra (L1). These vertebrae are the most susceptible because there is a greater range of mobility in the vertebral column in these areas. Injury can be categorized as primary (usually permanent) or secondary (nerve fibers swell and disintegrate as a result of ischemia, hypoxia, edema, and hemorrhagic lesions). Secondary injury may be reversible if treated within 4 to 6 hours of the initial injury.

RISK FACTORS

- Motor vehicle accidents (42%)
- Falls (26.7%)
- Sports injuries (7.6%)
- Violence (15%)
- Male between 16 and 30 years of age
- Substance abuse/use

CLINICAL MANIFESTATIONS AND ASSESSMENT

The consequences of SCI depend on the type and level of injury of the cord. Incomplete spinal cord lesions (the sensory, motor fibers, or both, are preserved below the lesion) are classified according to the area of spinal cord damage: central, lateral, anterior, or peripheral. The American Spinal Injury Association (ASIA) provides another standard classification of SCI according to the degree of sensory and motor function present after injury. SCI can result in paraplegia (paralysis of the lower body) or tetraplegia (formerly quadriplegia; paralysis of all four extremities). Complete SCI also includes loss of all spinal reflexes below the level of the lesion, loss of the ability to perspire below the level of the lesion, dysfunction of the bowel and bladder, and absence of visceral and somatic sensations below the level of the lesion.

- Patient usually complains of acute pain in the back or neck, which may radiate along the involved nerve; absence of pain does not rule out SCI.
- Respiratory dysfunction may occur; in high cervical cord injury, acute respiratory failure is the leading cause of death.

Ascending edema of the spinal cord in the acute phase of the injury may cause respiratory difficulty that requires immediate intervention. Therefore, the patient's respiratory status must be monitored frequently.

DIAGNOSTIC METHODS

- Detailed neurologic examination, X-ray examinations (lateral cervical spine X-rays), computed tomography (CT)
- Magnetic resonance imaging (MRI)
- Electrocardiogram (bradycardia and asystole are common in acute spinal injuries) is a common assessment and diagnostic method.
- Assessment is made for other injuries because spinal trauma often is accompanied by concomitant injuries, commonly to the head and chest.

EMERGENCY MANAGEMENT

- All patients involved in a motor vehicle accident, a diving or contact sports injury, a fall, or having any direct trauma to the head and neck are considered to have a SCI until such an injury has been ruled out.
- Rapid assessment, immobilization, extrication, stabilization or control of life-threatening injuries, and transportation to a regional spinal injury or trauma center is vital.
- Immobilize patient on a spinal (back) board, with head and neck in a neutral position, to prevent an incomplete injury from becoming complete. One member of the team must assume control of the patient's head to limit movement and maintain alignment during immobilization.

MEDICAL AND NURSING MANAGEMENT

The goals of management are to prevent further SCI and to observe for symptoms of progressive neurologic deficits.

Pharmacologic Therapy

- High-dose corticosteroids, specifically methylprednisolone (Solu-Medrol), seem to improve motor and sensory outcomes if given within 8 hours after injury. Although consistent evidence is inconclusive, steroids are justified in nondiabetic and nonimmunocomprised patients as no alternative therapies currently are available.
- Biologic agents are currently being investigated for the acute and chronic phases of SCI. Cell-based therapies, including stem cells and glial cells, are showing promise in animal trials.

Nonsurgical Management

- Treatment of SCI attempts to decompress, stabilize, and realign the spinal cord while preserving or improving neurologic function.
- Cervical fractures are reduced, and the cervical spine is aligned with some form of skeletal traction, such as skeletal tongs or calipers, or a halo device.
- A halo device may be used initially with traction. Consisting of a stainless-steel halo ring, it is fixed to the skull by four pins. Alternately, the ring may be attached to a removable halo vest, a device that suspends the weight of the unit circumferentially around the chest, permitting the patient increased mobility and ambulation.
- Thoracic and lumbar injuries are usually treated with surgical intervention followed by immobilization with a fitted brace.

Surgical Management

Surgery is performed to decompress the spinal cord, reduce the spinal fracture or dislocation, or to stabilize the spinal column.

- The most common procedure used to decompress or stabilize the spinal column is a laminectomy, which involves excision of the lamina (a portion of the posterior arch) and spinous processes of a vertebra.
- Various techniques (ie, fusion or fixation) are used to create a stable spinal column.

MONITORING AND MANAGING ACUTE COMPLICATIONS OF SPINAL CORD INJURY

Spinal and Neurogenic Shock

Spinal shock associated with SCI reflects a sudden depression of reflex activity in the spinal cord (areflexia) below the level of injury. The muscles innervated by the part of the spinal cord segment below the level of the lesion are without sensation, paralyzed, and flaccid.

- Intestinal decompression with a nasogastric (NG) tube is used to treat bowel distention and paralytic ileus caused by depression of reflexes.

  Neurogenic shock develops due to the loss of autonomic nervous system function below the level of the lesion. Symptoms include:

- Decreased cardiac output and venous pooling in the extremities
- Hypotension secondary to peripheral vasodilation.
- Bradycardia
- Warm flushed skin
- Lack of perspiration on paralyzed portion of body secondary to blocked sympathetic activity

Deep Vein Thrombosis

- Deep vein thrombosis (DVT) occurs in a high percentage (67% to 100%) of SCI patients, placing them at risk for pulmonary embolism (PE), the third leading cause of death in patients with SCI.
- Low-grade fever may be the first sign of DVT.
- Manifestations of PE include pleuritic chest pain, anxiety, and SOB.
- Thigh and calf measurements should be made daily. The patient is evaluated for the presence of DVT if the circumference of one extremity increases significantly.
- Diagnostic studies used to detect DVT and PE include Doppler ultrasound, radiocontrast venography, and ventilation–perfusion lung scans.

- Anticoagulation therapy to prevent DVT and PE is initiated once head injury and other systemic injuries have been ruled out and there is low risk for bleeding. Anticoagulant therapy should be continued for at least 6 to 12 weeks after injury.
- Elastic compression stockings or pneumatic compression devices, as well as range-of-motion (ROM) exercises, are important preventive measures that work to reduce venous pooling and promote venous return.
- Vena cava filters prevent emboli (dislodged clots) from migrating to the lungs and causing PE in patients who have developed clots despite receiving anticoagulation.

Orthostatic Hypotension

Following SCI, blood pressure tends to be unstable and quite low.

- Observe for orthostatic hypotension, a drop in systolic blood pressure of at least 20 mm Hg or a drop in diastolic pressure of at least 10 mm Hg, regardless of the patient's symptoms. Orthostasis is particularly common in patients with lesions above T7 and in those with tetraplegia.
- Closely monitor vital signs before and during position changes. Interventions for orthostasis include vasopressors to counteract vasodilation, elastic compression stockings to improve venous return, and abdominal binders to encourage venous return and provide diaphragmatic support.
- Plan activity in advance, allowing adequate time for slow progression of position changes.

Autonomic Dysreflexia

Also known as autonomic hyperreflexia, it is an acute emergency that occurs as a result of exaggerated autonomic responses to stimuli that are harmless in normal people.

- Common in individuals with cord lesions T6 and above
- Characterized by:
  - Severe pounding headache
  - Paroxysmal hypertension (HTN)
  - Bradycardia
  - Flushing
  - Profuse diaphoresis

- Nausea
- Nasal congestion
- Distended bladder is the most common trigger; also distention or contraction of the visceral organs, especially the bowel (from constipation, impaction), or stimulation of the skin (tactile, pain, thermal stimuli, pressure ulcer).
- Treatment consists of removing the cause of dysreflexia:
  - Elevate the head of bed to lower blood pressure.
  - Perform rapid assessment to identify and remove cause.
  - Empty bladder by ensuring patency of indwelling catheter; irrigate or replace with new catheter if necessary.
  - Examine rectum for fecal mass; use local anesthetic, such as lidocaine, 10 to 15 minutes prior to disimpaction.
  - Examine skin for any areas of pressure, irritation, or broken areas.
  - Observe for an object next to the skin or a draft of cold air, and remove.
  - If these measures do not relieve the HTN and headache continues, a ganglionic blocking agent (hydralazine hydrochloride [Apresoline]) is prescribed and administered slowly by the IV route.
  - Label the medical record or chart with a clearly visible note about the risk for autonomic dysreflexia.
  - Teach the patient about prevention and management measures, including the development of dysreflexia years after the initial injury.
- Complications: Rupture of cerebral vessels or increased intracerebral pressure (ICP)

NURSING PROCESS

The Patient With Acute Spinal Cord Injury

Assessment

- Observe breathing pattern; assess strength of cough; auscultate lungs.

(continues on page 642)

- Monitor patient closely for any changes in motor or sensory function and for symptoms of progressive neurologic damage. Record on flow sheet.
- Test motor ability by asking patient to spread fingers, squeeze examiner's hand, and move toes or turn the feet.
- Evaluate sensation by pinching the skin or touching it lightly with a tongue blade, starting at shoulder and working down both sides of the extremities; patient's eyes should be closed. Ask patient where sensation is felt.
- Decreased neurologic function is reported immediately.
- Assess for spinal shock, urinary retention, overdistention of the bladder, and paralytic ileus.

Diagnosis

Nursing Diagnoses

- Ineffective breathing patterns related to weakness or paralysis of abdominal and intercostal muscles and inability to clear secretions
- Ineffective airway clearance related to weakness of intercostal muscles
- Impaired bed and physical mobility related to motor and sensory impairment
- Disturbed sensory perception related to immobility and sensory loss
- Risk for impaired skin integrity related to immobility or sensory loss
- Impaired urinary elimination related to inability to void spontaneously
- Constipation related to presence of atonic bowel as a result of autonomic disruption
- Acute pain and discomfort related to treatment and prolonged immobility

Collaborative Problems/Potential Complications

- Deep vein thrombosis
- Orthostatic hypotension
- Autonomic dysreflexia

Planning and Goals

Major patient goals may include improved breathing pattern and airway clearance, improved mobility, improved sensory and perceptual awareness, maintenance of skin integrity, relief of urinary retention, improved bowel function, promotion of comfort, and absence of complications.

Nursing Interventions

Promoting Adequate Breathing and Airway Clearance

- Administer oxygen to maintain normal saturation level; hypoxemia can create or worsen a neurologic deficit. If endotracheal intubation is necessary, extreme care is taken to avoid flexing or extending the patient's neck, which can result in extension of a cervical injury.
- Detect potential respiratory failure by observing patient, noting rate and depth of respirations, assessing lung sounds and accessory muscle use, and monitoring oxygen saturation through pulse oximetry and ABG values.
- Prevent retention of secretions and resultant atelectasis with early and vigorous attention to clearing bronchial and pharyngeal secretions.
- Suction with caution because this procedure can stimulate the vagus nerve, producing bradycardia and cardiac arrest.
- Initiate chest physical therapy and assisted coughing to mobilize secretions if the patient cannot cough effectively.

Improving Mobility

- Maintain proper body alignment at all times.
- Reposition the patient frequently, and assist patient out of bed as soon as the spinal column is stabilized.
- Apply splints (various types) to prevent footdrop and trochanter rolls to prevent external rotation of the hip joints; reapply every 2 hours.
- Patients with lesions above the midthoracic level may tolerate changes in position poorly; monitor blood pressure when positions are changed.

(continues on page 644)

- Do not turn patient who is not on a rotating specialty bed unless the spine is stable and the provider indicates that it is safe to do so.
- Perform passive ROM exercises as soon as possible after injury to avoid complications such as contractures and atrophy.

Promoting Adaptation to Disturbed Sensory Perception

- Stimulate the area above the level of the injury through touch, aromas, flavorful food and beverages, conversation, and music.
- Provide prism glasses to enable patient to see from supine position.
- Encourage use of hearing aids, if applicable.
- Provide emotional support; teach patient strategies to compensate for or cope with sensory deficits.

Maintaining Skin Integrity

Up to 85% of patients with spinal cord disorders will develop pressure ulcers in their lifetime. In the spinal cord population, there is about an 8% mortality rate from pressure ulcers.

- Observe for ulcers over the ischial tuberosity, greater trochanter, sacrum, gluteal area, occiput, and under cervical collars.
- Change patient's position every 2 hours, and inspect the skin each time the patient is turned.
- Keep skin clean by washing with a mild soap, rinse well, and blot dry. Keep pressure-sensitive areas well lubricated and soft with bland cream or lotion.
- Teach patient about pressure ulcers and encourage participation in preventive measures.

Maintaining Urinary Elimination

- Perform intermittent catheterization to avoid overstretching the bladder and urinary tract infections (UTIs). If this is not feasible, insert an indwelling catheter temporarily.
- Teach family members how to catheterize, and encourage them to participate in this facet of care.
- Teach patient to record fluid intake, voiding pattern, characteristics of urine, and any unusual sensations.

Improving Bowel Function

- Provide a high-calorie, high-protein, high-fiber diet, gradually increasing the amount of food when bowel sounds return.
- Administer prescribed stool softener to counteract effects of immobility and analgesic agents.
- Institute a bowel program as early as possible.

Providing Comfort Measures

- Reassure patient in halo traction or with stabilization devices that he will adapt to the appearance of the device, feeling caged in, and hearing noises.
- Cleanse pin sites daily, and observe for redness, drainage, and pain; observe pins for loosening. If a pin becomes detached, stabilize the patient's head in a neutral position and have someone notify the neurosurgeon; keep a torque screwdriver readily available.
- Inspect the skin under the halo vest for excessive perspiration, redness, and skin blistering, especially on the bony prominences. Open vest at the sides to allow torso to be washed. Do not allow vest to become wet; change liner periodically.

Promoting Home- and Community-Based Care

Teaching Patients Self-Care

- Shift emphasis from surviving injury to learning strategies needed to develop skills necessary for activities of daily living.
- Initially, focus patient teaching on the injury and its effects on mobility, dressing, and bowel, bladder, and sexual function.
- As the patient and family acknowledge the consequences of the injury and the resulting disability, broaden the focus of teaching to address issues necessary for carrying out the tasks of daily living and taking charge of their lives.
- Teaching begins in the acute phase and continues throughout rehabilitation.

(continues on page 646)

- Interventions are aimed at increasing function, improving adjustment, increasing social integration, and reducing social stigma.

Continuing Care

- Support and assist patient and family to assume responsibility for increasing care, and provide assistance in dealing with psychological impact of SCI and its consequences.
- Coordinate interdisciplinary team, and serve as liaison with rehabilitation centers, home care agencies, health care providers, respiratory therapy, physical and occupational therapy, case management, and social services.
- Assist patient and family in dealing with psychological impact of injury.
- Assist patients with modifications of risk factors related to aging, including cardiovascular disease, diabetes, psychiatric disorders, and alcohol or substance abuse. Teach patients about healthy lifestyles, remind them of the need for health screenings, and make referrals as appropriate.

Evaluation

Expected Patient Outcomes

- Demonstrates improvement in gas exchange and clearance of secretions
- Moves within limits of dysfunction, and demonstrates completion of exercises within functional limitations
- Demonstrates adaptation to sensory and perceptual alterations
- Demonstrates optimal skin integrity
- Regains control of urinary bladder function
- Regains control of bowel function
- Reports absence of pain and discomfort
- Is free of complications

COMPLICATIONS

- Deep vein thrombosis/PE
- Autonomic dysreflexia
- Hypotension/orthostatic hypotension

For more information, see Chapter 45 in Pellico, L.H. (2013). *Focus on adult health: Medical-surgical nursing*. Philadelphia: Wolters Kluwer Health | Lippincott Williams & Wilkins.

Syndrome of Inappropriate Antidiuretic Hormone Secretion

The syndrome of inappropriate antidiuretic hormone (SIADH) secretion refers to excessive antidiuretic hormone (ADH) secretion from the pituitary gland even in the face of subnormal serum osmolality.

PATHOPHYSIOLOGY

Patients with increased levels of ADH cannot excrete properly dilute urine. This results in fluid retention and dilutional hyponatremia. SIADH is often of nonendocrine origin and may occur in patients with carcinomas (lung, pancreas, and lymphoma) that synthesize and release ADH.

RISK FACTORS

- Pituitary/brain tumor or surgery
- Central nervous system (CNS) infection
- Cancers
- Pulmonary diseases (pneumonia, pneumothorax)
- Medications (vincristine, phenothiazines, tricyclic antidepressants, thiazide diuretics, and nicotine)
- Physical or psychological stress

CLINICAL MANIFESTATIONS AND ASSESSMENT

- Hyponatremia (sodium <134 mEq/L)
- Serum osmolarity less than 280 mOsm/kg, increased urine osmolality, and urine sodium greater than 20 mEq/L
- Normal vital signs
- Moist mucous membranes, normal skin turgor, and lack of edema
- Confusion, lethargy, weakness, myoclonus, asterixis, depressed reflexes, generalized seizure, and coma relating to hyponatremia and cerebral edema

MEDICAL AND NURSING MANAGEMENT

SIADH is treated by eliminating the underlying cause where possible and restricting fluid intake. Diuretics, hypertonic saline, and fluid restriction treat severe hyponatremia.

Pharmacologic Management

- Furosemide (Lasix) to enhance water excretions
- Lithium or demeclocycline to antagonize the osmotic effect of ADH

Nursing Management

- Monitor fluid I & O, daily weight, urine and blood chemistries, and neurologic status.
- Serum sodium should not increase by more than 12 mEq/L in 24 hours, to avoid neurologic damage due to osmotic demyelination
- Assess neurological changes related to hyponatremia and osmotic demyelination.

NURSING ALERT

Institute seizure precautions to protect from injury and prevent aspiration. Keep oxygen and suctioning equipment at the bedside. Ensure side rails are padded. In the event of a seizure, place patient on side to prevent aspiration and protect the airway.

COMPLICATIONS

- Brain herniation
- Central pontine myelinolysis (CMP) is related to a too rapid rise in serum sodium.

For more information, see Chapters 4 and 31 in Pellico, L.H. (2013). *Focus on adult health: Medical-surgical nursing.* Philadelphia: Wolters Kluwer Health | Lippincott Williams & Wilkins.

Systemic Lupus Erythematosus

Systemic lupus erythematosus (SLE) is a chronic, inflammatory autoimmune disease with variable presentations, course, and prognosis, characterized by remissions and exacerbations.

PATHOPHYSIOLOGY

Systemic lupus erythematosus is a result of disturbed immune regulation that causes an exaggerated production of autoantibodies. The immune abnormalities that characterize SLE occur in five phases: susceptibility, abnormal innate and adaptive immune responses, autoantibodies immune complexes, inflammation, and damage. Abnormal B-cell and T-cell responses produce pathogenic autoantibodies and immune complexes that activate complement, form in tissue, and cause inflammation. Inflammation stimulates antigens, which in turn stimulate additional antibodies. The cycle repeats and, over time, leads to irreversible organ damage. Some individuals do not progress through all phases.

> ☼ **N U R S I N G A L E R T**
>
> Certain medications, such as hydralazine (Apresoline), procaina-
> mide (Pronestyl), isoniazid or INH (Nydrazid), chlorpromazine
> (Thorazine), and some antiseizure medications, have been impli-
> cated in chemical- or drug-induced SLE.

RISK FACTORS

- Females are affected more often than males
- African American, Hispanic, and Caucasian
- Medications (hydralazine, procainamide, INH, Thorazine, some anticonvulsants)

CLINICAL MANIFESTATIONS AND ASSESSMENT

Onset is insidious or acute; SLE can go undiagnosed for many years. The clinical course is one of exacerbations and remissions.

- Any body system can be affected.
- Fatigue and myalgias/arthralgias are most prevalent; may be mistaken for rheumatoid arthritis.
- Skin manifestations: Most characteristic is "butterfly-shaped" rash on bridge of nose and cheeks, and photosensitivity rashes, which worsen during flares and are provoked by sunlight or artificial ultraviolet (UV) light. Discoid lupus presents solely with coin-like lesions and alopecia.

> ☼ **N U R S I N G A L E R T**
>
> The nurse should teach patients with SLE to avoid sunlight or UV
> exposure and to protect themselves with sunscreen, with at least
> a sun protection factor of 30, and clothing.

- Neuropsychiatric presentations, manifested by subtle changes in behavior or cognitive ability or mood disorder, depression, or psychosis may occur.
- Pericarditis and pleuritis are the most common cardiopulmo-nary disorders; women are at risk for early atherosclerosis.

- Renal disease, such as glomerulonephritis, which may lead to HTN
- Weight loss

DIAGNOSTIC METHODS

Diagnosis is based on a complete history, physical examination, and diagnostic tests; diagnosis is difficult due to wide range of presenting signs and symptoms.

- Presence of 4 of the 11 criteria established by the American College of Rheumatology (ACR) is required to make the diagnosis of SLE.
- Elevated erythrocyte sedimentation rate (ESR), CBC showing anemia, thrombocytopenia, elevated creatinine, hematuria
- No single laboratory test confirms SLE. Elevated serum levels of antinuclear antibody (ANA) may be seen; small percent of patients will test negative for ANA but will have antibodies to the nuclear antigen anti-Ro.
- C-reactive protein, anti-double-stranded DNA (anti-ds DNA), anti-RNA, anti-Sm (Smith), and high-titer IgG antibodies may be present. The double-stranded DNA test, C3, and C4 indicate whether there is a genetic component.

MEDICAL AND NURSING MANAGEMENT

The goals of treatment include preventing progressive loss of organ function, reducing the likelihood of acute disease, minimizing disease-related disabilities, and preventing complications from therapy.

PHARMACOLOGIC THERAPY

- Corticosteroids are the single most important medication available for SLE; used orally or intravenously. Due to side effects, tapering dosage is a major concern.

- Nonsteroidal anti-inflammatory drugs (NSAIDs)
- Antimalarial drugs, such as hydroxychloroquine (Plaquenil), chloroquine (Aralen)
- Immunosuppressive agents (azathioprine, mycophenolate mofetil, methotrexate)
- Moderate to severe SLE consists of a period of intensive immunosuppressive therapy (induction therapy) followed by a longer period of less intensive maintenance therapy.
- B-cell depleting therapies such as the monoclonal antibodies rituximab (Rituxan) and epratuzumab (humanized anti-CD22 antibody) are the newest form of treatment for SLE; reserved for patients who have not responded to conservative therapies.

For more information, see Chapter 39 in Pellico, L.H. (2013). *Focus on adult health: Medical-surgical nursing.* Philadelphia: Wolters Kluwer Health | Lippincott Williams & Wilkins.

Thrombocytopenia

Thrombocytopenia refers to a low platelet count.

PATHOPHYSIOLOGY

Thrombocytopenia can result from various factors: decreased production of platelets within the bone marrow, increased destruction of platelets, or increased consumption of platelets. There are numerous causes of thrombocytopenia including malignancy, infection, medications, and disseminated intravascular coagulation. Another cause of thrombocytopenia is sequestration in the spleen.

RISK FACTORS

- Malignancy
- Infection
- Medications
- Disseminated intravascular coagulation (DIC)
- Autoimmune processes.
- Genetics

CLINICAL MANIFESTATIONS AND ASSESSMENT

- With platelet count below 50,000/mm^3, bleeding and petechiae occur.

- With platelet count below 20,000/mm^3, petechiae, along with nasal and gingival bleeding, excessive menstrual bleeding, and excessive bleeding after surgery or dental extractions occur.
- With platelet count below 10,000/mm^3, spontaneous, potentially fatal central nervous system hemorrhage or gastrointestinal (GI) hemorrhage may occur.
- If the platelets are dysfunctional due to disease (eg, myelodysplastic syndrome) or medications (eg, aspirin), the risk for bleeding may be much greater even when the actual platelet count is not significantly reduced.

DIAGNOSTIC FINDINGS

- Bone marrow aspiration and biopsy, if platelet deficiency is secondary to decreased production
- Increased megakaryocytes (the cells from which platelets originate) in bone marrow, and normal or increased platelet production as compensation, when platelet destruction is the cause.
- "Pseudothrombocytopenia" results when platelets aggregate and clump in the tube used for blood collection due to presence of ethylenediamine tetra-acetic acid (EDTA), the anticoagulant present in the tube.

MEDICAL AND NURSING MANAGEMENT

The management of thrombocytopenia is usually treatment of the underlying disease.

- Platelet transfusions are used to raise platelet count and stop bleeding or prevent spontaneous hemorrhage if platelet production is impaired.
- If excessive platelet destruction is the cause, the patient is treated as indicated for immune (formerly idiopathic) thrombocytopenia purpura (ITP).
- Splenectomy may be used for ITP; however, it is not an option for other patients with splenomegaly from certain causes (ie, portal hypertension related to cirrhosis).

Nursing Management

Nursing management focuses on prevention and treatment of bleeding.

- Avoid giving aspirin, aspirin-containing medications, or other medications that inhibit platelet function.
- Do not give intramuscular injections, insert indwelling catheters, or use the rectal route for medications or for temperatures.
- Use the smallest possible needles when performing venipuncture; apply pressure to venipuncture sites for 5 minutes or until bleeding has stopped.
- Avoid flossing teeth (for platelet count <20,000/ mm^3 or if gums are bleeding) and do not use commercial mouthwashes. Use soft-bristled tooth brush.
- Use stool softeners and oral laxatives to prevent constipation.
- Avoid tourniquets or overinflation of blood pressure cuffs.
- Avoid suctioning; if unavoidable, use only gentle suctioning.
- Discourage vigorous coughing or blowing the nose.
- Use only electric razor for shaving.
- Prevent falls by ambulating with patient as necessary and keeping the environment safe.
- Teach patient to avoid contact sports and sports with risk for falling or injury (such as biking or roller-blading).
- Teach patient to avoid sexual intercourse (both vaginal and anal) until platelet count is over 50,000/mm^3.

Control Bleeding

- Apply direct pressure with gauze over the source of bleeding.
- For epistaxis, sit patient up with body tilted forward and the mouth open; apply ice pack to the bridge of the nose and direct pressure to nose.
- Hemostatic agents, such as thromboplastin, absorbable gelatin, fibrin sealants, collagen, and alginate, can be used for hemostasis at wound sites and central venous access device sites that are bleeding.
- Notify health care provider for prolonged bleeding (eg, unable to stop within 10 minutes).
- Administer platelets, fresh frozen plasma, packed red blood cells, as prescribed.

For more information, see Chapters 19 and 20 in Pellico, L.H. (2013). *Focus on adult health: Medical-surgical nursing.* Philadelphia: Wolters Kluwer Health | Lippincott Williams & Wilkins.

Thyroiditis

Thyroiditis refers to the inflammation of the thyroid gland that may result in abnormalities in its functioning. The clinical classification of thyroiditis is based on the onset and duration of the disease such as acute, subacute, or chronic.

RISK FACTORS

- Infection by bacteria, fungi, mycobacteria, or parasites (*Staphylococcus aureus* most common)
- Chronic thyroiditis occurs frequently in women between 30 and 50 years.
- Cell-mediated immunity may play a role.
- Acute thyroiditis may follow a respiratory infection.

CLINICAL MANIFESTATIONS AND ASSESSMENT

Acute Thyroiditis

- Anterior neck pain lasting 1 to 2 months, then disappears
- Pharyngitis or pharyngeal pain
- Thyroid enlargement with warmth, erythema, and tenderness; overlying skin often warm and red
- Swallowing may be difficult and uncomfortable.
- Irritability, nervousness, insomnia, and weight loss (manifestations of hyperthyroidism) are common.

Subacute and Chronic Thyroiditis

- Palpable enlarged and painless firm mass over the thyroid gland
- Thyroid activity is normal or low rather than increased.

MEDICAL AND NURSING MANAGEMENT

Acute Thyroiditis

- Antimicrobial agents and fluid replacement
- Surgical incision and drainage if abscess is present

Subacute Thyroiditis

- Control of inflammation; nonsteroidal anti-inflammatory drugs (NSAIDs) to relieve neck pain. Avoid ASA, which displaces thyroid hormone from the binding site and increases circulating hormone, thus worsening the condition.
- Oral corticosteroids relieve pain and reduce swelling in severe cases.
- Beta-blocking agents control symptoms of hyperthyroidism.
- Thyroid hormone therapy if temporary hypothyroidism develops

Chronic Thyroiditis

- Thyroid hormone therapy reduces thyroid activity and the production of thyroglobulin, as well as treats symptoms of hypothyroidism.
- Surgery may be used if symptoms persist.

Nursing Management

- Educate patient about the condition and pain management.

For more information, see Chapter 31 in Pellico, L.H. (2013). *Focus on adult health: Medical-surgical nursing.* Philadelphia: Wolters Kluwer Health | Lippincott Williams & Wilkins.

Thyrotoxicosis or Thyroid Storm

The term thyrotoxicosis refers to *symptomatic* hyperthyroxinemia. The patient with thyroid storm or crisis is critically ill and requires astute observation and aggressive and supportive nursing care during and after the acute stage of illness.

PATHOPHYSIOLOGY

Thyrotoxic crisis or thyroid storm is a life-threatening complication of hyperthyroidism in which profound hypermetabolism involves multiple systems. Although thyrotoxicosis can be caused by hyperthyroidism, other examples of thyrotoxicosis are associated with thyroid gland inflammation or ingestion of thyroid hormone, in which there is an increased release of stored thyroid hormone or increased exogenous hormone ingestion, not accelerated synthesis.

RISK FACTORS

- Stress such as injury infection, thyroid surgery, insulin reaction, diabetic ketoacidosis (DKA)
- Pregnancy
- Abrupt withdrawal of antithyroid medications
- Vigorous palpation of the thyroid
- Thyroid gland inflammation
- Ingestion of thyroid hormone
- Multinodular goiter

CLINICAL MANIFESTATIONS AND ASSESSMENT

- Fever (hyperpyrexia) above 38.5°C (101.3°F)
- Extreme tachycardia (more than 130 beats/min)
- Electrocardiogram (ECG) may show sinus tachycardia or atrial fibrillation

- Exaggerated symptoms of hyperthyroidism with disturbances of a major system, such as GI (weight loss, diarrhea, abdominal pain) or cardiovascular (edema, chest pain, dyspnea, palpitations)
- Altered neurologic or mental state, which frequently appears as delirium psychosis, somnolence, or coma

MEDICAL AND NURSING MANAGEMENT

Immediate objectives are to reduce body temperature and heart rate and prevent vascular collapse.

- A hypothermia mattress or blanket, ice packs, cool environment, hydrocortisone, and acetaminophen (Tylenol)
- Humidified oxygen to improve tissue oxygenation and meet high metabolic demands; arterial blood gases (ABGs) or pulse oximetry to monitor respiratory status
- Intravenous fluids containing dextrose are administered to replace glycogen stores.

Pharmacologic Management

- Hydrocortisone is given to treat shock or adrenal insufficiency.
- Iodine is administered to decrease output of thyroxine (T_4) from thyroid gland.
- Propylthiouracil (PTU) or methimazole is given to impede formation of thyroid hormone.
- Propranolol, combined with digitalis, has been effective in reducing cardiac symptoms.

NURSING ALERT

Salicylates are not used in the management of thyroid storm because they displace thyroid hormone from binding proteins and worsen the hypermetabolism.

Nursing Management

Care provided for the patient with hyperthyroidism is the basis for nursing management of patients with thyroid storm.

See Chapter H, pages 401–408 for more information on hyperthyroidism.

For more information, see Chapter 31 in Pellico, L.H. (2013). *Focus on adult health: Medical-surgical nursing*. Philadelphia: Wolters Kluwer Health | Lippincott Williams & Wilkins.

Toxic Epidermal Necrolysis and Stevens–Johnson Syndrome

Toxic epidermal necrolysis (TEN) and Stevens–Johnson syndrome (SJS) are potentially fatal skin disorders and the most severe forms of erythema multiforme. Both conditions are triggered by medications.

PATHOPHYSIOLOGY

These diseases are mucocutaneous reactions that constitute a spectrum of reactions, with TEN being the most severe. Most patients with TEN have an abnormal metabolism of the medication; the mechanism leading to TEN seems to be a cell-mediated cytotoxic reaction. The complete body surface may be involved, with widespread areas of erythema and blisters. Sepsis and keratoconjunctivitis are possible complications.

The mortality rate from TEN is 30% to 35%. Both TEN and SJS are triggered by a reaction to medications. Although the incidence of TEN and SJS is about 2 to 3 cases per 1 million people, the risk associated with sulfonamides in HIV-positive individuals may approach 1 case per 1,000.

RISK FACTORS

- Antibiotics, particularly sulfonamides
- Antiseizure agents

- Nonsteroidal anti-inflammatory drugs
- Immunosuppressed
- Incidence increased in older individuals
- Possible genetic predisposition to erythema multiforme

CLINICAL MANIFESTATIONS AND ASSESSMENT

- Initial signs are conjunctival burning or itching, cutaneous tenderness, fever, headache, cough, sore throat, extreme malaise, and myalgias (aches and pains).
- Rapid onset of erythema follows, involving much of the skin surface and mucous membranes, including oral mucosa, conjunctiva, and genitalia.
- Large, flaccid bullae in some areas; in other areas, large sheets of epidermis are shed, exposing underlying dermis. Fingernails, toenails, eyebrows, and eyelashes may all be shed, along with surrounding epidermis.
- Excruciatingly tender skin and loss of skin lead to a weeping surface similar to that of a total body partial-thickness burn; this condition may be referred to as *scalded skin syndrome.* Skin loss may approach 100% of total body surface area.
- In severe cases of mucosal involvement, there may be danger of damage to the larynx, bronchi, and esophagus from ulcerations.

DIAGNOSTIC METHODS

- Histologic studies of frozen skin cells from fresh lesions
- Cytodiagnosis of cells from a freshly denuded area
- Immunofluorescent studies for atypical epidermal autoantibodies

MEDICAL AND NURSING MANAGEMENT

Treatment goals include control of fluid and electrolyte balance, prevention of sepsis, and prevention of ophthalmic complications. Supportive care is the mainstay of treatment.

- All nonessential medications are discontinued immediately.
- If possible, patient is treated in a regional burn center.
- Surgical débridement or hydrotherapy may be performed to remove involved skin.
- Tissue samples from the nasopharynx, eyes, ears, blood, urine, skin, and unruptured blisters are used to identify pathogens.
- Intravenous fluids are prescribed to maintain fluid and electrolyte balance. Fluids are administered via nasogastric tube or orally as soon as possible, as IV catheters are potential sources of infection.
- Systemic corticosteroid use is controversial due to risk of infection and poor wound healing; however, they may be used in TEN caused by medication reactions. Monitor closely for adverse effects.
- Topical antibacterial and anesthetic agents are used to prevent wound sepsis.
- Temporary biologic dressings (pigskin, amniotic membrane) or plastic semipermeable dressings (Vigilon) are applied to reduce pain, decrease evaporation, and prevent secondary infection.
- Meticulous oropharyngeal and eye care is essential when there is severe involvement of mucous membranes and eyes.
- Teach patient and family members procedures for wound care, dressing changes, pain management, nutrition, measures to increase mobility, and detect infection as the patient improves and transitions to rehabilitation or outpatient care.

COMPLICATIONS

- Sepsis secondary to pseudomonas, *Klebsiella, E. coli, Serratia,* and *Candida.*
- Conjunctival retraction, scars, and corneal lesions
- Keratoconjunctivitis

For more information, see Chapter 52 in Pellico, L.H. (2013). *Focus on adult health: Medical-surgical nursing.* Philadelphia: Wolters Kluwer Health | Lippincott Williams & Wilkins.

Tuberculosis, Pulmonary

Tuberculosis (TB), an infectious disease primarily affecting the lung parenchyma, is caused primarily by *Mycobacterium tuberculosis.* Tuberculosis is a worldwide public health problem, and mortality and morbidity rates continue to rise. *M. tuberculosis* infects an estimated one-third of the world's population and remains the leading cause of death from infectious disease in the world.

PATHOPHYSIOLOGY

Tuberculosis spreads from person to person by droplet transmission via talking, coughing, sneezing, laughing, or singing. Inhaled bacteria are transmitted to the alveoli, where macrophages ingest the bacilli. If the bacilli escape the antimicrobial activities of the macrophages, an infection begins. Phagocytes (neutrophils and macrophages) engulf many of the bacteria, and TB-specific lymphocytes destroy the bacilli along with normal tissue. This tissue reaction results in the accumulation of exudate in the alveoli, causing bronchopneumonia to occur 2 to 10 weeks after exposure.

The material (bacteria and macrophages) becomes necrotic, forming a cheesy mass, which may become calcified. At this point, the bacteria become dormant, and there is no further progression of active disease. Approximately 10% of people who are initially infected develop active disease. Some people develop reactivation TB. This type of TB results from a breakdown of the host defenses.

RISK FACTORS

- Birth in country with high prevalence of TB or travel abroad to endemic areas (Asia, Haiti)
- Homeless, impoverished, overcrowded and substandard housing
- Minorities, particularly children younger than 15 years and young adults 15 to 44 years

- Resident or employee of corrections center, homeless shelter, long-term care facility
- Health care worker caring for high-risk patients or performing high-risk activities (ie, suctioning, sputum induction, bronchoscopy, intubation)
- Substance abuse
- Immunocompromised
- Malnutrition, gastric or intestinal bypass
- Chronic illness; diabetes, chronic kidney disease

CLINICAL MANIFESTATIONS AND ASSESSMENT

The signs and symptoms of pulmonary TB are insidious; most patients have:

- Low-grade fever, cough, night sweats, fatigue, and weight loss
- Nonproductive cough, which may progress to mucopurulent sputum with hemoptysis
- Dyspnea and chest pain as the disease progresses
- Systemic and the pulmonary symptoms are chronic and may have been present for weeks to months.
- Elderly patients usually present with less pronounced symptoms than do younger patients.
- Extrapulmonary disease occurs in up to 16% of cases. In patients with AIDS, extrapulmonary disease is more prevalent and is manifested by neurologic deficits, bone pain, meningitis symptoms, and dysuria.

DIAGNOSTIC METHODS

- Tuberculosis skin test (Mantoux test). Note: A positive reaction does not necessarily mean that active disease is present; reaction indicates past exposure to *M. tuberculosis* or vaccination with Bacille Calmette-Guérin (BCG) vaccine.

- A negative skin test does not exclude TB infection or disease; patients who are immunosuppressed cannot develop an immune response that is adequate to produce a positive skin test.
- QuantiFeron-TB Gold (QFT-G) test (not affected by prior vaccination with BCG)
- Chest X-ray
- Sputum for acid-fast bacillus (AFB) smear and culture

Gerontologic Considerations

Elderly patients may have atypical manifestations, such as unusual behavior or disturbed mental status, fever, anorexia, and weight loss. In many elderly patients, the tuberculin skin test produces no reaction due to loss of immunologic memory or delayed reactivity for up to 1 week (recall phenomenon). A second skin test is performed in 1 to 2 weeks.

MEDICAL AND NURSING MANAGEMENT

- Pulmonary TB is treated primarily with antituberculosis agents, as either active disease treatment or prophylactic treatment for persons exposed to and at risk for developing the disease. Increasing prevalence of drug resistance emphasizes the need to begin TB treatment with four or more medications, to ensure completion of therapy, and to develop and evaluate new anti-TB medications.
- A prolonged treatment duration is necessary to ensure eradication of the organisms and to prevent relapse.

Pharmacologic Therapy

- First-line medications: Isoniazid or INH, rifampin, pyrazinamide, and ethambutol; combination medications and medications taken twice weekly are available to improve adherence.
- Second-line medications: Capreomycin, ethionamide, para-aminosalicylate sodium, and cycloserine
- Additional medications include other aminoglycosides, quinolones, rifabutin, clofazimine, and combinations of medications.

- The total number of doses taken, not simply the duration of treatment, more accurately determines whether a course of therapy has been completed.
- Vitamin B (pyridoxine) is usually administered with INH to prevent INH-associated peripheral neuropathy.

Side Effects of Medication Therapy

- Assess medication side effects, because they are often a reason why patients fail to adhere to the prescribed medication regimen.
- Instruct the patient to take the medication on an empty stomach or at least 1 hour before meals as food interferes with medication absorption.
- Patients taking INH should avoid foods that contain tyramine and histamine (tuna, aged cheese, red wine, soy sauce, yeast extracts); a food–drug interaction with INH may result in headache, flushing, hypotension, lightheadedness, palpitations, and diaphoresis.
- Rifampin can increase the metabolism of certain other medications, making them less effective. These medications include beta blockers, oral anticoagulants (eg, warfarin), digoxin, quinidine, corticosteroids, oral hypoglycemic agents, oral contraceptives, theophylline, and verapamil.
- Inform the patient that rifampin may discolor contact lenses and that the patient may want to wear eyeglasses during treatment.
- Monitor for other side effects of anti-TB medications, including hepatitis, neurologic changes (hearing loss, neuritis), and rash.
- Monitor renal and hepatic function tests, as well as sputum AFB closely.
- Monitor vital signs and observe for spikes in temperature or changes in the patient's clinical status. Changes in the patient's respiratory status are reported to the primary health care provider.
- Emphasize the risk of drug resistance if the medication regimen is not strictly and continuously followed.
- Directly observed therapy (DOT) can be implemented to ensure that patients are compliant with medications regimens.

Patient Teaching

- Education is related to halting the spread of the infection and its complex drug regimens.
- Patients should be instructed to cover their mouths and noses when they cough or sneeze, dispose of facial tissues in plastic bags, and wear a mask when in public until sputum samples are documented as free of AFB.
- To counter effects of inadequate nutrition, collaborate with the dietitian, provider, social worker, family, and patient to identify strategies to ensure an adequate intake of high-calorie, nutritious foods.
- Identifying facilities (eg, shelters, soup kitchens, Meals on Wheels) that provide meals in the patient's neighborhood may increase the likelihood that the patient with limited resources and energy will have access to a more nutritious intake.

For more information, see Chapter 10 in Pellico, L.H. (2013). *Focus on adult health: Medical-surgical nursing.* Philadelphia: Wolters Kluwer Health | Lippincott Williams & Wilkins.

Ulcerative Colitis

Ulcerative colitis is a recurrent ulcerative and inflammatory disease of the mucosal and submucosal layers of the colon and rectum.

PATHOPHYSIOLOGY

Ulcerative colitis affects the superficial mucosa of the colon and is characterized by multiple ulcerations, diffuse inflammations, and desquamation or shedding of the colonic epithelium. Bleeding, edema, inflammation, and abscesses develop. The lesions are contiguous, occurring one after the other. Ulcerative colitis usually begins in the rectum and spreads proximally to the entire colon. Eventually, the bowel narrows, shortens, and thickens because of muscular hypertrophy and fat deposits. It is a serious disease, accompanied by systemic complications and a high mortality rate. Approximately 5% of patients with ulcerative colitis develop colon cancer.

RISK FACTORS

Caucasians and those of Jewish heritage are most at risk.

CLINICAL MANIFESTATIONS AND ASSESSMENT

The clinical course is usually one of intermittent exacerbations and remissions.

- Predominant symptoms: Diarrhea, left lower quadrant abdominal pain, intermittent tenesmus, and rectal bleeding
- Bleeding may be mild or severe; pallor, anemia, and fatigue result.
- Anorexia, weight loss, fever, vomiting, dehydration, cramping, and feeling an urgent need to defecate (may report passing 10 to 20 liquid stools daily) is common.
- Hypocalcemia may occur.
- Rebound tenderness in right lower quadrant is present.
- Extraintestinal manifestations include skin lesions (eg, erythema nodosum), eye lesions (eg, uveitis), joint abnormalities (eg, arthritis), and liver disease.
- Tachycardia, hypotension, tachypnea, fever, and pallor may be present.
- Examine abdomen for bowel sounds, distention, and tenderness to determine severity of the disease.
- Assess level of hydration and nutritional status.

DIAGNOSTIC METHODS

- Stool may be positive for blood.
- Blood studies demonstrate low hematocrit and hemoglobin, high white blood cell count, decreased albumin level, and electrolyte imbalance.
- Abdominal X-rays are performed to determine cause of symptoms.
- Barium enema may show mucosal irregularities, focal strictures or fistulas, shortening of the colon, and dilation of bowel loops.
- Colonoscopy may reveal friable, inflamed mucosa with exudate and ulcerations.
- Computed tomography (CT), magnetic resonance imaging (MRI), and ultrasound can identify abscesses and perirectal involvement.
- Leukocyte scanning, using the patient's WBCs, which are labeled with a radiopharmaceutical agent and reinjected, is helpful for localization of acute abscess formation; useful when severe colitis prohibits the use of colonoscopy to determine the extent of inflammation.

- Stool examination for parasites and other microbes to rule out dysentery caused by common intestinal organisms, especially *Entamoeba histolytica* and *Clostridium difficile*.

MEDICAL AND NURSING MANAGEMENT

Medical treatment for both regional enteritis and ulcerative colitis is aimed at reducing inflammation, suppressing inappropriate immune responses, providing rest for a diseased bowel so that healing may take place, improving quality of life, and preventing or minimizing complications.

Nutritional Therapy

- Oral fluids and a low-residue, high-protein, high-calorie diet with supplemental vitamins iron replacement are prescribed.
- Fluid and electrolyte imbalances are corrected with IV therapy or orally if outpatient.
- Foods that exacerbate diarrhea are avoided. Milk may contribute to diarrhea in those with lactose intolerance.
- Cold foods and smoking are avoided because both increase intestinal motility.
- Parenteral nutrition may be indicated.

Pharmacologic Therapy

- Sedative, antidiarrheal, and antiperistaltic medications
- Aminosalicylates: Sulfasalazine (Azulfidine) is effective for mild or moderate inflammation. Sulfa-free aminosalicylates (eg, mesalamine [Asacol, Pentasa]) are effective in preventing and treating recurrence of inflammation.
- Corticosteroids (eg, oral: Prednisone [Deltasone]; parenteral: Hydrocortisone [Solu-Cortef]; topical: Budesonide [Entocort]) are used to treat severe and fulminant disease and can be administered orally or parenterally. When the dosage of corticosteroids is reduced or stopped, the symptoms of disease may return.

- Topical (ie, rectal administration) corticosteroids (eg, hydrocortisone enema, budesonide [Entocort]) are also widely used.
- Antibiotics (eg, metronidazole [Flagyl]) are used for secondary infections, particularly for purulent complications such as abscesses, perforation, and peritonitis.
- Immunomodulator agents (eg, azathioprine [Imuran, 6-mercaptopurine [6-MP], methotrexate, and cyclosporine) have been used in severe disease when other therapies have failed.
- Monoclonal antibodies are being studied, including natalizumab (Tysabri) for treating Crohn's disease) and infliximab (Remicade) for treating ulcerative colitis.

Surgical Management

The most common indications for surgery are medically intractable disease, poor quality of life, or complications from the disease or its treatment.

- Laparoscope-guided strictureplasty is performed commonly to widen a blocked or narrowed section of intestine.
- Bowel resection is performed in some cases, with the remaining segments anastomosed.
- In severe cases, total colectomy or proctocolectomy with ileostomy may be performed. If the rectum can be preserved, restorative proctocolectomy with ileal pouch anal anastomosis (IPAA) is the procedure of choice. Fecal diversions may be needed.

COMPLICATIONS

- Toxic megacolon
- Perforation
- Bleeding
- Risk of osteoporotic fractures due to decreased bone mineral density.

For more information, see Chapter 24 in Pellico, L.H. (2013). *Focus on adult health: Medical-surgical nursing.* Philadelphia: Wolters Kluwer Health | Lippincott Williams & Wilkins.

Urolithiasis and Nephrolithiasis

Urolithiasis and nephrolithiasis refer to stones (calculi) in the urinary tract and kidney, respectively. Urinary stones account for more than 320,000 hospital admissions each year.

PATHOPHYSIOLOGY

Stones are formed in the urinary tract when the urinary concentrations of substances such as calcium oxalate, calcium phosphate, and uric acid increases. Stones may be found anywhere from the kidney to the bladder, and may vary in size from minute granular deposits, called sand or gravel, to those the size of an orange.

Stone formation is not clearly understood; one theory is a deficiency of substances that normally prevent crystallization in the urine, such as citrate, magnesium, nephrocalcin, and uropontin. Another theory relates to fluid volume status of the patient; stones tend to occur more often in dehydrated patients. Certain factors favor stone formation; however, in many patients, no cause may be found.

When stones block the flow of urine, obstruction develops, producing an increase in hydrostatic pressure, distending the renal pelvis and proximal ureter. Some stones cause few symptoms while slowly destroying the nephrons of the kidney; others cause excruciating pain and discomfort.

RISK FACTORS

- Third to fifth decade of life
- Men are affected more often than women
- Anatomical structure of urinary tract
- Hyperparathyroidism
- Hyperuricemia (gout)
- Genetic predisposition (familial renal tubule acidosis)
- Spring and summer (ostensibly due to dehydration)

CLINICAL MANIFESTATIONS AND ASSESSMENT

Manifestations depend on the presence of obstruction, infection, and edema. Symptoms range from mild to excruciating pain and discomfort.

Stones in Renal Pelvis

- Intense, deep ache in costovertebral region
- Hematuria and pyuria
- Pain that radiates anteriorly and downward toward bladder in women and toward testes in men
- Sudden acute pain indicates renal colic; patient displays nausea, vomiting, costovertebral area tenderness.
- Abdominal discomfort, diarrhea may occur.

Ureteral Stones (Stones Lodged in Ureter)

- Acute ureteral colic, excruciating wave-like pain, radiating down the thigh to the genitalia
- Frequent desire to void, but little urine passed; urine usually contains blood because of the abrasive action of the stone

Stones Lodged in Bladder

- Symptoms of irritation associated with urinary tract infection (UTI) and hematuria
- Urinary retention, if stone obstructs bladder neck

DIAGNOSTIC METHODS

- Diagnosis is confirmed by X-rays of the kidneys, ureters, and bladder (KUB) or by ultrasonography, IV urography, or retrograde pyelography.
- Blood chemistries and a 24-hour urine test for measurement of calcium, uric acid, creatinine, sodium, pH, and total volume are done.

- Dietary and medication histories and family history of renal stones are obtained to identify factors predisposing the patient to the formation of stones.
- Chemical analysis is performed to determine stone composition.

MEDICAL MANAGEMENT

Basic goals are to eradicate the stone, determine the stone type, prevent nephron destruction, control infection, and relieve any obstruction that may be present.

- Hot baths or moist heat to the flank may be useful.

Pharmacologic Therapy

- Relive pain using opioid analgesic agents and nonsteroidal anti-inflammatory drugs (NSAIDs); NSAIDs inhibit synthesis of prostaglandin E, reducing swelling, and facilitating passage of the stone.
- Fluids are encouraged to increase hydrostatic pressure behind the stone and assist its passage downward.

Nutritional Therapy

- Encourage the patient to drink eight to ten 8-ounce glasses of water daily or administer IV fluids to keep the urine dilute. A urine output exceeding 2 L a day is advisable.

Procedures for Treatment of Stone Disease

- Ureteroscopy: Stones are fragmented with use of laser, electro-hydraulic lithotripsy, or ultrasound and then removed.
- Extracorporeal shock wave lithotripsy (ESWL)
- Endourologic percutaneous nephrostomy
- Chemolysis (stone dissolution): Alternative for those who are poor risks for other therapies, refuse other methods, or have easily dissolved stones (struvite)
- Surgical removal is performed in only 1% to 2% of patients who do not respond to other forms of treatment and to correct anatomic abnormalities to improve urinary drainage.

- Nephrolithotomy incision into the kidney for removal of the stone
- Nephrectomy, if the kidney is nonfunctional secondary to infection or hydronephrosis
- Pyelolithotomy removes stones in the renal pelvis, ureterolithotomy removes stones in the ureter, and cystostomy removes stones in the bladder. Cystolitholapaxy removes a stone in the bladder using an instrument inserted through the urethra; the stone is usually crushed before removal.

NURSING PROCESS

The Patient With Kidney Stones

Assessment

- Assess for pain and discomfort, including severity, location, and radiation of pain.
- Assess for associated symptoms, including nausea, vomiting, diarrhea, and abdominal distention.
- Observe for signs of UTI and obstruction.
- Observe urine for blood; strain for stones or gravel.
- Focus history on factors that predispose patient to urinary tract stones or that may have precipitated current episode of renal or ureteral colic.
- Assess patient's knowledge about renal stones and measures to prevent recurrence.

Diagnosis

Nursing Diagnoses

Appropriate nursing diagnoses of the patient with kidney stones may include:

- Pain, acute, related to inflammation, obstruction, and abrasion of the urinary tract
- Knowledge, deficient, regarding prevention of recurrence of renal stones
- Knowledge, deficient, regarding role of diet in the treatment of renal stones

(continues on page 676)

- Urinary elimination, impaired due to presence of renal stones

Potential Complications

Potential complications may include the following:

- Infection and urosepsis (from UTI and pyelonephritis)
- Obstruction of the urinary tract by a stone or edema, with subsequent acute renal failure

Planning

Major goals may include relief of pain and discomfort, prevention of recurrence of renal stones, and absence of complications.

Nursing Interventions

Relieving Pain

- Administer opioid analgesics with NSAID as prescribed.
- Encourage and assist patient to assume a position of comfort.
- Assist patient to ambulate if this brings pain relief.
- Monitor pain closely and promptly report increases in severity.

Monitoring and Managing Potential Complications

- Encourage increased fluid intake and ambulation.
- Begin IV fluids if patient cannot take adequate oral fluids.
- Monitor total urine output and patterns of voiding.
- Encourage ambulation as a means of moving the stone through the urinary tract.
- Strain all urine; crush any blood clots passed in urine, and inspect sides of urinal and bedpan for clinging stones.
- Instruct patient to report decreased urine volume, bloody or cloudy urine, fever.
- Instruct patient to report any increase in pain that may indicate obstruction.
- Monitor vital signs for early indications of infection; infections should be treated with the appropriate antibiotic agent before efforts are made to dissolve the stone.

- Provide education about the causes of kidney stones and recommendations to prevent their recurrence, with emphasis on fluid intake of greater than 2,000 mL/day.

Continuing Care

- Monitor patient closely with follow-up care to ensure that treatment has been effective and that no complications, such as obstruction, infection, renal hematoma, or hypertension, have developed.
- The patient's ability to monitor urinary pH and interpret the results is assessed during follow-up visits to the clinic or health care provider's office.
- Ensure patient's understanding of signs and symptoms of stone formation, obstruction, and infection, and the importance of reporting these signs promptly.
- If medications are prescribed for the prevention of stone formation, the actions and importance of the medications are explained to the patient.

Evaluation

Expected patient outcomes may include

- Reports relief of pain
- States increased knowledge of health-seeking behaviors to prevent recurrence
- Experiences no complications

For more information, see Chapter 28 in Pellico, L.H. (2013). *Focus on adult health: Medical-surgical nursing.* Philadelphia: Wolters Kluwer Health | Lippincott Williams & Wilkins.

V

Venous Disorders: Venous Thrombosis and Deep Vein Thrombosis

Venous blood flow is reduced by a thrombus or embolus obstructing a vein, by incompetent venous valves, or by a reduction of the pumping action effectiveness of surrounding muscles. Decreased venous blood flow causes increased venous pressure, which increases capillary hydrostatic pressure, facilitating filtration of fluid out of the capillaries into the interstitial space, with resultant development of tissue edema. Edematous tissue does not receive adequate nutrition from the blood and is more susceptible to breakdown, injury, and infection. Thus, the nurse is aware that edematous tissue is fragile tissue.

VENOUS THROMBOSIS

The terms venous thrombosis, deep vein thrombosis (DVT), thrombophlebitis, and phlebothrombosis do not necessarily reflect identical disease processes, but they are grouped together for clinical purposes.

PATHOPHYSIOLOGY

The exact cause of venous thrombosis remains unclear. Three factors, known as Virchow's triad, are believed to play a significant role in the development of venous thrombosis. This triad includes hypercoagulability, venous stasis and endothelial injury. Some hypercoagulable states are hereditary.

Upper extremity venous thrombosis is not as common as lower extremity thrombosis. However, it may occur in patients with IV catheters (IV lines or wires from pacemaker leads, chemotherapy ports, dialysis catheters, or parenteral nutrition lines) or in patients with an underlying hypercoagulation disorder. Effort thrombosis is caused by repetitive motion (as in competitive swimmers, tennis players, and construction workers) that irritates the vessel wall, causing inflammation and subsequent thrombosis.

Venous thrombi are aggregates of platelets attached to the vein wall. They have a tail-like appendage containing fibrin, white blood cells, and many red blood cells, which can propagate as successive layers of thrombus form. Venous thrombosis is dangerous as fragments may embolize to the lung. After an episode of acute DVT, recanalization of the lumen of the vessel occurs; however, the venous valves remain open and are ineffective. Reverse venous flow contributes to chronic venous insufficiency. Over time, postphlebitic syndrome occurs, manifested by skin and tissue changes.

RISK FACTORS

- History of varicose veins, hypercoagulation, neoplastic disease, cardiovascular disease, or recent major surgery or injury
- Obesity
- Immobility
- Elderly
- Oral contraceptive use

CLINICAL MANIFESTATIONS AND ASSESSMENT

- Signs and symptoms are nonspecific, with the exception of phlegmasia cerulea dolens (massive iliofemoral venous thrombosis), in which the entire extremity becomes massively swollen, tense, painful, and cool to the touch.
- Edema and swelling of the extremity resulting from obstruction of the deep veins of the leg; circumferential measurement of

the extremities, comparing one extremity with the other at the same level, will reveal swelling. The affected extremity may feel warmer than the unaffected extremity.

- Skin over the affected leg may become warmer; superficial veins may become more prominent (cordlike venous segment).
- Tenderness occurs later and is detected by gently palpating the leg.
- Homans' sign (pain in the calf after sharp dorsiflexion of the foot) is not considered reliable and is no longer used.
- In some cases, signs of a pulmonary embolus (PE) are the first indication of DVT.
- Low-grade fever may be present.
- Superficial vein thrombus produces pain or tenderness, redness, and warmth in the involved area; many dissolve spontaneously.
- Recognize that, although NSAIDs provide analgesia, they may obscure clinical evidence of thrombus propagation.

DIAGNOSTIC METHODS

- History revealing risk factors as cited
- D-dimer assay

N u r s i n g   A l e r t

The D-dimer blood assay is a marker of coagulation activity. When a clot lyses, fibrin degradation occurs and the D-dimer is positive. Elevation of the D-dimer can be associated with a variety of disorders including recent surgery, hemorrhage, trauma, cancer, myocardial infarction, pneumonia, and sepsis; however, a negative D-dimer decreases the likelihood that DVT or PE is present.

- Doppler ultrasonography, duplex ultrasonography

PREVENTION

Prevention includes identifying at-risk individuals and using the following measures: elastic compression stockings, intermittent pneumatic compression devices, and body positioning and exercise. Medications to prevent thrombosis include anticoagulant therapy with subcutaneous unfractionated or low-molecular-weight heparin (LMWH).

MEDICAL AND NURSING MANAGEMENT

Objectives of management are to prevent the thrombus from growing and fragmenting, resolve the current thrombus, and prevent recurrence.

Pharmacologic Therapy

Heparins

Anticoagulant therapy is effective prophylaxis; however, anticoagulants do not dissolve a thrombus that has already formed.

Unfractionated Heparin

- Unfractionated heparin is administered subcutaneously to prevent development of DVT.
- Intravenous infusion of heparin prevents the extension of a thrombus and the development of new thrombi; provides rapid anticoagulant effects (may be administered subcutaneously).
- Unfractionated heparin is administered via an infusion pump to carefully control the rate.
- Dosage is weight-based; possible bleeding tendencies are detected by a pretreatment clotting profile.
- Periodic coagulation tests and hematocrit levels are obtained.

N U R S I N G   A L E R T

Heparin is in the effective, or therapeutic, range when the activated partial thromboplastin time (aPTT) is 1.5 times to 2.5 times the baseline control. Normal aPTT level is 21 to 35 seconds. If the PTT is greater than 100 seconds, the risk for hemorrhage is significant!

- The nurse is aware that heparin has a half-life of about 60 minutes; therefore, in an emergency, heparin is discontinued for a period of at least 1 hour.
- Coumadin, an oral anticoagulant, is administered soon after initiating heparin therapy, since Coumadin may require 3 to 5 days to achieve a therapeutic effect; until a therapeutic international normalized ratio (INR) is achieved, both medications are administered concurrently.
- Medication dosage is regulated by monitoring the activated partial thromboplastin time (aPTT) for heparin, the INR for

Coumadin, and the platelet count, to assess heparin-induced thrombocytopenia (HIT), discussed later in this chapter.

Low-Molecular-Weight Heparin (LMWH)

- Subcutaneous LMWH is an effective treatment for some cases of DVT; due to a longer half-life than that of unfractionated heparin, doses can be given once or twice daily.
- Doses are weight-based; LMWH prevents the extension of a thrombus and development of new thrombi. Low-molecular-weight heparin is associated with fewer bleeding complications and lower risks of HIT than is unfractionated heparin.
- Because LMWH is cleared almost entirely by the kidneys, clearance can be variable in patients with renal insufficiency, thus longer half-life may be expected.
- The cost of LMWH is higher than that of unfractionated heparin; however, LMWH may be used safely in pregnant women.

Thrombolytic Therapy

- Thrombolytic (fibrinolytic) therapy lyses and dissolves thrombi; it is most effective if given within the first 3 days after acute thrombosis.
- The advantages of thrombolytic therapy are less long-term damage to the venous valves, and less likelihood of post thrombotic syndrome and chronic venous insufficiency.
- An increase in bleeding complications occurs with thrombolytics as opposed to heparin. If bleeding occurs, the thrombolytic agent may be discontinued.

Oral Anticoagulants

- Warfarin is a vitamin K antagonist used for extended anticoagulant therapy.
- Routine coagulation monitoring of the INR is essential to ensure that a therapeutic response is obtained and maintained over time.
- Drug–food and drug–medication interactions (such as those containing vitamin K) can reduce or enhance the anticoagulant effects of warfarin.
- Warfarin has slow onset of action; the full anticoagulant effect of warfarin may take 3 to 5 days, during which heparin administration continues until the INR is therapeutic.

- A normal INR is approximately 1. The target INR for DVT or atrial fibrillation is 2 to 3, with a goal of 2.5. Once INR is stable, levels are checked weekly for 2 to 4 weeks, progressing to monthly thereafter.

Surgical Management

- Surgery is necessary for DVT when anticoagulant or thrombolytic therapy is contraindicated, the danger of PE is likely, or the venous drainage is so severely compromised that permanent damage to the extremity is likely.
- Thrombectomy (removal of the thrombosis) is the procedure of choice.
- A vena cava filter may be placed to trap large emboli and prevent PE. The filter does not prevent other thrombi from forming.
- Balloon angioplasty and stent placement are being used in the iliac veins.

Nursing Management

Monitoring Drug Therapy

- When the patient is receiving anticoagulant therapy, the nurse frequently monitors the aPTT, prothrombin time (PT), INR, activated coagulation time (ACT), hemoglobin and hematocrit values, platelet count, and fibrinogen level, depending on prescribed medication.
- Observe for spontaneous bleeding anywhere in the body. Observe for microscopic hematuria, often the first sign of excessive dosage, bruises, nosebleeds, and bleeding gums.
- To promptly reverse the effects of heparin, protamine sulfate may be administered. Risks of protamine administration include bradycardia and hypotension, which can be minimized by slow administration. Protamine sulfate is less effective with LMWH than with unfractionated heparin.
- Plan to reverse warfarin with vitamin K and/or infusion of fresh-frozen plasma or prothrombin concentrate.
- Monitor for HIT, which is defined as a sudden decrease in the platelet count by at least 30% of baseline levels in patients receiving heparin.

V

NURSING ALERT

A normal adult platelet count is 140 to $400 \times 10^3/mm^3$. A platelet count of less than $20 \times 10^3/mm^3$ is associated with bleeding from gums, injection sites; epistaxis (nose bleed), ecchymosis (bruising), and petechiae may be noted. When the platelet count drops to less than $10 \times 10^3/mm^3$, spontaneous intracranial hemorrhage becomes a significant risk

- Patients at greatest risk for bleeding are those receiving unfractionated heparin for a long period of time (ie, several days or weeks); therefore, it is preferable to avoid unfractionated heparin over the long term. Warfarin may be used instead.
- Recognize that HIT is thought to result from an autoimmune mechanism that causes destruction of platelets. If the process is not arrested, platelets may aggregate, initiating inappropriate clotting and thrombosis throughout the body; prognosis is extremely guarded.
- Note early signs of complications associated with anticoagulants, including decreasing platelet count, the need for increasing doses of heparin to maintain the therapeutic level, and thromboembolic or hemorrhagic complications such as skin necrosis at the injection site, at distal sites of thromboses, skin discoloration consisting of hemorrhagic areas, hematomas, purpura, and blistering.
- Lepirudin (Refludan) and argatroban are direct thrombin inhibitors used for anticoagulation in patients who have developed HIT. Monitor the aPTT or ACT.
- Be aware of interactions of oral anticoagulants with many other medications and herbal and nutritional supplements; check to see if any medications or supplements the patient is taking are contraindicated with warfarin.

Providing Comfort

- Elevate affected extremity, apply elastic compression stockings, and administer analgesics as adjuncts to therapy.
- Bed rest may be required for a few days after the diagnosis; early ambulation may decrease risk of thrombus extension with risk of PE. Follow institutional protocol until further research clarifies this.

- Apply warm, moist packs to the affected extremity to reduce discomfort.

Applying Compression Therapy

- Elastic compression stockings are prescribed for patients with chronic venous insufficiency to exert a sustained, graduated compression of superficial veins, to minimize venous blood pooling, and promote flow toward the deep veins.
- Short, stretch elastic wraps may be applied from the toes to the knee in a 50% spiral overlap.
- Intermittent pneumatic compression devices can be used with elastic compression stockings to prevent DVT and to reduce edema during bedrest.
- Other types of compression include the Unna boot, which consists of a gauze roll impregnated with glycerin, gelatin, and sometimes zinc oxide or calamine.

Body Positioning and Exercise

- Elevate feet and lower legs periodically above heart level when on bed rest.
- Perform active and passive leg exercises, particularly those involving calf muscles, to increase venous flow.
- Provide early ambulation to help prevent venous stasis.
- Encourage deep-breathing exercises that increase negative pressure in the thorax, promoting emptying of the large veins.
- Once ambulatory, instruct the patient to avoid sitting for more than 2 hours at a time and to perform active and passive leg exercises during long car, train, and plane trips when ambulation is not possible.

V

For more information, see Chapter 18 in Pellico, L.H. (2013). *Focus on adult health: Medical-surgical nursing.* Philadelphia: Wolters Kluwer Health | Lippincott Williams & Wilkins.

APPENDIX

Selected Lab Values

Blood Chemistry

Test	Conventional Units	SI Units
Alanine aminotransferase (ALT, formerly SGPT)	Males: 10–40 U/mL Females: 8–35 U/mL	Males: 0.17–0.68 μkat/L Females: 0.14–0.60 μkat/L
Alkaline phosphatase	50–120 U/L	50–120 U/L
Ammonia (plasma)	15–45 μg/dL (varies with method)	11–32 μmol/L
Amylase	60–160 Somogyi U/dL	111–296 U/L
Aspartase amino transferase (AST, formerly SGOT)	Males: 10–40 U/L Females: 15–30 U/L	Males: 0.34–0.68 μkat/L Females: 0.25–0.51 μkat/L
Bicarbonate	24–31 mEq/L	24–31 mmol/L
Bilirubin (total)	0.3–1.0 mg/dL	5–17 μmol/L
Direct	0.1–0.4 mg/dL	1.7–3.7 μmol/L
Indirect	0.1–0.4 mg/dL	3.4–11.2 μmol/L
Blood urea nitrogen (BUN)	8–20 mg/dL	2.9–7.1 mmol/L
B-type Natriuretic Peptide	<100 pg/mL	<100 mg/L
Calcium	8.6–10.2 mg/dL	2.5–2.55 mmol/L
Carbon dioxide, arterial (whole blood) partial pressure ($PaCO_2$)	35–45 mm Hg	4.66–5.99 kPa
Chloride	97–107 mEq/L	97–107 mmol/L
Creatinine (serum)	0.7–1.4 mg/dL[†]	64–124 μmol/L[†]
Gamma-glutamyl-transpeptidase (GGT)	Males: 20–30 U/L Females: 1–24 U/L	0.03–0.5 μkat/L 0.02–0.4 μkat/L
Glucose (blood)	Fasting: 60–110 mg/dL	3.3–6.05 mmol/L
	Postprandial (2 h): 65–140 mg/dL	3.58–7.7 mmol/L

(continued on page 688)

Blood Chemistry

Test	Conventional Units	SI Units
Glycosylated hemoglobin (HbA_{1c}) (non diabetic)	4.4%–6.4%	
Lactate dehydrogenase (LDH)	90–176 mU/mL	90–176 U/L
Lipids		
Cholesterol	<200 mg/dL (desirable)	<5.2 mmol/L
Triglycerides	<165 mg/dL	<1.65 g/L
Lipase	0–160 U/L[†]	0.266 µkat/L[†]
Magnesium	1.3–2.3 mg/dL	0.62–0.95 mmol/L
Myoglobin	5-70 ng/mL	5–70 mcrograms/mL
Osmolality	275–300 mOsm/kg	275–300 mmol/L
Phosphorus (inorganic)	2.5–4.5 mg/dL	0.8–1.45 mmol/L
Potassium	3.5–5.0 mEq/L	3.5–5.0 mmol/L
Prostate-specific antigen (PSA)	0–4 ng/mL	0–4 µg/L
Protein total	6.0–8.0 g/dL	60–80 g/L
Albumin	3.5–5.5 g/dL	40–55 g/L
Globulin	1.7–3.3 g/dL	17–33 g/L
A/G ratio	1.0–2.2	1.0–2.2
Thyroid Tests		
Thyroxine (T_4) total	5.0–11.0 µg/dL	65–138 mmol/L
Thyroxine, free (FT_4)	0.8–2.7 ng/dL	10.3–35 pmol/L
Triiodothyronine (T_3) total	70–204 ng/dL	1.08–3.14 nmol/L
Thyroid-stimulating hormone (TSH)	0.4–6.0 µU/mL	0.4–4.2 mIU/L
Thyroglobulin	3–42 ng/mL	3–42 µg/L
Troponin 1 (MI)	<0.35 ng/mL	<0.35 mg/L
Sodium	135–145 mEq/L	135–145 mmol/L
Uric acid	2.5–8 mg/dL	0.15–0 mmol/L

U, units.

[†] Laboratory and/or method specific.

[‡] Varies with age and muscle mass.

Hematology

Test	Conventional Units	SI Units
Erythrocyte count (RBC count)	Males: 4.6–6.2 million/mm^3 Females: 4.2–5.4 million/mm^3	Males: 4.6–6.2 × 10^{12}/L Females: 4.2–5.4 × 10^{12}/L
Hematocrit (Hct)	Males: 42%–52% Females: 35%–47%	
Hemoglobin (Hb)	Males: 13–18 g/dL Females: 12–16 g/dL	
Mean corpuscular hemoglobin (MCH)	28–33 micromicrogram/cell	
Mean corpuscular hemoglobin concentration (MCHC)	33%–35%	
Mean corpuscular volume (MCV)	84–96 µg^3	84–96 fL
Reticulocyte count	0.5%–1.5% total RBC	
Leukocyte count (WBC count)	4,500–11,000 cells/mm^3	4.5–11. × 10^9/L
Basophils	0%–4%	
Eosinophils	0%–4%	
Lymphocytes	20%–40%	
Monocytes	2%–8%	
Neutrophils (segmented [Segs])	45%–73%	
Neutrophils (bands)	0%–4%	
Prothrombin Time (PT)	9.5–12 seconds INR 1.0	
Activated Partial Thromboplastin Time (APTT)	25–39 seconds	

(continued on page 690)

Hematology

Test	Conventional Units	SI Units
Arterial Blood Gases	**Reference Values** pH 7.35–7.45 pCO_2 35–45 mm Hg pO_2 85–95 mm Hg HCO^{3-} 18–24 mEq/L O_2 Saturation 95%–99% Base Excess (–2)–(+3) mEq/L	

Normal reference values may vary. Always follow the guidelines of your institution.

INDEX